ACP | MKSAP® 18

Medical Knowledge Self-Assessment Program®

Pulmonary and Critical Care Medicine

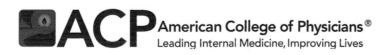

ACP American College of Physicians®
Leading Internal Medicine, Improving Lives

Welcome to the Pulmonary and Critical Care Medicine Section of MKSAP 18!

In these pages, you will find updated information on pulmonary diagnostic testing; airways disease; diffuse parenchymal lung disease; occupational lung disease; pleural disease; pulmonary vascular disease; lung tumors; sleep medicine; high-altitude–related illnesses; principles of ventilation in critical care; common ICU conditions such as upper airway emergencies, respiratory failure, sepsis, anaphylaxis, and toxicologic emergencies; and other clinical challenges. All of these topics are uniquely focused on the needs of generalists and subspecialists *outside* of pulmonary and critical care medicine.

The core content of MKSAP 18 has been developed as in previous editions—all essential information that is newly researched and written in 11 topic areas of internal medicine—created by dozens of leading generalists and subspecialists and guided by certification and recertification requirements, emerging knowledge in the field, and user feedback. MKSAP 18 also contains 1200 all-new peer-reviewed, psychometrically validated, multiple-choice questions (MCQs) for self-assessment and study, including 103 in Pulmonary and Critical Care Medicine. MKSAP 18 continues to include *High Value Care* (HVC) recommendations, based on the concept of balancing clinical benefit with costs and harms, with associated MCQs illustrating these principles and HVC Key Points called out in the text. Internists practicing in the hospital setting can easily find comprehensive *Hospitalist*-focused content and MCQs, specially designated in blue and with the 🄷 symbol.

If you purchased MKSAP 18 Complete, you also have access to MKSAP 18 Digital, with additional tools allowing you to customize your learning experience. MKSAP Digital includes regular text updates with new, practice-changing information, 200 new self-assessment questions, and enhanced custom-quiz options. MKSAP Complete also includes more than 1200 electronic, adaptive learning–enhanced flashcards for quick review of important concepts, as well as an updated and enhanced version of Virtual Dx, MKSAP's image-based self-assessment tool. As before, MKSAP 18 Digital is optimized for use on your mobile devices, with iOS- and Android-based apps allowing you to sync between your apps and online account and submit for CME credits and MOC points online.

Please visit us at the MKSAP Resource Site (mksap.acponline.org) to find out how we can help you study, earn CME credit and MOC points, and stay up to date.

On behalf of the many internists who have offered their time and expertise to create the content for MKSAP 18 and the editorial staff who work to bring this material to you in the best possible way, we are honored that you have chosen to use MKSAP 18 and appreciate any feedback about the program you may have. Please feel free to send any comments to mksap_editors@acponline.org.

Sincerely,

Patrick Alguire

Patrick C. Alguire, MD, FACP
Editor-in-Chief
Senior Vice President Emeritus
Medical Education Division
American College of Physicians

Pulmonary and Critical Care Medicine

Committee

Craig E. Daniels, MD, Section Editor[2]
Associate Professor of Medicine
Division of Pulmonary and Critical Care Medicine
Mayo Clinic College of Medicine and Science
Rochester, Minnesota

Rendell Ashton, MD, FACP[1]
Program Director, Pulmonary and Critical Care Fellowship
Associate Director, Medical Intensive Care Unit
Cleveland Clinic Lerner College of Medicine of Case Western
    Reserve University
Cleveland, Ohio

Sean M. Caples, DO, MS[2]
Associate Professor of Medicine
Division of Pulmonary and Critical Care Medicine
Mayo Clinic College of Medicine and Science
Rochester, Minnesota

Neal Chaisson, MD[2]
Program Director, Critical Care Medicine Fellowship
Assistant Professor of Medicine
Cleveland Clinic Lerner College of Medicine of Case Western
    Reserve University
Cleveland, Ohio

C. Jessica Dine, MD, MSHPR, FACP[2]
Assistant Professor of Medicine
Perelman School of Medicine at the University
    of Pennsylvania
Perelman Center for Advanced Medicine
Philadelphia, Pennsylvania

Melissa B. King-Biggs, MD[1]
Assistant Professor of Medicine
Department Chair HealthPartners Medical Group
    Lung and Sleep Health
University of Minnesota Medical School
Minneapolis, Minnesota

Eduardo Mireles-Cabodevila, MD[2]
Director, Medical Intensive Care Unit
Assistant Professor of Medicine
Cleveland Clinic Lerner College of Medicine of Case
    Western Reserve University
Cleveland, Ohio

Darlene R. Nelson, MD[1]
Associate Program Director of PCCM fellowship
Assistant Professor of Medicine
Division of Pulmonary and Critical Care Medicine
Mayo Clinic College of Medicine and Science
Rochester, Minnesota

Timothy Whelan, MD[2]
Professor of Medicine
Medical Director of Lung Transplantation
Medical University of South Carolina
Charleston, South Carolina

Consulting Editor

Steven Weinberger, MD, MACP[2]
Executive Vice President and CEO Emeritus
American College of Physicians
Adjunct Professor of Medicine
Perelman School of Medicine at the University
    of Pennsylvania
Philadelphia, Pennsylvania

Editor-in-Chief

Patrick C. Alguire, MD, FACP[2]
Senior Vice President Emeritus, Medical Education
American College of Physicians
Philadelphia, Pennsylvania

Deputy Editor

Denise M. Dupras, MD, PhD, FACP[1]
Associate Program Director
Department of Internal Medicine
Associate Professor of Medicine
Mayo Clinic College of Medicine
Rochester, Minnesota

Pulmonary and Critical Care Medicine Reviewers

Mahmoud Amarna, MD, FACP[1]
Sameh G. Aziz, MD, FACP[1]
Thomas Bice, MD[1]
Martin M. Cearras, MD[1]

Sanjay Chawla, MD, FACP[2]
Jacob F. Collen, MD, FACP[1]
Oleg Epelbaum, MD, FACP[1]
Leila Hashemi, MD, FACP[1]
Ankur Kalra, MD, FACP[1]
Amay Parikh, MD, FACP[1]

Hospital Medicine Pulmonary and Critical Care Medicine Reviewers

Shashi K Bellam, MD FACP[2]
Ehab G. Daoud, MD, FACP[1]

Pulmonary and Critical Care Medicine ACP Editorial Staff

Chuck Emig[1], Staff Editor
Margaret Wells[1], Director, Self-Assessment and Educational Programs[1]
Becky Krumm[1], Managing Editor, Self-Assessment and Educational Programs[1]

ACP Principal Staff

Davoren Chick, MD, FACP[2]
Senior Vice President, Medical Education

Patrick C. Alguire, MD, FACP[2]
Senior Vice President Emeritus, Medical Education

Sean McKinney[1]
Vice President, Medical Education

Margaret Wells[1]
Director, Self-Assessment and Educational Programs

Becky Krumm[1]
Managing Editor

Valerie Dangovetsky[1]
Administrator

Ellen McDonald, PhD[1]
Senior Staff Editor

Megan Zborowski[1]
Senior Staff Editor

Jackie Twomey[1]
Senior Staff Editor

Randy Hendrickson[1]
Production Administrator/Editor

Julia Nawrocki[1]
Digital Content Associate/Editor

Linnea Donnarumma[1]
Staff Editor

Chuck Emig[1]
Staff Editor

Joysa Winter[1]
Staff Editor

Kimberly Kerns[1]
Administrative Coordinator

1. Has no relationships with any entity producing, marketing, reselling, or distributing health care goods or services consumed by, or used on, patients.

2. Has disclosed relationship(s) with any entity producing, marketing, reselling, or distributing health care goods or services consumed by, or used on, patients.

Disclosure of Relationships with any entity producing, marketing, reselling, or distributing health care goods or services consumed by, or used on, patients.

Patrick C. Alguire, MD, FACP
Royalties
UpToDate

Shashi K. Bellam, MD FACP
Speakers Bureau
Genentech

Sean M. Caples, DO, MS
Consultantship
Zephyr Labs

Neal Chaisson, MD
Consultantship
Actelion Pharmaceuticals, Putnam Associates, Schlesinger Associates, Bayer
Speakers Bureau
Bayer, Gilead

Sanjay Chawla, MD, FACP
Stock Options/Holdings
Pfizer

Davoren Chick, MD, FACP
Royalties
Wolters Kluwer Publishing
Consultantship
EBSCO Health's DynaMed Plus
Other: Owner and sole proprietor of Coding 101, LLC; research consultant (spouse) for Vedanta Biosciences Inc.

Craig E. Daniels, MD
Research Grants/Contracts
Boehringer, Genentech/Roche
Patent Holder
Sanovas Inc.

C. Jessica Dine, MD, MSHPR, FACP
Consultantship
National Board of Medical Examiners

iv

Eduardo Mireles-Cabodevila, MD
Co-Patent Owner
Co-owners Robert Chatburn and Cleveland Clinic:
   Ventilator Control System Utilizing a Mid-Frequency
   Ventilation Pattern

Steven Weinberger, MD, MACP
Royalties
Elsevier, Wolters Kluwer Publishing, UpToDate

Timothy Whelan, MD
Consultantship
Gilead Sciences, Boehringer Ingelheim, Sharing Hope SC,
   Genentech, France Foundation, RockPointe, Inc.
Research Grants/Contracts
Gilead Sciences, Boehringer Ingelheim, Genetech, Global
   Blood Therapeutics, Kadmon, National Institute of
   Health, Pulmonary Fibrosis Foundation, Celgene,
   Galapagos
Board Member
Sharing Hope SC

Acknowledgments

The American College of Physicians (ACP) gratefully
acknowledges the special contributions to the development and production of the 18th edition of the Medical
Knowledge Self-Assessment Program® (MKSAP® 18) made
by the following people:

Graphic Design: Barry Moshinski (Director, Graphic
Services), Michael Ripca (Graphics Technical
Administrator), and Jennifer Gropper (Graphic
Designer).

Production/Systems: Dan Hoffmann (Director, Information
Technology), Scott Hurd (Manager, Content Systems),
Neil Kohl (Senior Architect), and Chris Patterson (Senior
Architect).

MKSAP 18 Digital: Under the direction of Steven Spadt
(Senior Vice President, Technology), the digital version
of MKSAP 18 was developed within the ACP's Digital
Products and Services Department, led by Brian
Sweigard (Director, Digital Products and Services). Other
members of the team included Dan Barron (Senior Web
Application Developer/Architect), Chris Forrest (Senior
Software Developer/Design Lead), Kathleen Hoover
(Senior Web Developer), Kara Regis (Manager, User
Interface Design and Development), Brad Lord (Senior
Web Application Developer), and John McKnight (Senior
Web Developer).

The College also wishes to acknowledge that many
other persons, too numerous to mention, have contrib-
uted to the production of this program. Without their
dedicated efforts, this program would not have been
possible.

MKSAP Resource Site (mksap.acponline.org)

The MKSAP Resource Site (mksap.acponline.org) is a continually updated site that provides links to MKSAP 18 online answer
sheets for print subscribers; access to MKSAP 18 Digital; Board
Basics® e-book access instructions; information on Continuing
Medical Education (CME), Maintenance of Certification (MOC),
and international Continuing Professional Development (CPD)
and MOC; errata; and other new information.

International MOC/CPD

For information and instructions on submission of international MOC/CPD, please go to the MKSAP Resource Site
(mksap.acponline.org).

Continuing Medical Education

The American College of Physicians is accredited by the
Accreditation Council for Continuing Medical Education
(ACCME) to provide continuing medical education for
physicians.

The American College of Physicians designates this endur-
ing material, MKSAP 18, for a maximum of 275 *AMA PRA
Category 1 Credits*™. Physicians should claim only the
credit commensurate with the extent of their participation
in the activity.

Up to 25 *AMA PRA Category 1 Credits*™ are available from
December 31, 2018, to December 31, 2021, for the MKSAP 18
Pulmonary and Critical Care Medicine section.

Learning Objectives

The learning objectives of MKSAP 18 are to:

- Close gaps between actual care in your practice and pre-
  ferred standards of care, based on best evidence
- Diagnose disease states that are less common and some-
  times overlooked and confusing
- Improve management of comorbid conditions that can
  complicate patient care
- Determine when to refer patients for surgery or care by
  subspecialists
- Pass the ABIM Certification Examination
- Pass the ABIM Maintenance of Certification Examination

Target Audience

- General internists and primary care physicians
- Subspecialists who need to remain up to date in internal
  medicine
- Residents preparing for the certifying examination in
  internal medicine
- Physicians preparing for maintenance of certification in
  internal medicine (recertification)

ABIM Maintenance of Certification

Check the MKSAP Resource Site (mksap.acponline.org) for the latest information on how MKSAP tests can be used to apply to the American Board of Internal Medicine (ABIM) for Maintenance of Certification (MOC) points following completion of the CME activity.

Successful completion of the CME activity, which includes participation in the evaluation component, enables the participant to earn up to 275 medical knowledge MOC points in the ABIM's MOC program. It is the CME activity provider's responsibility to submit participant completion information to ACCME for the purpose of granting MOC credit.

Earn Instantaneous CME Credits or MOC Points Online

Print subscribers can enter their answers online to earn instantaneous CME credits or MOC points. You can submit your answers using online answer sheets that are provided at mksap.acponline.org, where a record of your MKSAP 18 credits will be available. To earn CME credits or to apply for MOC points, you need to answer all of the questions in a test and earn a score of at least 50% correct (number of correct answers divided by the total number of questions). Please note that if you are applying for MOC points, you must also enter your birth date and ABIM candidate number.

Take either of the following approaches:

1. Use the printed answer sheet at the back of this book to record your answers. Go to mksap.acponline.org, access the appropriate online answer sheet, transcribe your answers, and submit your test for instantaneous CME credits or MOC points. There is no additional fee for this service.

2. Go to mksap.acponline.org, access the appropriate online answer sheet, directly enter your answers, and submit your test for instantaneous CME credits or MOC points. There is no additional fee for this service.

Earn CME Credits or MOC Points by Mail or Fax

Pay a $20 processing fee per answer sheet and submit the printed answer sheet at the back of this book by mail or fax, as instructed on the answer sheet. Make sure you calculate your score and enter your birth date and ABIM candidate number, and fax the answer sheet to 215-351-2799 or mail the answer sheet to Member and Customer Service, American College of Physicians, 190 N. Independence Mall West, Philadelphia, PA 19106-1572, using the courtesy envelope provided in your MKSAP 18 slipcase. You will need your 10-digit order number and 8-digit ACP ID number, which are printed on your packing slip. Please allow 4 to 6 weeks for your score report to be emailed back to you. Be sure to include your email address for a response.

If you do not have a 10-digit order number and 8-digit ACP ID number, or if you need help creating a user-name and password to access the MKSAP 18 online answer sheets, go to mksap.acponline.org or email custserv@acponline.org.

Disclosure Policy

It is the policy of the American College of Physicians (ACP) to ensure balance, independence, objectivity, and scientific rigor in all of its educational activities. To this end, and consistent with the policies of the ACP and the Accreditation Council for Continuing Medical Education (ACCME), contributors to all ACP continuing medical education activities are required to disclose all relevant financial relationships with any entity producing, marketing, re-selling, or distributing health care goods or services consumed by, or used on, patients. Contributors are required to use generic names in the discussion of therapeutic options and are required to identify any unapproved, off-label, or investigative use of commercial products or devices. Where a trade name is used, all available trade names for the same product type are also included. If trade-name products manufactured by companies with whom contributors have relationships are discussed, contributors are asked to provide evidence-based citations in support of the discussion. The information is reviewed by the committee responsible for producing this text. If necessary, adjustments to topics or contributors' roles in content development are made to balance the discussion. Further, all readers of this text are asked to evaluate the content for evidence of commercial bias and send any relevant comments to mksap_editors@acponline.org so that future decisions about content and contributors can be made in light of this information.

Resolution of Conflicts

To resolve all conflicts of interest and influences of vested interests, ACP's content planners used best evidence and updated clinical care guidelines in developing content, when such evidence and guidelines were available. All content underwent review by peer reviewers not on the committee to ensure that the material was balanced and unbiased. Contributors' disclosure information can be found with the list of contributors' names and those of ACP principal staff listed in the beginning of this book.

Hospital-Based Medicine

For the convenience of subscribers who provide care in hospital settings, content that is specific to the hospital setting has been highlighted in blue. Hospital icons (🄷) highlight where the hospital-only content begins, continues over more than one page, and ends.

High Value Care Key Points

Key Points in the text that relate to High Value Care concepts (that is, concepts that discuss balancing clinical benefit with costs and harms) are designated by the HVC icon [**HVC**].

Educational Disclaimer

The editors and publisher of MKSAP 18 recognize that the development of new material offers many opportunities for error. Despite our best efforts, some errors may persist in print. Drug dosage schedules are, we believe, accurate and in accordance with current standards. Readers are advised, however, to ensure that the recommended dosages in MKSAP 18 concur with the information provided in the product information material. This is especially important in cases of new, infrequently used, or highly toxic drugs. Application of the information in MKSAP 18 remains the professional responsibility of the practitioner.

The primary purpose of MKSAP 18 is educational. Information presented, as well as publications, technologies, products, and/or services discussed, is intended to inform subscribers about the knowledge, techniques, and experiences of the contributors. A diversity of professional opinion exists, and the views of the contributors are their own and not those of the ACP. Inclusion of any material in the program does not constitute endorsement or recommendation by the ACP. The ACP does not warrant the safety, reliability, accuracy, completeness, or usefulness of and disclaims any and all liability for damages and claims that may result from the use of information, publications, technologies, products, and/or services discussed in this program.

Publisher's Information

Disclaimer Regarding Direct Purchases from Online Retailers

Unauthorized Use of This Book Is Against the Law

MKSAP 18 ISBN: 978-1-938245-47-3
(Pulmonary and Critical Care Medicine)
ISBN: 978-1-938245-58-9

Printed in the United States of America.

For order information in the U.S. or Canada call 800-ACP-1915. All other countries call 215-351-2600 (Monday to Friday, 9 AM – 5 PM ET). Fax inquiries to 215-351-2799 or email to custserv@acponline.org.

Errata

Errata for MKSAP 18 will be available through the MKSAP Resource Site at mksap.acponline.org as new information becomes known to the editors.

Table of Contents

Lung Tumors

Sleep Medicine

High-Altitude-Related Illnesses

Critical Care Medicine: ICU Utilization

Principles of Critical Care

Common ICU Conditions

Pulmonary and Critical Care Medicine High Value Care Recommendations

The American College of Physicians, in collaboration with multiple other organizations, is engaged in a worldwide initiative to promote the practice of High Value Care (HVC). The goals of the HVC initiative are to improve health care outcomes by providing care of proven benefit and reducing costs by avoiding unnecessary and even harmful interventions. The initiative comprises several programs that integrate the important concept of health care value (balancing clinical benefit with costs and harms) for a given intervention into a broad range of educational materials to address the needs of trainees, practicing physicians, and patients.

HVC content has been integrated into MKSAP 18 in several important ways. MKSAP 18 includes HVC-identified key points in the text, HVC-focused multiple choice questions, and, for subscribers to MKSAP Digital, an HVC custom quiz. From the text and questions, we have generated the following list of HVC recommendations that meet the definition below of high value care and bring us closer to our goal of improving patient outcomes while conserving finite resources.

High Value Care Recommendation: A recommendation to choose diagnostic and management strategies for patients in specific clinical situations that balance clinical benefit with cost and harms with the goal of improving patient outcomes.

Below are the High Value Care Recommendations for the Pulmonary and Critical Care Medicine section of MKSAP 18.

- Spirometry before and after workplace exposures is a cost-effective way to confirm a suspected diagnosis of occupational asthma.
- A sputum culture is not routinely used to assess COPD exacerbations as it rarely affects management.
- The diagnosis of diffuse parenchymal lung disease can often be made based on high-resolution CT without a lung biopsy.
- Avoid mechanical ventilation for patients with idiopathic pulmonary fibrosis if lung transplantation is not an option.
- Uvulopalatopharyngoplasty and similar procedures are ineffective for treatment of obstructive sleep apnea.
- Do not routinely use haloperidol or atypical antipsychotics for the prevention of delirium.
- Do not routinely measure gastric residuals in critically ill malnourished patients because it delays achievement of feeding goals and may increase the risk of aspiration.
- Do not order diagnostic tests at regular intervals but rather in response to specific clinical questions.
- Do not use parenteral nutrition in adequately nourished critically ill patients within the first 7 days of an ICU stay.
- Adjunctive therapies for severe asthma exacerbation, including anesthetics with bronchodilator properties, inhalation of a helium-oxygen mixture, mucolytics, and leukotriene receptor antagonists lack evidence of clear efficacy.
- Pulmonary artery catheters have no benefit, and in some cases increase risk to patients when used to guide therapy for shock.
- Given the relative expense of colloids, crystalloid administration for distributive shock is generally preferred.
- There is no role for procalcitonin measurement in sepsis that is likely due to infection.
- There is no role for glucocorticoids in sepsis without shock.
- Home sleep testing is preferred in a patient with a high probability of obstructive sleep apnea without underlying cardiopulmonary or neuromuscular disease (see Item 4).

Pulmonary and Critical Care Medicine

Pulmonary Diagnostic Tests

Pulmonary Function Testing

Pulmonary function testing is an essential tool to diagnose obstructive and restrictive pathophysiology and to quantify the severity of the abnormality. Pulmonary function testing can include spirometry, bronchial challenge testing, lung volume testing, and measurement of diffusion capacity of the lung for carbon monoxide (D_{LCO}). These findings are compared to age, sex, height, and race-adjusted population norms and expressed as a percent of the predicted value (**Table 1**). Values below 80% of the predicted value are considered reduced. Recent American Thoracic Society guidelines alternatively use the lower limit of normal (below the fifth percentile of healthy never-smokers) as a cutoff, but in most cases this is very similar to 80% of the predicted value.

KEY POINT

- Pulmonary function test results below 80% of predicted or below the lower limit of normal are indicative of pulmonary impairment.

H Spirometry

Measurement of expiratory airflow and volume is an essential diagnostic and management test for patients with lung diseases. Spirometry measures the maximal volume and flow of air during a best-effort, forced exhalation; reported values include the FEV_1, the FVC, and the FEV_1/FVC ratio. Measurement of maximal expiratory flow by peak flow meter is commonly used at home and in office settings to follow and manage patients with asthma, but is not considered a valid diagnostic tool for airways disease. Spirometry correlates with hand-held peak expiratory flow-meter measurements, but is more reliable, provides more data, and is used in both diagnosis and management of airways disease. Although spirometry is easily performed in the outpatient setting, technical test validation and patient factors—including poor effort, coughing, and failure to exhale for a minimum of 6 seconds—may result in suboptimal test performance and misinterpretation. H

Bronchial Challenge Testing

Bronchial challenge testing is used to identify bronchial hyperresponsiveness, a diagnostic feature of asthma. This is particularly helpful in patients whose symptoms are suggestive of asthma but for whom other pulmonary function test results are normal. Patients inhale increasing doses of a substance known to induce bronchospasm, such as methacholine or histamine, in a stepwise fashion. This is followed by repeated measurements of FEV_1; if FEV_1 falls by 20% or more from the baseline value, the test is considered positive. Bronchial challenge testing has a high negative predictive value for diagnosing asthma; however, a positive test can be caused by other conditions including COPD, smoking, upper respiratory infections, allergic rhinitis, bronchiectasis, and cystic fibrosis.

KEY POINT

- Bronchial challenge testing is a helpful diagnostic tool in patients whose symptoms are suggestive of asthma but for whom other pulmonary function test results are normal.

Lung Volumes and D_{LCO}

Measures of lung volume include total lung capacity (TLC), vital capacity (VC), and residual volume (RV). D_{LCO} measurement estimates the amount of gas transfer through the alveolar/capillary unit and is proportional to the surface area of functional lung. D_{LCO} is measured by inhalation of a gas mixture containing carbon monoxide and helium; the resulting value is corrected for hemoglobin level.

Pulmonary Function Testing Interpretation H

The purpose of pulmonary function testing interpretation is to classify abnormal results as an obstructive, a restrictive, or a mixed obstructive/restrictive pattern and to assess the severity of

TABLE 1. Characterization of Impairment Severity in Pulmonary Function Tests

Severity of Impairment	% of Predicted
FEV_1	
Mild	79-70
Moderate	60-69
Moderately severe	50-59
Severe	35-49
Very severe	<35
D_{LCO}	
Mild	<LLN but >60
Moderate	40-60
Severe	<40

LLN = lower limit of normal; below the fifth percentile of healthy never-smokers.

Reproduced with permission from ©ERS 2018. Pellegrino R, Viegi G, Brusasco V, Crapo RO, Burgos F, Casaburi R, et al. Interpretative strategies for lung function tests. Eur Respir J. 2005;26:948-68. [PMID: 16264058] doi: 10.1183/09031936.05.00035205

impairment (**Figure 1**). The initial step is to review the results of spirometry. An FEV_1/FVC ratio below 0.70 is consistent with obstruction, and the severity is determined based on the measured FEV_1 as a percent of the predicted value (see Table 1). Reversibility of obstruction is determined by the response to a short-acting inhaled bronchodilator. An increase from baseline in FEV_1, FVC, or both of at least 12% and at least 200 mL indicates a positive bronchodilator response (reversibility). The TLC is normal or even increased in pure obstructive disease. Elevation of TLC and residual volume (120% or greater of predicted) can be observed in obstruction and generally is indicative of hyperinflation and air trapping, a common pattern in severe COPD or asthma.

If FEV_1 or FVC is reduced and the FEV_1/FVC ratio is 0.70 or greater, then the pattern may be interpreted as restrictive, but measurement of TLC is needed to confirm this. If the TLC is below 80% of predicted (or the lower limit of normal) a restrictive pattern is present.

Some patients may present with coexisting obstructive and restrictive pulmonary disorders, such as a COPD patient who develops an interstitial lung disease. In these cases, a low FEV_1/FVC ratio (obstructive pattern) and a low TLC (restrictive pattern) are both present.

DLCO is reduced in conditions where functioning alveolar capillary units are destroyed (COPD), infiltrated (interstitial lung diseases), removed (lung resection), or their function is compromised (pulmonary parenchymal and vascular disorders). Conditions that increase pulmonary capillary blood volume, such as pulmonary alveolar hemorrhage, left-to-right shunt, or asthma, can cause an elevation in DLCO.

The flow-volume loop is a graphic representation of maximally forced inspiratory and expiratory flow (on the Y-axis) against volume (on the X-axis). The shape of the spirometric flow-volume loop is also useful in differentiating obstructive from restrictive patterns (**Figure 2**).

KEY POINTS

- The purpose of pulmonary function testing interpretation is to classify abnormal results as either an obstructive or restrictive pattern and to assess the severity of impairment.
- The FEV_1/FVC ratio is the primary measurement that defines obstructive disease, and total lung capacity is the primary measurement to confirm restrictive disease.

6-Minute Walk Test

The 6-minute walk test provides a valid and reliable measurement of exercise capacity in patients with lung disease. Patients walk at their own pace along a course for 6 minutes,

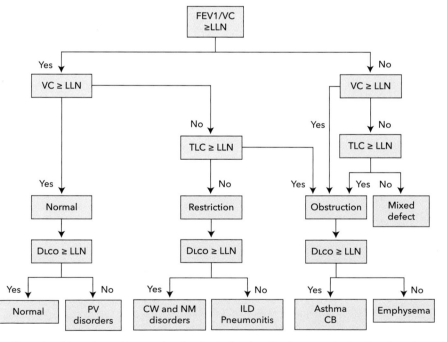

FIGURE 1. A simplified algorithm such as this may be used to assess lung function in clinical practice. It presents classic patterns for various pulmonary disorders. As in any such diagram, patients may or may not present with the classic patterns, depending on their illnesses, severity, and lung function prior to the disease onset (for example, did they start with a vital capacity [VC] close to the upper or lower limit of normal [LLN]?). The decisions about how far to follow this diagram are clinical, and will vary depending on the questions being asked and the clinical information available at the time of testing. The FEV_1/VC ratio and VC should be considered first. Total lung capacity (TLC) is necessary to confirm or exclude the presence of a restrictive defect when VC is below the LLN. The algorithm also includes DLCO measurement with the predicted value adjusted for hemoglobin. In the mixed defect group, the DLCO patterns are the same as those for restriction and obstruction. This flow chart is not suitable for assessing the severity of upper airway obstruction. CB = chronic bronchitis; CW = chest wall; ILD = interstitial lung diseases; NM = neuromuscular; PV = pulmonary vascular.

Reproduced with permission from ©ERS 2018. Pellegrino R, Viegi G, Brusasco V, Crapo RO, Burgos F, Casaburi R, et al. Interpretative strategies for lung function tests. Eur Respir J. 2005;26:948-68. [PMID: 16264058] doi: 10.1183/09031936.05.00035205

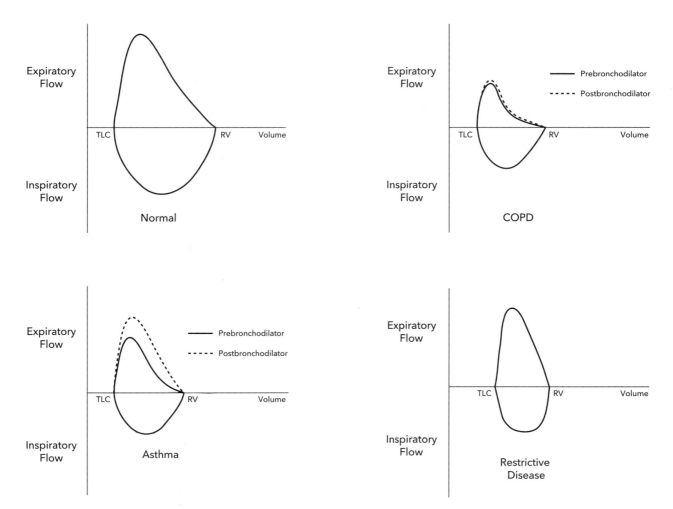

FIGURE 2. Pulmonary function test flow-volume patterns. RV = residual volume; TLC = total lung capacity.

and the total distance walked is recorded. Lower 6-minute walk test distances correlate with increased mortality in several lung diseases, including COPD, interstitial lung disease, and pulmonary arterial hypertension. Serial 6-minute walk testing may be used to assess response to therapy in patients with chronic respiratory disorders, especially pulmonary arterial hypertension.

Pulse Oximetry

Pulse oximetry provides a readily available noninvasive measurement of oxygen-bound hemoglobin in the circulation. Oximeters work by calculating the differential between absorption of infrared light by oxygenated and deoxygenated blood. A normal hemoglobin saturation measured by pulse oximetry is 95% to 100% and values below 90% indicate hypoxemia. Substances in the blood that absorb infrared light may cause erroneous readings, including carboxyhemoglobin (present in carbon monoxide poisoning), methemoglobin (caused by nitrates), methylene blue, and some topical anesthetics. More commonly, patient factors such as cool extremities, poor circulation, and motion artifact result in erroneous

readings. In these cases, alternative methods of measuring oxygenation are needed.

Imaging and Bronchoscopy
Imaging
Chest Radiography

Conventional chest radiographs are indicated as the initial imaging procedure for most patients with significant respiratory symptoms. Posteroanterior and lateral views should be obtained. Advantages are the availability of testing and low dose of radiation exposure for the patient. Limitations of chest radiographs include patient factors such as the need to take a deep inspiration, breath holding, image resolution, and the 2-dimensional nature of the images.

Computed Tomography

CT of the thorax allows detailed, high-resolution imaging of the lungs and options for both static and dynamic imaging techniques. Helical scanners allow rapid scanning, but may require patients to hold their breath at full inspiration for 30 or

CONT. more seconds. Reconstruction can include sagittal and coronal images, which result in 3-dimensional representation of the extent and distribution of disease. More specialized techniques reformat the data to highlight imaging of specific structures, such as maximum intensity projection (MIP), which focuses on the vasculature, and minimum intensity projection (MINIP), which focuses on the airways. Additional variables in CT imaging including slice thickness and interval; contrast enhancement may be used to augment the value of imaging based on the underlying disease.

The choice of examination will depend on the clinical context and information sought. For most patients, a routine (slice thickness of 2 or 2.5 mm) noncontrast CT is sufficient to provide the needed information. For patients suspected of having interstitial lung disease, a high-resolution (slice thickness of 1 mm) study should be ordered. Addition of expiratory views can evaluate for air trapping and further inform the diagnosis of small airways disease. However, because the slice interval (the distance between individual slices) with high-resolution CT is larger than with conventional CT, this technique "skips" interval sections of the lung and should not be used to evaluate lung nodules. Use of intravenous contrast dye helps delineate mediastinal structures and is particularly useful in patients with suspected lymphadenopathy or vascular pathology. CT angiography is used for detection of pulmonary embolism and utilizes a rapid, timed bolus of intravenous contrast.

CT scanning exposes the patient to a much higher dose of radiation than traditional chest radiographs, and CT is currently the primary source of imaging radiation exposure for patients. Efforts to reduce radiation doses are ongoing, and low-dose CT scanning of the chest is now the recommended choice for lung cancer screening in the United States (see Lung Tumors).

KEY POINT

- High-resolution CT techniques are preferred for evaluation of interstitial lung disease, conventional noncontrast CT is used to evaluate lung nodules, and CT angiography is used for detection of pulmonary embolism.

Positron Emission Tomography Scanning
PET scans utilize the radionuclide 18-fluoro-2-deoxyglucose, which accumulates within highly metabolically active cells such as cancer cells, and can be visualized as discrete areas of uptake. Integrated PET/CT scanning allows improved localization of the metabolic activity. PET scans are widely used to evaluate risk of malignancy in lung nodules, to stage known thoracic tumors, and to evaluate for metastatic disease from other non-thoracic malignancies. False positive PET scans can occur in other hypermetabolic conditions where cells accumulate fluorodeoxyglucose, such as infection or inflammation. False negatives can occur when tumors have low rates of metabolic activity, such as carcinoid, adenocarcinoma in situ, and, rarely, metastatic kidney,

prostate, or testicular cancer. PET scanning is not useful for determination of malignant potential in lung nodules less than 8 mm in size.

Bronchoscopy and Endobronchial Ultrasound
Bronchoscopy is a diagnostic and therapeutic tool for patients with lung disorders (**Table 2**). It is used for the diagnosis of localized and diffuse pulmonary diseases. It is important in the diagnostic evaluation for pulmonary infections, particularly in the immunocompromised host, and also has various therapeutic uses (**Table 3**). The addition of endobronchial ultrasound (EBUS) to visualize mediastinal and hilar lymph nodes for needle aspiration has made EBUS bronchoscopy the initial procedure of choice for obtaining tissue from mediastinal and hilar lymph nodes in the diagnosis and staging of patients with known or suspected thoracic malignancy.

KEY POINT

- Endobronchial ultrasound (EBUS) is the initial procedure of choice for obtaining tissue from mediastinal and hilar lymph nodes in the staging of patients with known or suspected thoracic malignancy.

Airways Disease
Asthma
Epidemiology and Natural History
Asthma is an inflammatory disorder of the airways characterized by cough, wheezing, chest tightness, dyspnea, and variable airflow obstruction. Asthma is a major health burden throughout the world, and approximately 7.4% of the U.S. population has been diagnosed with asthma, accounting for more than 10 million office visits per year. Prevalence is increased among patients older than 65 years, women, blacks, and persons below the poverty level. Mortality in asthma is significant, causing 10.3 deaths per million Americans in 2015, with significantly higher mortality among patients who are black or are older than 65 years.

The onset of asthma can occur at any age, and the natural history varies with the duration and severity of symptoms, sex, and response to therapy. Children often have a family history of atopy, or exposure to sensitizing allergens such as dust mites or cockroaches. Childhood asthma may improve or resolve during teen and adult years, particularly in males. New-onset asthma in adults may have occupational exposures known to induce bronchial hyperreactivity. Those with severe symptoms generally have a more persistent course, lower pulmonary function, and increased risks of developing fixed airway obstruction. Diagnosis and treatment of asthma in older adults is often challenged by symptom overlap with other conditions (COPD, heart failure) and the normal effects of aging on pulmonary physiology.

TABLE 2. Bronchoscopic Diagnostic Procedures

Technique	Description	Examples of Indications
Airway inspection	Visualization of the tracheobronchial tree to the level of segmental airways	Hemoptysis Localized wheeze Persistent atelectasis Diagnosis of tracheobronchomalacia Inhalational injury
Bronchial washings	Samples from large airways	Diagnosis of infections
Bronchoalveolar lavage	Samples from small bronchi and alveoli	Diagnosis of infections Cell counts in diagnosis of parenchymal lung disease Alveolar hemorrhage Cytology for malignancy
Bronchial brushings	Brushings of the endobronchial mucosa for cells	Endobronchial lesions
Endobronchial biopsy	Biopsy within the airway lumen	Endobronchial mass or lesion
Transbronchial lung biopsy	Biopsy of the lung parenchyma or lung nodules/masses using small forceps; often aided by guidance technology including electromagnetic navigation and radial ultrasound	Diffuse lung disease Persistent infiltrates Lung nodules/masses Posttransplant rejection
Transbronchial needle aspiration	Aspiration of a lymph node or mass adjacent to the airway	Lymphadenopathy Pulmonary mass Mediastinal mass
Endobronchial ultrasound	Use of an ultrasound probe at the distal end of the bronchoscope to guide transbronchial needle aspiration	Lymphadenopathy Pulmonary mass Mediastinal mass
Electromagnetic navigation	Images from a recent CT are "linked" with the bronchoscope. An electromagnetic guidance system at the bronchoscope creates a map of the airways and guides the physician to the area of interest.	Pulmonary mass or nodule

TABLE 3. Bronchoscopic Therapeutic Procedures

Technique	Description	Examples of Indications
Flexible bronchoscopy	Large airway suctioning Basket and forceps Balloon tamponade of airway	Lobar atelectasis from mucus plugs Foreign body Bleeding
Bronchial thermoplasty	Radiofrequency energy ablation of proximal airway smooth muscle	Severe asthma
Endobronchial stent placement	Bronchoscopic placement of silicon and metal prostheses to expand and support the airways	Malignant obstruction Benign strictures Tracheomalacia or bronchomalacia Anastomotic dehiscence
Airway ablative therapies	Laser therapy Electrocautery Argon plasma coagulation Cryotherapy Brachytherapy	Malignant airway obstruction Benign airway obstruction Airway tumor ablation
Endobronchial valve placement	Airway placement of one-way valves	Bronchopleural fistula Emphysema
Balloon dilation	Targeted endobronchial balloon inflation	Benign or malignant airway stricture

- Approximately 7.4% of the U.S. population has been diagnosed with asthma, and prevalence is increased among patients older than 65 years, women, blacks, and persons below the poverty level.

Pathogenesis

The pathophysiologic mechanisms of asthma include chronic airway inflammation, airway narrowing due to edema, subepithelial fibrosis, smooth muscle hypertrophy, and mucus hypersecretion, in addition to airway smooth muscle constriction causing bronchial hyperreactivity in response to various stimuli. The airway cellular inflammatory profile is variable; persists even during the absence of symptoms; and includes eosinophils, T lymphocytes, mast cells, and neutrophils. Eosinophilic inflammation is commonly recognized in allergic asthma, but patients may have other cellular profiles, with neutrophilic inflammation increasingly recognized in older patients. Bronchial hyperreactivity that causes airway obstruction is typically episodic and triggered by stimuli that would not induce symptoms in healthy people. Common triggers include allergens, dusts, fumes, exercise, extremes of temperature, and viral respiratory infections.

Risk Factors

Risk factors for asthma include both host and environmental factors. Genes predisposing to atopy, bronchial hyperreactivity, and airway inflammation have been identified, but genetic predisposition is thought to interact with additional factors, including exposure to indoor allergens (mites, furred animals, cockroaches, molds) and outdoor allergens (pollens, molds), tobacco smoke, occupational sensitizers and allergens, viral respiratory infections, and air pollution. In addition, obesity is an important risk factor for asthma.

Asthma is heterogeneous, but distinct phenotypes are recognized and have implications for underlying mechanisms, treatment, and outcomes. Although specific phenotypes are not yet broadly accepted, many are commonly described. Clinically recognizable groups include allergic, nonallergic, late-onset, adult onset eosinophilic, and obesity-associated asthma. These subsets tend to have different cellular compositions of airway inflammation and may respond variably to anti-inflammatory therapies.

- Genetic predisposition to asthma is thought to interact with additional factors, including exposure to indoor allergens (mites, furred animals, cockroaches, molds) and outdoor allergens (pollens, molds), tobacco smoke, occupational sensitizers and allergens, viral respiratory infections, and air pollution.

Symptoms and Clinical Evaluation

Common symptoms of asthma are cough, wheezing, chest tightness, and shortness of breath that are intermittent and occur in response to various potential stimuli, including allergens, infections, dusts, fumes, and exercise. Symptoms often have a diurnal variation, worsening in the evening and early morning. Viral respiratory infections are a particularly robust trigger for most patients. Variability of symptoms (both improvement and worsening of symptoms over time) is a key diagnostic feature of asthma.

History taking should establish whether the patient has ever smoked tobacco or other products, has pets, or has had environmental exposures (either recreationally or in the work place) to dust, fumes, or particulate matter known to cause bronchial hyperreactivity. A personal or family history of atopy or allergic sinus disease may be present. In particular, the presence of nasal polyps, sensitivity to aspirin, and wheezing is known as the "asthmatic triad." The physical examination may demonstrate wheezing, reduced airflow, or a prolonged expiratory phase. However, patients may also have a completely normal respiratory exam, particularly when they are symptom-free.

Confirmation of reversible airflow obstruction is a cornerstone of asthma diagnosis and can be assessed by spirometry, with measurement of forced expiratory volume in one second (FEV_1), forced vital capacity (FVC), and the FEV_1/FVC ratio, or by serial measurement of peak expiratory flow rates. Airway obstruction that improves with bronchodilators, on subsequent measurements, or after 4 weeks of anti-inflammatory treatment supports a diagnosis of asthma. For adults, a significant change in FEV_1 is an increase from baseline of at least 12% and at least 200 mL. For some patients, airflow obstruction is not present during the initial evaluation, and demonstration of bronchial hyperreactivity with bronchial challenge testing is indicated. This is usually performed with inhaled methacholine, although other stimuli (exercise, mannitol) have been validated. If a bronchial challenge test is negative, it is unlikely that a patient has asthma. A positive challenge test confirms bronchial hyperreactivity, but is not sufficient to confirm asthma because other disorders may demonstrate this finding. Therefore, clinical correlation of this finding with symptoms and other testing is needed.

A chest radiograph is helpful in many patients to rule out other diagnoses, such as COPD, heart failure, parenchymal lung disorders, central airway obstruction, and bronchiectasis. This is especially important in older adults, in whom asthma is often underrecognized and undertreated.

- Common symptoms of asthma are cough, wheezing, chest tightness, and shortness of breath that are intermittent and occur in response to various potential stimuli, including allergens, infections, dusts, fumes, and exercise.
- Confirmation of reversible airflow obstruction with bronchodilators is a cornerstone of asthma diagnosis and can be assessed by spirometry, with measurement of FEV_1, FVC, and the FEV_1/FVC ratio showing an increase from baseline of ≥12% and ≥200 mL.

(Continued)

- In patients with clinical symptoms suggestive of asthma but with normal spirometry, bronchial challenge testing (such as with methacholine) may be helpful to evaluate for asthma. A negative test excludes asthma, whereas a positive test requires clinical correlation and may require additional testing.

Asthma Syndromes

Allergic Asthma

Identifying the presence of atopy can identify an allergic asthma phenotype in a patient with respiratory symptoms. The most common tests are allergy skin prick tests, which may be administered in the outpatient setting by qualified personnel, or laboratory measurement of allergen-specific IgE in serum. Results of each method are generally concordant. Skin testing is more sensitive but subject to errors related to administration, whereas serum tests are more specific but have higher costs. Measurement of total serum IgE is not useful because a normal level does not preclude clinical allergies. However, IgE is a therapeutic target for advanced treatments such as omalizumab (monoclonal antibody targeting IgE in severe atopic asthma), so measurement of IgE can help guide the use of these agents.

Identifying eosinophilic airway inflammation through either elevated serum or sputum eosinophil counts, or measurement of exhaled nitric oxide levels, may help phenotype patients. A phenotype of severe adult-onset asthma with significant eosinophilia has been recognized, often without a significant component of allergies or atopy. These patients often require treatment with systemic glucocorticoids and may be appropriate for advanced anti-interleukin therapies such as mepolizumab.

Cough-Variant Asthma

Patients with asthma whose primary symptom manifestation is chronic cough without other symptoms are considered to have cough-variant asthma. Diagnosis requires documentation of bronchial hyperreactivity, as most patients will have normal baseline spirometry. Recommended therapies are the same as those for other types of asthma. Other causes of chronic cough should be investigated, including gastroesophageal reflux and upper airway cough syndrome due to rhinitis. Frequently, these etiologies coexist and require concomitant therapy (see MKSAP 18 General Internal Medicine).

Exercise-Induced Bronchospasm

Exercise-induced bronchospasm (EIB) refers to acute, measurable airway obstruction that occurs in response to exercise. EIB is one of the most common triggers of symptoms in patients with known asthma, and also occurs in patients without asthma, typically elite athletes, during periods of high-intensity exercise. Environmental factors play a key role in precipitating symptoms. Exercise in cold, dry air, such as

during winter or in indoor ice rinks; exposure to high levels of trichloramines in swimming pools; and inhalation of airborne particulates and ozone have all been implicated.

Other disorders, such vocal cord dysfunction and cardiac disorders, can mimic EIB; therefore, establishing the presence of bronchial hyperreactivity is crucial to make an accurate diagnosis. For most patients this entails bronchial challenge testing with inhaled agents or, ideally, exercise. Initial pharmacologic therapy should consist of administration of an inhaled short-acting β2-agonist (SABA) 15 minutes before exercise. If patients require use of a SABA every day, or have inadequate symptom control, a second controller agent (inhaled glucocorticoid or a leukotriene receptor antagonist) should be added. Nonpharmacologic measures including preexercise warm-up and warming cold air before inhalation (such as a mask or scarf) are also recommended.

- Initial pharmacologic therapy for exercise-induced bronchospasm should consist of administration of a short-acting β2-agonist 15 minutes before exercise.

Occupational Asthma

A careful occupational history is an essential part of asthma evaluation, as it is estimated that 15% of adult asthma is work-related. Occupational asthma includes asthma directly caused by exposure to sensitizing or irritant substances in the workplace, as well as preexisting asthma that is exacerbated by these same factors. Typical sensitizing agents are high molecular weight substances, such as proteins, that induce an IgE-mediated immunologic response. Examples include animal and plant allergens, latex, grains, and diisocyanates. Once sensitized, patients may subsequently react to very low levels of exposure. Those at risk include farmers and animal workers, health care workers, latex glove users, bakers, and manufacturers of polyurethane products. A key clinical indicator is the relationship of symptoms to work exposures; patients often improve during weekends and time away from work. Spirometry before and after workplace exposures is a cost-effective way to confirm a suspected diagnosis of occupational asthma. Alternatively, demonstration of bronchial hyperreactivity through bronchial challenge testing or serial peak flow measurements can be used. Treatment consists of reducing exposure to the offending agent through workplace modifications or removing patients from the workplace entirely, in addition to pharmacologic therapy. The overriding principle of treatment should be prevention, which includes workplace interventions to avoid exposures and monitoring for early identification of disease.

- A key clinical indicator of occupational asthma is symptom improvement during weekends and time away from work; spirometry before and after workplace exposures is a cost-effective way to confirm a suspected diagnosis. **HVC**

Reactive Airways Dysfunction Syndrome

Reactive airways dysfunction syndrome is a well-described subset of irritant-induced occupational asthma. This syndrome occurs in patients without preexisting asthma following a single, high-level exposure to fumes, gases, or vapors; usually the exposure is severe enough to prompt immediate medical evaluation. The diagnosis requires evidence of asthmatic symptoms for at least 3 months following the exposure and is confirmed by airway obstruction or bronchial hyperreactivity.

Aspirin-Exacerbated Respiratory Disease

Aspirin-exacerbated respiratory disease describes asthma and rhinosinusitis that are precipitated by exposure to aspirin or other NSAIDs that inhibit cyclooxygenase-1. Clinical characteristics include an onset in adulthood; airway and peripheral eosinophilia; inflammatory sinusitis with polyposis; and persistent, often severe asthma. Ingestion of triggering substances can cause life-threatening bronchospasm within minutes to hours, sometimes accompanied by rhinorrhea, conjunctival injection, and flushing. Chronic management, in addition to the usual stepped asthma care includes discontinuing all NSAIDs and use of leukotriene-receptor antagonists that target the increased leukotriene production implicated in the mechanism of this particular asthma. Aspirin desensitization can improve control in a significant percentage of patients but requires specialized expertise.

Allergic Bronchopulmonary Aspergillosis

Allergic bronchopulmonary aspergillosis is an ongoing immunologic response to inhaled *Aspergillus* species that leads to persistent eosinophilic airway inflammation, increased IgE levels (both total and *Aspergillus* specific), and eventually tissue damage with airway remodeling. Patients present with difficult-to-control asthma, productive cough, and expectoration of brownish mucus plugs. Radiographs may demonstrate pulmonary infiltrates and bronchiectasis. The diagnostic criteria are debated but include the presence of asthma, elevated IgE levels, positive skin tests to *Aspergillus* antigens, increased pulmonary *Aspergillus*-specific IgE and IgG levels, and either central bronchiectasis or infiltrates. Management is aimed at suppressing the enhanced immunologic response with systemic glucocorticoids and reducing the fungal antigenic burden with antifungal agents.

Common Comorbidities

Comorbidities in asthma are common and should be considered and actively managed to reduce symptoms and potentially improve asthma control.

Gastroesophageal Reflux Disease

Gastroesophageal reflux disease frequently coexists in asthma patients, and may be an independent cause of respiratory symptoms such as cough and chest pain. In patients with active gastroesophageal reflux disease symptoms, an empiric trial of a proton pump inhibitor for 2 months is indicated. Patients whose reflux symptoms do not improve should be considered for further testing such as endoscopy and 24-hour esophageal pH monitoring (see MKSAP 18 Gastroenterology and Hepatology).

Sinus Disease

Disease of the upper airway, including rhinitis and sinusitis, is extremely common in patients with asthma and is associated with more severe asthma symptoms. Allergic rhinitis is an IgE-driven inflammatory response to sensitizing allergens, and is characterized by rhinorrhea, nasal obstruction, itching, and sneezing. Symptoms can be seasonal, intermittent, or perennial (usually caused by persistent exposure to indoor allergens such as dust mites). Patients with chronic rhinosinusitis have endogenous, ongoing inflammation of both the nose and paranasal sinuses, with additional symptoms of facial pain, sinus pressure, and sometimes anosmia. Those that develop nasal polyposis have more-difficult-to-control asthma. Guidelines suggest treating with intranasal glucocorticoids; more severe cases may require combined use of intranasal glucocorticoid and intranasal H1-antihistamines, oral antileukotrienes, oral glucocorticoids, biologics targeting IgE, and immunotherapy.

Obstructive Sleep Apnea

Symptomatic obstructive sleep apnea (OSA) and polysomnographic evidence of OSA are more common in patients with asthma compared to those without asthma. The association becomes stronger with increasing severity of asthma. The presence of OSA also worsens asthma control, increases asthma-related health care utilization, and reduces quality of life. Although nocturnal worsening of asthma symptoms is common, patients should also be asked about snoring, excessive daytime sleepiness, and witnessed apneas, which are typical symptoms of OSA. If present, diagnostic testing to confirm the presence of OSA is indicated because treatment of OSA improves asthma outcomes, including symptoms, quality of life, bronchodilator use, and peak flow rates.

Vocal Cord Dysfunction

Vocal cord dysfunction refers to paradoxical adduction of the vocal cords during inspiration, leading to functional upper airway obstruction. This entity is important as its symptoms mimic those of asthma. Vocal cord dysfunction should be considered in the differential diagnosis of asthma, particularly if patients complain of prominent inspiratory breathlessness, with throat tightness or voice dysfunction during attacks. Symptoms are often triggered by exercise, exposure to fumes or irritants, and stress. Patients with vocal cord dysfunction do not respond to standard asthma therapy. Vocal cord dysfunction also can coexist with asthma. The gold standard diagnosis is demonstration of the paradoxical vocal cord adduction using direct laryngoscopy during a symptomatic episode. However, patients are generally asymptomatic when evaluated or unable to tolerate the maneuver during an acute episode. Therefore, in patients with suggestive symptoms, a trial of treatment is often indicated. Management includes addressing factors known to worsen vocal cord dysfunction (gastroesophageal reflux disease, postnasal drip), but the mainstay of treatment is speech therapy, which employs cognitive-behavioral techniques to self-identify triggers and symptoms and to reduce the functional obstruction.

> **KEY POINT**
>
> - Vocal cord dysfunction should be considered in the differential diagnosis of asthma, particularly if patients complain of prominent inspiratory breathlessness, with throat tightness or voice dysfunction during attacks.

Obesity

Obese patients have a higher prevalence of asthma and poorer control of symptoms. Increased BMI appears to influence asthma through mechanisms related to both systemic inflammation and respiratory mechanics. Obese patients with asthma do not respond as well to standard controller therapies as nonobese patients, possibly because of an alternate inflammatory profile or the presence of comorbidities associated with obesity, such as gastroesophageal reflux disease and OSA. Asthma may be overdiagnosed and underdiagnosed in obese patients because of the overlap of symptoms of breathlessness and exertional wheezing. Therefore, it is important to measure BMI in all patients undergoing asthma evaluation and to objectively document reversible airway obstruction through pulmonary function testing. In patients with obesity-related asthma, weight loss has been demonstrated to improve asthma control and lung function and should be considered an essential part of the treatment plan. In some patients, bariatric surgery may be indicated because greater amounts of weight loss correlate with better outcomes, including reduction in asthma exacerbations, improved quality of life, improved lung function, and decreased systemic and bronchial inflammation (see MKSAP 18 General Internal Medicine).

Management of Chronic Asthma

The goals of longitudinal asthma management are to control chronic asthma symptoms, prevent acute exacerbations, and minimize risks of developing fixed airway obstruction. This should be accomplished by assessing asthma severity, controlling symptoms on an ongoing basis, and then modifying therapies appropriately using a stepwise approach (**Figure 3**). There are three essential components to the management of asthma:

1. Assessment of symptom control and risk—Standardized, validated questionnaires that can discriminate between well-controlled and inadequately controlled asthma based on patient symptoms include the Asthma Control Test and the Asthma Control Questionnaire. Patients with daytime symptoms less than twice weekly and nocturnal symptoms less than twice monthly during the preceding 4 weeks are considered well controlled. Risk is based on measured lung function and the potential for future exacerbations, which is related to the presence of comorbidities and historical features known to predict future exacerbations.

2. Treatment—Once symptoms and risk are established, therapy should be initiated. All patients with asthma should be provided with rescue medication to use as needed for symptoms. Controller medications are used as a maintenance therapy to control symptoms and prevent exacerbations. A critical component of this therapy is teaching and assessing proper inhaler technique, as patients require skill and training to effectively use these devices. Use of a spacer can be helpful with compatible inhaler devices.

3. Review response and adjust therapy—After initiation of asthma therapies, patients should be reassessed after several months for their level of control and tolerance of medications. Controller medications can be stepped up or down with the goal to maintain symptom control and minimize medication exposure.

> **KEY POINTS**
>
> - Control of asthma should be assessed with the use of validated questionnaires.
> - Inhaler skills training and adherence are essential for successful treatment.

Quick Relief Medications

All patients with asthma should be provided with quick relief, or rescue, therapy. Short-acting β_2-agonists (SABAs) are the preferred medications to quickly reverse bronchospasm and relieve acute asthma symptoms (**Table 4**). These inhaled agents have a rapid onset of action and deliver medications directly through the airways, reducing systemic side effects; SABAs are generally well tolerated. Their main mechanism of action is induction of airway smooth muscle relaxation using stimulation of β_2-agonist receptors. SABAs should be used as needed for symptoms and are generally not administered on a scheduled basis. They may also be used before exercise to prevent EIB. Albuterol is the most commonly used SABA in the United States. Use of SABAs as single-agent asthma therapy is only indicated for patients with symptoms occurring not more than twice weekly, normal lung function between exacerbations, and nocturnal symptoms not more than twice monthly. For all others, rescue therapy is used in conjunction with controller therapy.

Short-acting inhaled anticholinergics are less effective than SABAs at relieving acute bronchospasm; however, they may be used as adjunctive therapy to SABA treatment in the management of acute exacerbations in the emergency department; this combination has been shown to reduce hospital admission rates. **H**

> **KEY POINTS**
>
> - All patients with asthma should be provided with quick relief, or rescue, therapy.
> - Short-acting β_2-agonists are the preferred medications to quickly reverse bronchospasm and relieve acute asthma symptoms.

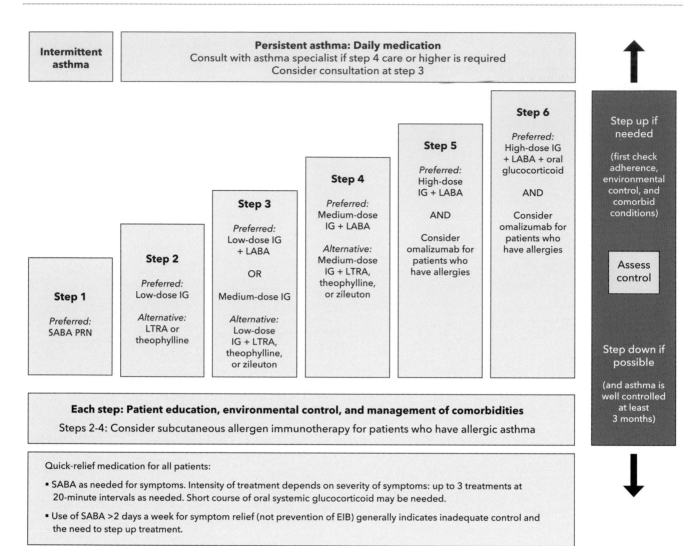

FIGURE 3. Stepwise approach to asthma therapy. EIB = exercise-induced bronchospasm; IG = inhaled glucocorticoid; LABA = long-acting β_2-agonist; LTRA = leukotriene receptor antagonist; PRN = as needed; SABA = short-acting β_2-agonist.

Source: National Heart, Lung, and Blood Institute; National Institutes of Health; U.S. Department of Health and Human Services. National Asthma Education and Prevention Program. Expert Panel Report 3 (EPR-3): Guidelines for the Diagnosis and Management of Asthma. www.nhlbi.nih.gov/files/docs/guidelines/asthsumm.pdf. Published 2007. Accessed May 9, 2018.

Controller Medications

Controller medications are used to provide ongoing symptom relief and to prevent asthma exacerbations. Several different classes of controllers exist that target different mechanisms of the asthmatic profile; therefore, medications can be effectively combined to achieve good control. The choice of therapy generally depends on the assessment of risk as described in **Management of Chronic Asthma**, and adjusted based on symptom response and patient tolerance (see Figure 3 and Table 4).

Inhaled glucocorticoids are the most effective class of asthma controller medications. These agents alleviate several pathologic processes that comprise the asthmatic response, including airway mucosal edema, mucus hypersecretion, and airway inflammation. Many strengths and formulations are available, and because individual patient response can vary, it is reasonable to try an alternate brand if the therapeutic response is not adequate. Side effects are dose-related and vary with the steroid formulation. Side effects relate to local deposition (oral candidiasis, dysphonia) and can sometimes be generalized due to some degree of systemic absorption. Systemic adverse effects such as adrenocortical suppression, reduced bone mineral density, and cataracts do not generally occur at doses below 400 µg of inhaled budesonide daily or equivalent doses of other inhaled glucocorticoid formulations. An increased rate of pneumonia is found with high-dose and high-potency formulations. Despite these risks, use of inhaled glucocorticoids to prevent the need for oral glucocorticoids should outweigh these potential adverse effects. In active smokers, the effectiveness of these medications is diminished, and higher dosing may be required.

Inhaled long-acting β_2-agonists (LABAs) that provide sustained airway dilation with just once- or twice-daily dosing are an important tool for asthma treatment. When added to inhaled glucocorticoids, they provide improved control and

TABLE 4. Asthma Medications		
Drug	**Formulations**	**Side Effects**
Short-Acting β₂-Agonists		
Albuterol	HFA-MDI, nebulizer solution	Tachycardia and hypokalemia
Levalbuterol	HFA-MDI, nebulizer solution	
Short-Acting Anticholinergics (Muscarinic Antagonists)		
Ipratropium bromide	HFA-MDI, nebulizer solution	Dry mouth, tachycardia, acute narrow angle glaucoma (rare)
Albuterol/ipratropium bromide	HFA-MDI, nebulizer solution	Same and combined effects of both drug classes
Long-Acting β₂-Agonists		
Formoterol	DPI	Tremor, tachycardia; black box warning for use in asthma
Salmeterol	DPI	
Arformoterol	Nebulizer solution	
Formoterol fumarate	Nebulizer solution	
Olodaterol	SMI	
Indacaterol maleate	DPI	
Long-Acting Muscarinic Antagonists (Anticholinergics)		
Tiotropium	DPI, SMI	Dry mouth, tachycardia, urinary retention, acute narrow angle glaucoma (rare)
Aclidinium bromide	DPI	
Umeclidinium	DPI	
Glycopyrrolate	DPI	
Inhaled Glucocorticoids		
Beclomethasone	HFA-MDI	Dysphonia, oral candidiasis, skin bruising, pneumonia, side effects of oral glucocorticoids (rare)
Budesonide	DPI, nebulizer solution	
Fluticasone propionate	HFA, DPI	
Fluticasone furoate	DPI	
Mometasone	DPI	
Ciclesonide	HFA-MDI	
Flunisolide	HFA-MDI	
Inhaled Glucocorticoid and Long-Acting β₂-Agonist		
Budesonide and formoterol	HFA	Same as combined effects of both drug classes
Fluticasone and salmeterol	HFA, DPI	
Mometasone furoate and formoterol fumarate	HFA	
Fluticasone furoate and vilanterol	DPI	
Oral Glucocorticoids		
Prednisone	Tablet, liquid	Bruising, adrenal suppression, osteoporosis, glaucoma, diabetes mellitus, opportunistic infection, insomnia, cataracts, hypertension
Prednisolone	IV infusion, tablet	
Long-Acting Muscarinic Antagonist and Long-Acting β₂-Agonist		
Tiotropium and olodaterol	SMI	Same as combined effects of both drug classes
Umeclidinium and vilanterol	DPI	
Glycopyrrolate and formoterol	MDI	
Indacaterol and glycopyrrolate	DPI	

(Continued on the next page)

TABLE 4. Asthma Medications (*Continued*)

Drug	Formulations	Side Effects
Leukotriene-Receptor Antagonists		
Montelukast	Tablet	Headache, liver disease (rare)
Zafirlukast	Tablet	
Zileuton (5-lipoxygenase inhibitor)	Tablet	
Biologic Agents		
Omalizumab (Anti-IgE)	Subcutaneous injection	Anaphylaxis, increased risk of malignancy
Mepolizumab (Anti-IL5)	Subcutaneous injection	
Reslizumab (Anti-IL5)	IV infusion	
Other		
Theophylline	Tablet, capsule, liquid	Tachycardia, nausea, overdose can be fatal

DPI = dry powder inhaler; HFA = hydrofluoroalkane; IV = intravenous; MDI = metered dose inhaler; SMI = soft mist inhaler.

decrease risk of exacerbation. For patients whose asthma is not adequately controlled by moderate-strength inhaled glucocorticoids, addition of a LABA as combined therapy with inhaled glucocorticoids in a single inhaler device is the recommended next step. Administration in a single inhaler is preferred because of greater adherence and reduced cost compared with administration of each drug in a separate inhaler. Single-agent use of LABAs is not recommended because of the demonstrated increased risk of asthma-related death when used without a simultaneous controller medication, which led the FDA to place a black box warning on all medications containing these agents. However, the FDA recently removed the black box warning from combination inhaled glucocorticoids and LABA inhalers because five large clinical trials have shown that LABAs, when used with inhaled glucocorticoids, do not significantly increase the risk of asthma-related hospitalization, intubation, or death compared to inhaled glucocorticoids alone and result in significantly fewer asthma exacerbations.

Leukotriene-receptor antagonists have a modest bronchodilation effect and treat upper airway conditions such as allergic rhinitis. Patients with aspirin-exacerbated respiratory disease often respond well to these agents.

Oral glucocorticoids are a cornerstone of therapy for treatment of acute asthma exacerbations, but long-term use exposes patients to the well-known side effects of these agents (see Table 4).

Long-acting muscarinic antagonists (LAMAs) provide sustained airway dilation, and when added to therapy in patients not controlled with inhaled glucocorticoid/LABA combination therapy, tiotropium has been shown to improve lung function and reduce exacerbations. For patients with excessive side effects from LABAs, a LAMA can reasonably be substituted. However, there is not substantial evidence that LAMAs should be the first choice for long-acting airway dilation instead of LABAs.

Newer but expensive antibody therapies directed against specific mediators of the asthmatic response can be used in patients with severe asthma not adequately controlled on standard therapy. Currently, two types of biologic therapies are available: those targeting IgE and those targeting eosinophils through the interleukin-5 pathway. Anti-IgE therapy (such as omalizumab) is indicated for use in patients with elevated levels of IgE and sensitivity to allergens, as documented by skin testing or elevated serum allergen-specific IgE. Mepolizumab and reslizumab are anti-interleukin-5 monoclonal antibodies that act to reduce eosinophil levels in airway and sputum by blocking the action of interleukin-5, a cytokine that plays a significant role in eosinophil recruitment and maturation. These agents are effective in patients with eosinophil levels above 150 cells/μL (0.15×10^9/L), regardless of IgE level. Both anti-IgE and anti-interleukin-5 therapies reduce symptoms, need for oral glucocorticoids, and exacerbations in eligible patients with moderate or severe persistent asthma.

Although expensive, omalizumab reduces emergency department visits and may be cost-effective in eligible patients with moderate to severe atopic asthma not well controlled with other therapies.

KEY POINTS

- Inhaled glucocorticoids are the most effective class of asthma controller medications.
- For patients whose asthma is not adequately controlled by moderate strength inhaled glucocorticoids, addition of a long-acting β_2-agonist as combined therapy with an inhaled glucocorticoid in a single inhaler device is the recommended next step.
- Single-agent use of long-acting β_2-agonists is not recommended because of the demonstrated increased risk of asthma-related death when used without another controller medication.
- Targeting elevated IgE or eosinophil levels with antibody therapies in eligible patients with severe persistent allergic asthma despite standard therapy reduces symptoms, need for oral glucocorticoids, and exacerbations.

Nonpharmacologic Therapy

Comprehensive asthma-care strategies include avoidance of triggers with allergen management (mold abatement, pest control, air filters), reduced exposure to environmental tobacco smoke, and a healthy diet and exercise program to promote weight loss.

Bronchial thermoplasty is a radiofrequency airway treatment administered using bronchoscopy that can reduce exacerbations and improve quality of life. Candidates are patients with an FEV_1 above 60% and severe asthma that is poorly controlled despite high-dose inhaled glucocorticoid/LABA combination therapy.

Management of Asthma Exacerbations

Asthma exacerbation refers to an acute worsening in symptoms or lung function from baseline that necessitates a step-up in therapy (see Figure 3). Prompt recognition and treatment of asthma exacerbations are needed to relieve symptoms and prevent hospitalizations. All asthma patients should have a written asthma management plan that helps them to recognize the symptoms of an exacerbation and begin self-treatment. Clinicians should screen for patient factors that contribute to an increased risk of death from asthma and counsel patients appropriately (Table 5). Self-treatment of an exacerbation consists of frequent use of reliever medications; increasing the dose, frequency, or both of controller medications; and adding a short course of oral glucocorticoids (typically 5 to 7 days of prednisone 40-50 mg/day). Patients who do not improve with self-care or who have signs that indicate a severe attack should be evaluated in an acute care facility. Management there should include close monitoring of dyspnea, work of breathing, and vital signs; treatment should include frequent inhaled SABA administration, prompt glucocorticoid therapy, and administration of supplemental oxygen to maintain oxygen saturation above 93%. For further discussion of severe asthma exacerbations, see Common ICU Conditions.

KEY POINT

- All asthma patients should have a written asthma management plan that helps them recognize the symptoms of an exacerbation and begin self-treatment.

Severe Refractory Asthma

Severe refractory asthma is present in patients who require high doses of inhaled glucocorticoids plus a second controller and/or oral steroids to prevent worsening, or who experience 2 or more exacerbations within one year that require emergency department visits or hospitalization. This group of patients consumes most asthma-related health care resources. It is important to verify the diagnosis in these patients, document medication compliance, and correct inhaler technique before considering additional therapies. Additionally, comorbidities should be aggressively managed, and the possibility of coexisting vocal cord dysfunction should be considered. Treatment guided by specific phenotypes can be helpful in this group, such as biologic agents for patients with high IgE or high eosinophil levels, and leukotriene-receptor antagonists for patients with aspirin sensitivity. Referral to a team of subspecialists is often indicated.

Asthma in Pregnancy

Pregnant patients should be advised that the advantages of treatment are significantly greater than the potential risk to the fetus from asthma therapies or exacerbations. Pregnancy can affect asthma control, leading to either worsening or improvement, and patients should be closely monitored for signs of exacerbation, which occurs most frequently during the second trimester. Inhaled glucocorticoids, oral glucocorticoids, SABAs, leukotriene-receptor antagonists (montelukast, zafirlukast), and LABAs have all been used extensively during pregnancy without data to suggest fetal harm.

Chronic Obstructive Pulmonary Disease

Definition

Chronic obstructive pulmonary disease (COPD) is a chronic lung disease defined by persistent respiratory symptoms and airflow limitation or obstruction that is not fully reversible.

Epidemiology

COPD is a common disorder that currently affects 5% of the U.S. population. The worldwide prevalence continues to rise, and the World Health Organization predicts that by 2020 COPD will become the fifth most prevalent disorder and the third leading cause of death. COPD is associated with a high

TABLE 5. Severe Asthma Exacerbation Risk Factors and Signs
Risk Factors
History of near-fatal asthma attack or intubation
Emergency department or hospital visit in the last 12 months
Poor asthma medication adherence
Recent treatment with oral glucocorticoid
Psychosocial stressors or psychiatric disease
Signs
Unable to speak in full sentences
Use of accessory muscles of respiration
Respiration rate >30/min, heart rate >120/min
SpO_2 <90% on ambient air
Agitation, confusion, or drowsiness

SpO_2 = oxygen saturation as measured by pulse oximetry.

Data from Prasad Kerlin M. In the clinic. Asthma. Ann Intern Med. 2014;160: ITC3 2-15; quiz ITC3 16-9. [PMID: 24737276] doi:10.7326/0003-4819-160-5-201403040-01003 and Most Recent Asthma Data. Centers for Disease Control and Prevention Web site. www.cdc.gov/asthma/most_recent_data.htm. Updated February 27, 2017. Accessed May 9, 2018.

morbidity and mortality, and is the third leading cause of death in the United States.

Pathophysiology

COPD is an inflammatory condition. Cigarette smoke and other irritants activate both macrophages and epithelial cells within the respiratory tract. The epithelial cells then release several neutrophil chemotactic factors. Macrophages and neutrophils release proteases that cause destruction of lung parenchyma. Proteases are typically inactivated by antiproteases, such as α_1-antitrypsin, which may also be reduced in COPD. Oxidative stress from irritants and inflammatory cells may lead to additional inflammation and tissue destruction. Ultimately, patients develop fibrosis of the small airways and reduced elastic recoil of the lungs leading to static hyperinflation. As the degree of inflammation increases, airflow obstruction worsens and the ability to fully exhale decreases. Inhalation is initiated before exhalation is completed, resulting in dynamic hyperinflation, termed air trapping, which is seen as increased anteroposterior diameter of the chest and flattening of the diaphragm on chest radiographs. The diaphragmatic flattening limits the ability to increase breath volume during exertion. Compensatory use of accessory muscles, which increases tidal volume, and increased respiration rate augment minute ventilation. These changes increase the work of breathing and contribute to the sensation of dyspnea in patients with COPD.

Risk Factors

Exposure to cigarette smoke (both first- and second-hand exposure) is the most important risk factor for COPD. Genetic predisposition seems to explain some of the variation in susceptibility to developing COPD when exposed to cigarette smoke. Long-term exposure to other irritants can also result in COPD. This includes exposure to air pollution (both indoor and outdoor) and occupational chemicals and dusts. An important example of indoor air pollution is the use of biomass fuel for cooking inside the home. Although it is uncommon in the United States, use of biomass fuel indoors is a common risk factor for COPD in the developing world. A family history of COPD is also considered a risk factor for the disease, as is a genetic condition that results in a deficiency of α_1-antitrypsin.

> **KEY POINT**
> - Exposure to cigarette smoke is the most important risk factor for COPD.

Heterogeneity of COPD

COPD is a heterogeneous condition. Some patients present predominately with a chronic productive cough due to mucus hypersecretion, whereas others present predominately with progressive dyspnea secondary to hyperinflation. The heterogeneity extends beyond clinical symptoms. Phenotypic heterogeneity has been characterized on the basis of clinical, physiologic, molecular, and radiographic variables. For example, eosinophilia has been associated with increased responsiveness to glucocorticoids. There also appears to be a subgroup of patients who are more prone to developing acute exacerbations. Understanding such variables could potentially improve the accurate assessment of prognosis and individualize patient care. Because of the heterogeneity of the disease and its presentation, tools have been developed to aid in determining prognosis and best treatment strategies. Several staging assessments exist. For example, the Global Initiative for Chronic Obstructive Lung Disease (GOLD) system combines the degree of airflow obstruction obtained from spirometry with the number of previous exacerbations as well as symptoms to help determine treatment. The BODE index uses the variables of body mass index (B), airflow obstruction (O), dyspnea (D), and exercise capacity (E) to predict outcomes and response to therapy. Airflow obstruction is determined using the post-bronchodilator FEV_1 percent of predicted for age, gender, height, and race. The index uses the Modified British Medical Research Council (mMRC) questionnaire to grade perceived dyspnea ranging from dyspnea only with strenuous exercise to dyspnea even when getting dressed. The exercise capacity is determined by the walking distance on a 6-minute walk test. This index provides better prognostic information than the FEV_1 alone and has been used to approximate 4-year survival and risk of hospitalization for COPD.

Comorbid Conditions

Patients with COPD often suffer from comorbid conditions that further increase morbidity and mortality. Some conditions, like cardiovascular disease, share common risk factors, but others seem to be independently associated with COPD or a consequence of treatment of COPD. These include muscle loss with associated weakness and weight loss, osteoporosis, and depression.

> **KEY POINT**
> - COPD is a heterogeneous condition, and patients present with variable symptoms including cough, sputum production, and dyspnea.

Diagnosis

The possibility of COPD should be considered and spirometry should be performed in patients 40 years of age or older with progressive dyspnea, chronic cough, or chronic sputum production, particularly in the presence of known risk factors for the disease, especially smoking. The role of screening spirometry in asymptomatic individuals with risk factors is controversial. The USPSTF guideline and the joint guideline developed by ACP/ATS/ACCP/ERS recommend against screening for COPD in asymptomatic adults, whereas GOLD advocates performing screening spirometry in individuals with risk factors for COPD. The diagnosis of COPD is made using spirometric measurement to document airflow obstruction. COPD is confirmed by a post-bronchodilator FEV_1/FVC ratio of less than 0.70. This

CONT.

differs from the finding in asthmatic patients, whose airflow obstruction is fully reversible with bronchodilator therapy.

Some patients have bronchial inflammation with features of both asthma and COPD, referred to as asthma-COPD overlap syndrome. A GOLD and the Global Initiative for Asthma (GINA) consensus statement characterizes asthma-COPD overlap syndrome as persistent airflow limitation with several features usually associated with asthma and several features usually associated with COPD. Measuring lung volumes and diffusing capacity is not required to diagnose COPD but may help in determining the severity of disease. Clinicians should rule out other causes of chronic respiratory symptoms including heart failure, bronchiectasis, obliterative bronchiolitis, tuberculosis, and diffuse panbronchiolitis.

KEY POINTS

HVC
- There is no role for spirometric screening for COPD in asymptomatic individuals.
- COPD is defined as a post-bronchodilator FEV_1/FVC ratio of less than 0.70.

Disease Assessment

After a diagnosis of COPD has been established, the initial assessment focuses on disease severity, which is determined using a combination of symptoms, degree of airflow obstruction on spirometry, history of acute exacerbations, and presence of comorbid conditions. Several validated tools are available to assess patients' symptoms, including the COPD Assessment Test (CAT), the Clinical COPD Questionnaire (CCQ), and the mMRC scale (**Table 6**). The GOLD criteria use the CAT or mMRC scale to determine symptom severity, whereas the BODE index requires the use of the mMRC scale. The CCQ is often used to screen patients for symptoms of COPD. Symptoms are then combined with the results from spirometry (**Table 7**) to determine disease severity (**Table 8**).

Patients who have had two or more acute exacerbations within the last year, who have an FEV_1 of less than 50% of predicted, or who have ever been hospitalized for an acute exacerbation are considered to be at high risk for recurrent acute exacerbations. Clinicians should determine if the patient suffers from any of the common comorbid conditions associated with COPD that indicate a higher morbidity and mortality and treat appropriately.

Pulse oximetry at rest and at exertion should be used to determine the need of supplemental oxygen. Arterial blood gases should be measured to assess for underlying hypercapnia in patients with a low FEV_1, change in mental status, an acute exacerbation, an elevated level of serum bicarbonate, or oxygen saturation of less than 92% on pulse oximetry.

An α_1-antitrypsin level should be obtained in patients with COPD under the age of 45 who have a strong family history of COPD or who are without identifiable COPD risk factors. A pattern of basilar emphysema, associated liver disease

TABLE 6. Modified Medical Research Council Dyspnea Scale

Score	Description of Dyspnea	Severity
0	I get breathless only with strenuous exercise.	None
1	I get short of breath when hurrying on level ground or walking up a slight hill.	Mild
2	On level ground, I walk slower than other people my age because of breathlessness, or I have to stop for breath when walking at my own pace.	Moderate
3	I stop for breath after walking approximately 100 yards or after a few minutes on level ground.	Severe
4	I am too breathless to leave the house or breathless when dressing.	Very severe

Used with the permission of the Medical Research Council.

TABLE 7. Classification of COPD Severity by Spirometry[a]

Category	Severity	Spirometry
GOLD 1	Mild	$FEV_1 \geq 80\%$ of predicted
GOLD 2	Moderate	$50\% \leq FEV_1 < 80\%$ of predicted
GOLD 3	Severe	$30\% \leq FEV_1 < 50\%$ of predicted
GOLD 4	Very severe	$FEV_1 < 30\%$ of predicted

[a]In Patients with FEV_1/FVC less than 70%.

Reprinted from Vogelmeier CF, Criner GJ, Martinez FJ, Anzueto A, Barnes PJ, Bourbeau J, et al. Global strategy for the diagnosis, management, and prevention of chronic obstructive lung disease 2017 report. GOLD executive summary. Am J Respir Crit Care Med. 2017;195:557-582. [PMID: 28128970] doi:10.1164/rccm.201701-0218PP

TABLE 8. GOLD Model for Classifying Severity of Disease in COPD[a]

Patient Category	Characteristics	Exacerbations Per Year	CAT Score	mMRC Score
A	Low risk, fewer symptoms	≤1	<10	0-1
B	Low risk, more symptoms	≤1	≥10	≥2
C	High risk, fewer symptoms	≥2	<10	0-1
D	High risk, more symptoms	≥2/≥1 with hospital admission	≥10	≥2

CAT = COPD Assessment Test; mMRC = Modified Medical Research Council.

[a]See Table 7 for definitions of spirometric classifications.

Data from Vogelmeier CF, Criner GJ, Martinez FJ, Anzueto A, Barnes PJ, Bourbeau J, et al. Global strategy for the diagnosis, management, and prevention of chronic obstructive lung disease 2017 report. GOLD executive summary. Am J Respir Crit Care Med. 2017;195:557-582. [PMID: 28128970] doi:10.1164/rccm.201701-0218PP

or panniculitis, or a strong family history of emphysema in patients with COPD should also prompt consideration of α_1-antitrypsin deficiency in middle-aged and older patients. Some guidelines even recommend that all patients with COPD regardless of age be tested for α1-antitrypsin deficiency after weighing the risks and benefits of testing.

KEY POINTS

- After a diagnosis of COPD has been established, the initial assessment focuses on disease severity, which is determined using a combination of symptoms, degree of airflow obstruction on spirometry, history of acute exacerbations, and presence of comorbid conditions.

- Patients who have had two or more acute exacerbations within the last year, who have an FEV_1 of less than 50% of predicted, or who have ever been hospitalized for an acute exacerbation are considered to be at high risk for recurrent acute exacerbations.

Management of COPD

A management plan for COPD should include the identification and reversal of risk factors, especially ongoing exposure to cigarette smoke. The severity of a patient's COPD should guide the choice of therapy (**Table 9**). No currently available treatments can prevent long-term decline in lung function, so patients should be monitored for evidence of disease progression that may guide additional therapy. The goals of therapy are to reduce symptoms, improve exercise tolerance and quality of life, as well as prevent and treat exacerbations, prevent disease progression, and decrease mortality.

Smoking Cessation

Smoking cessation is essential in the management of COPD, as it can slow the decline of FEV_1. Providers should encourage patients to quit smoking and be aware that the success rates for smoking cessation increase when counseling is combined with medication therapy. Effective medications for cessation

---

TABLE 9. Pharmacologic Management of COPD

Patient Group	Recommended Therapy	Alternative Therapy	Other Considerations
A	Short-acting bronchodilator *or* Long-acting bronchodilator	Evaluate effect of therapy and continue, stop, or try alternative bronchodilator as appropriate	All patients in Group A should receive bronchodilator therapy based on its effect on dyspnea; therapy should be continued if symptomatic benefit is documented.
B	Long-acting bronchodilator (LABA or LAMA) *or* Combination therapy with two bronchodilators may be considered for patients with severe dyspnea.	If symptoms persist after one long-acting bronchodilator, try combined therapy with LABA and LAMA	Long-acting inhaled bronchodilators are superior to short-acting bronchodilators taken as needed. There is no evidence to support use of one class of long-acting bronchodilators over another for initial relief of symptoms for patients in Group B. In the individual patient, the choice should depend on the patient's perception of symptom relief. Patients in Group B are likely to have comorbidities that affect symptoms and prognosis, and these should be investigated.
C	LAMA; if further exacerbations, LAMA and LABA	LABA and inhaled glucocorticoids	LABA and LAMA is preferred to LABA and inhaled glucocorticoids because inhaled glucocorticoids increase the risk of developing pneumonia in some patients.
D	LABA and LAMA; if further exacerbations, add inhaled glucocorticoids	If exacerbations continue, consider: roflumilast (patients with an FEV_1 <50% of predicted and chronic bronchitis, particularly if they have experienced at least one hospitalization for an exacerbation in the previous year); *or* macrolide therapy (the best available evidence exists for the use of azithromycin)	Initial therapy with LABA and inhaled glucocorticoids may be appropriate in some patients, including those with a history or findings suggestive of asthma-COPD overlap.

LABA = long-acting β_2-agonist; LAMA = long-acting muscarinic agent.

Data from Vogelmeier CF, Criner GJ, Martinez FJ, Anzueto A, Barnes PJ, Bourbeau J, et al. Global strategy for the diagnosis, management, and prevention of chronic obstructive lung disease 2017 report. GOLD executive summary. Am J Respir Crit Care Med. 2017;195:557-582. [PMID: 28128970] doi:10.1164/rccm.201701-0218PP

include nicotine replacement, varenicline, and bupropion (see MKSAP 18 General Internal Medicine). H

> **KEY POINT**
> - Smoking cessation is essential in the management of COPD, as it can slow the decline of FEV_1.

Pharmacologic Therapy

Pharmacologic therapies in COPD are used to reduce symptoms, improve quality of life, and reduce the frequency and severity of exacerbations (**Table 10**). Bronchodilators are mainstays of therapy in COPD irrespective of the severity of the disease. Any time bronchodilators or other inhalers are prescribed, the clinician should ensure that the patient receives education on proper inhaler technique. Initial management is outlined in Table 9.

Bronchodilators

Inhaled bronchodilators include β_2-agonists and anticholinergics/antimuscarinic agents. Both are available as short-acting and long-acting inhalers and improve symptoms and expiratory airflow. Short-acting β_2-agonists and muscarinic antagonists result in similar bronchodilation, and either can be used as monotherapy. However, dual treatment results in a greater degree of bronchodilation and expiratory airflow, which may lead to symptom benefit in select patients.

If short-acting bronchodilators are insufficient to control symptoms in patients with more severe disease, a long-acting bronchodilator, either a LABA or a LAMA, can be added. Choosing the appropriate long-acting bronchodilator inhaler requires consideration of patient and physician preference, potential side effects, and cost. If symptoms persist on monotherapy, addition of a second long-acting bronchodilator from the alternate bronchodilator class may result in clinical improvement. Long-acting bronchodilators alone should not be used in patients with an asthma component to their COPD (asthma-COPD overlap syndrome) unless an inhaled glucocorticoid is also prescribed because of the potential for increased risk of mortality in this patient population when a LABA is used without an inhaled glucocorticoid.

Inhaled Glucocorticoids

Inhaled glucocorticoids are typically used only in combination with a long-acting bronchodilator for treatment of COPD (see Table 9). Inhaled glucocorticoids are not used alone unless a patient is not able to use long-acting bronchodilators (see Table 10). Inhaled glucocorticoids, used alone and in combination with long-acting bronchodilators, improve lung function and reduce symptoms and exacerbations in patients with moderate to severe COPD, but are associated with an increased risk of pneumonia. In patients with severe COPD, triple inhaler therapy with a LABA, a LAMA, and an inhaled glucocorticoid may provide additional symptom benefit. H

> **KEY POINT**
> - Bronchodilators are mainstays of therapy in COPD irrespective of the severity of the COPD; any time bronchodilators or other inhalers are prescribed, the clinician should ensure that the patient receives education on proper inhaler technique.

Systemic Glucocorticoids

Systemic glucocorticoids are recommended for short-duration treatment of acute exacerbations of COPD. (See Acute Exacerbations: Goals and Therapeutic Management section.) However, long-term use of systemic glucocorticoids should be avoided due to the risk of significant side effects, including diabetes and osteoporosis. H

Methylxanthines

The methylxanthines (aminophylline and theophylline) are now rarely used to treat COPD. Theophylline has been shown to improve functional capacity and reduce the number of exacerbations. However, it has a narrow window between therapeutic and toxic dosages and is therefore only used for patients with advanced COPD who have refractory symptoms not controlled by standard therapy. Studies of the use of either aminophylline or theophylline during acute exacerbations have shown no benefit.

Roflumilast

Roflumilast is a selective phosphodiesterase-4 inhibitor that is used to reduce chronic symptoms and the frequency of exacerbations in patients with severe COPD who have either primarily symptoms of chronic bronchitis or frequent exacerbations. H

α_1-Antitrypsin Augmentation Therapy

Antiproteases, including α_1-antitrypsin, typically inactivate proteases that may lead to permanent lung injury. In patients with α_1-antitrypsin deficiency, replacing this enzyme with augmentation therapy may slow the progression of related emphysema. However, it is costly, has not been shown to decrease exacerbations or the rate of FEV_1 decline, and is not effective for treatment of patients whose COPD is not caused by α_1-antitrypsin deficiency.

Other Agents

Macrolide antibiotics have inflammatory and antimicrobial effects. Long-term macrolide therapy may reduce the frequency of exacerbations when prescribed to patients with severe COPD and a history of frequent exacerbations. Mucolytics and antitussives are not routinely used in the management of COPD but may provide some symptomatic relief in patients with significant sputum production. H

Immunization

Immunizations can prevent infections in patients with COPD. Because infections are the most common trigger of

TABLE 10. Drug Treatment for COPD		
Agent	**Side Effects**	**Notes**
Bronchodilators		
Inhaled short-acting β_2-agonists (albuterol, fenoterol, levalbuterol, metaproterenol, pirbuterol, terbutaline)	Tachycardia and hypokalemia (usually dose dependent), but generally well tolerated by most patients	Generally used as needed for mild disease with few symptoms
Inhaled short-acting anticholinergic agents (ipratropium)	Dry mouth, mydriasis on contact with eye, tachycardia, tremors, rarely acute narrow angle glaucoma; this drug class has been shown to be safe in a wide range of doses and clinical settings	Generally used as needed for mild disease with few symptoms; avoid using both short- and long-acting anticholinergics
Inhaled long-acting anticholinergic agents (tiotropium, aclidinium, umeclidinium, glycopyrronium)	Dry mouth, mydriasis on contact with eye, tachycardia, tremors, rarely acute narrow angle glaucoma	Not to be used with ipratropium; use when short-acting bronchodilators provide insufficient control of symptoms for patients with an FEV_1 <60% of predicted
Inhaled long-acting β_2-agonists (salmeterol, formoterol, arformoterol, indacaterol, olodaterol)	Sympathomimetic symptoms such as tremor and tachycardia; overdose can be fatal	Use as maintenance therapy when short-acting bronchodilators provide insufficient control of symptoms for patients with an FEV_1 <60% of predicted; not intended to be used for treatment of exacerbations of COPD or acute bronchospasm
Methylxanthines (theophylline, aminophylline; sustained and short-acting)	Tachycardia, nausea, vomiting, and disturbed sleep; narrow therapeutic index; overdose can be fatal with seizures and arrhythmias	Used as maintenance therapy; generally use only after long-acting bronchodilator treatment to provide additional symptomatic relief of exacerbations; may also improve respiratory muscle function
Oral β_2-agonists (albuterol, metaproterenol, terbutaline)	Sympathomimetic symptoms such as tremor and tachycardia	Used as maintenance therapy; rarely used because of side effects but may be beneficial for patients who cannot use inhalers
Oral Phosophodiesterase-4 Inhibitor		
Roflumilast	Diarrhea, nausea, backache, decreased appetite, dizziness	Used to reduce risk for exacerbations in patients with severe COPD (blood levels not required) with chronic bronchitis and history of exacerbations; roflumilast should not be used with methylxanthines owing to potential toxicity; very expensive and should be used only in select patients
Anti-Inflammatory Agents		
Inhaled glucocorticoids (fluticasone, budesonide, mometasone, ciclesonide, beclomethasone)	Dysphonia, skin bruising, oral candidiasis, rarely side effects of oral glucocorticoids (see below)	Most effective in patients with a history of frequent exacerbations and when used in conjunction with long-acting bronchodilators
Oral glucocorticoids (prednisone, prednisolone)	Skin bruising, adrenal suppression, glaucoma, osteoporosis, diabetes mellitus, systemic hypertension, pneumonia, cataracts, opportunistic infection, insomnia, mood disturbance	Use for significant exacerbations of COPD; avoid, if possible, in stable COPD to limit glucocorticoid toxicity; consider inhaled glucocorticoids to facilitate weaning of systemic glucocorticoids
Combination Agents		
Combined inhaled long-acting β_2-agonist and inhaled glucocorticoid in a single inhaler (fluticasone/salmeterol, budesonide/formoterol)	Same/combined effects of both drug classes	Fluticasone/salmeterol is approved by the FDA as maintenance therapy and for prevention of exacerbations; budesonide/formoterol metered-dose inhaler is approved by the FDA as maintenance therapy; combinations are not to be used for treatment of acute bronchospasm
Combined short-acting β_2-agonist plus short-acting anticholinergic in a single inhaler (fenoterol/ipratropium, salbutamol/ipratropium)	Same/combined effects of both drug classes	Generally used as needed for mild disease with few symptoms; avoid using both short- and long-acting anticholinergics; this combination therapy may be used for maintenance therapy only if patients have well-controlled disease on this combination treatment and do not require rescue therapy if/when expense is a determining factor
Combined inhaled glucocorticoid and ultra–long-acting β_2-agonist in a single inhaler (fluticasone/vilanterol)	Same/combined effects of both drug classes	Not to be used for treatment of acute bronchospasm
Combined long-acting anticholinergic plus ultra–long-acting β_2-agonist in a single inhaler (umeclidinium/vilanterol)	Same/combined effects of both drug classes	Not to be used for treatment of acute bronchospasm. Avoid using both short- and long-acting anticholinergics.

acute exacerbations, routine immunizations are recommended for all patients with COPD. Patients should receive annual influenza immunization and the pneumococcal polysaccharide vaccine (PPSV23). Those above the age of 65 should also receive the pneumococcal conjugate vaccine (PCV13).

KEY POINTS

- Systemic glucocorticoids are recommended for short-duration treatment of acute exacerbations of COPD; long-term use of systemic glucocorticoids should be avoided.

- All COPD patients should have annual influenza immunization and the pneumococcal polysaccharide vaccine; those above the age of 65 should also receive the pneumococcal conjugate vaccine.

Nonpharmacologic Therapy
Pulmonary Rehabilitation
Pulmonary rehabilitation is a comprehensive program that combines exercise training, nutritional support, education, and social support for patients with chronic lung conditions. It has been shown to relieve symptoms, improve quality of life, and decrease frequency of hospitalizations in patients with COPD. Clinicians should consider adding this to appropriate medical therapy in symptomatic patients with an FEV_1 of less than 50% of predicted and to patients recovering from COPD exacerbation; particularly those recently hospitalized or treated with systemic steroids would benefit from pulmonary rehabilitation.

Oxygen Therapy
The use of supplemental oxygen has been shown to improve quality of life and decrease mortality in patients with COPD and resting hypoxemia with an arterial Po_2 of 55 mm Hg or less, or oxygen saturation as measured by pulse oximetry of 88% or less. Patients with cor pulmonale, heart failure, or erythrocytosis should be offered the use of supplemental oxygen if the Po_2 is 59 mm Hg or less or the oxygen saturation is 89% or less. Some patients may not qualify for oxygen at rest but may desaturate during sleep, exertion, or air travel. Supplemental oxygen is typically prescribed if the oxygen saturation as measured by pulse oximetry falls below 89% in these situations, but the benefits are less defined.

Noninvasive Mechanical Ventilation
Noninvasive mechanical ventilation (NIV), also termed noninvasive positive pressure ventilation (NIPPV), can be used for acute and chronic respiratory failure. For patients with a COPD exacerbation and acute hypercapnic respiratory failure with acidosis, NIV improves symptoms and reduces intubation rates, length of hospital stay, and mortality. It may also be beneficial in COPD patients with pneumonia, to help with discontinuing mechanical ventilation, and for palliative care. It does not replace intubation and mechanical ventilation in critically ill patients, comatose patients, or patients who have sustained a cardiac arrest. NIV is generally well tolerated, and improvement of the pH and Pco_2 within 1 to 2 hours predicts success. The benefit of using NIV in the treatment of chronic respiratory failure or in the outpatient setting is less clear. It may, especially if used at night, provide additional symptomatic relief when added to medical therapy in patients with severe COPD. **H**

Prognosis and Goals of Care
The current GOLD initiative recommends combining the degree of airflow limitation using the post-bronchodilator FEV_1 with the number of exacerbations and the patient's symptoms to classify the severity of disease. This will allow the clinician to guide escalation or de-escalation of medical therapies as appropriate.

The BODE index can be used as a prognostic indicator for patients with COPD. Using the BMI, the post-bronchodilator FEV_1 percent of predicted, dyspnea as defined using the mMRC scale (see Table 6), and the distance walked on a 6-minute walk test, it is possible to approximate the patient's 4-year survival. In patients with severe disease with an overall poor prognosis, referral for hospice and palliative care can provide significant improvements in symptom burden.

Palliative care can significantly aid in symptom management in patients with COPD at any stage of disease. Patients experience not only dyspnea, but also anxiety and depression, which may also be addressed. Opioids are commonly used to treat dyspnea that persists despite medical therapy. Current guidelines suggest a patient with severe COPD — defined by disabling symptoms despite medical therapy, progression of disease as evidenced by increasing emergency department evaluations or hospitalizations, and hypoxemia or hypercapnia — should be considered for hospice care. **H**

KEY POINT

- Current guidelines suggest a patient with severe COPD (defined by disabling symptoms despite medical therapy, progression of disease as evidenced by increasing emergency department evaluations or hospitalizations, and hypoxemia or hypercapnia), should be considered for hospice care.

Lung Volume Reduction Therapy
The National Emphysema Treatment Trial (NETT) demonstrated that patients with upper lobe–predominant and significant exercise limitations even after participation in a pulmonary rehabilitation program had improved quality of life, exercise tolerance, pulmonary function, and survival with lung volume reduction surgery. A key finding from NETT was that patient selection was critical to success and that patients with an FEV_1 of less than 20% of predicted, a diffusing capacity of less than 20% of predicted, or non–upper lobe predominant disease had a high operative mortality and should not be offered lung volume reduction surgery. The procedure should be considered in patients with upper lobe–predominant who have low exercise tolerance despite

maximal medical therapy and completion of a pulmonary rehabilitation program. Nonsurgical lung volume reduction procedures, including bronchoscopic placement of endobronchial one-way valves, plugs, or coils; administration of biologic sealants; and thermal ablation of the airway are being studied for treatment of emphysematous changes in patients with COPD. Early results suggest patients with severe air trapping and hyperinflation may get the most benefit from these new techniques.

Lung Transplantation

Referral for lung transplantation can be considered in patients with severe COPD. The decision to refer should depend on the patient's life expectancy, quality of life, and patient preferences. In general, patients at high risk of dying in less than 2 years who have a high probability of 90-day postoperative survival are candidates. Patients with an elevated BODE index (5 or 6), resting hypoxemia, hypercapnia, an FEV_1 of less than 25% of predicted, or significant exercise limitation despite medical therapy, smoking cessation, and participation in a pulmonary rehabilitation program may be referred for evaluation for lung transplantation. Transplantation improves quality of life, and the median life expectancy is 5.7 years.

Acute Exacerbations

Definition

An acute exacerbation of COPD is a change in a patient's typical symptoms that leads to a change in medical therapy or requires hospitalization. Most commonly, exacerbations are manifested by an increase in the severity or frequency of cough, worsening dyspnea, and an increase in the amount or change in the character of sputum produced. Most exacerbations are triggered by a respiratory infection (either viral or bacterial), smoking, and environmental exposures. An exacerbation can be triggered by other causes, but in some cases no trigger is ever identified. Studies suggest that exacerbations are underreported by patients and result in adverse outcomes. **H**

KEY POINT

- An acute exacerbation of COPD is a change in a patient's typical symptoms that leads to a change in medical therapy or hospitalization; the most common exacerbations are manifested by an increase in the severity or frequency of cough, worsening dyspnea, and an increase in the amount or change in the character of sputum produced.

Prevention

Acute exacerbations of COPD can have substantial effects on quality of life and health care costs, and may accelerate the decline in lung function and increase mortality. It is therefore important to prevent exacerbations whenever possible. Strategies to prevent exacerbations include smoking cessation, participating in pulmonary rehabilitation programs when appropriate, receiving recommended immunizations, and ensuring proper inhaler technique and use of medications. Long-term use of azithromycin or roflumilast has also been shown to prevent future exacerbations in patients who have a history of frequent exacerbations. **H**

KEY POINT

- Strategies to prevent COPD exacerbations include smoking cessation, participating in pulmonary rehabilitation programs when appropriate, receiving recommended immunizations, and ensuring proper inhaler technique and use of medications.

Initial Assessment and Setting of Care

The first steps in managing a patient with a presumed COPD exacerbation are to confirm the diagnosis and determine the severity of the exacerbation for accurate triaging. A mild exacerbation is one that can be managed solely by increasing the dose of the regular medications the patient is already on. A moderate exacerbation requires treatment with antibiotics, steroids, or both; a severe exacerbation is defined by the need for an evaluation in the emergency department or hospitalization. Patients with respiratory distress or who are at risk of developing respiratory distress should be hospitalized; additional testing, including a chest radiograph, electrocardiogram, complete blood count, and basic metabolic panel, should be obtained to rule out other causes or comorbidities contributing to the acute presentation. Oxygen saturation should be measured by pulse oximetry. Arterial blood gas measurement is recommended for patients with a severe exacerbation to determine the presence of hypercapnia or hypoxemia. A sputum culture is not routinely used to assess COPD exacerbations as it rarely affects management. Patients with mild symptoms may not require any additional testing. **H**

KEY POINTS

- Patients who have COPD and respiratory distress or who are at risk of developing respiratory distress should be hospitalized and evaluated with a chest radiograph, electrocardiogram, complete blood count, basic metabolic panel, and oxygen saturation; arterial blood gas measurements can determine the presence of hypercapnia or hypoxemia.
- A sputum culture is not routinely used to assess COPD exacerbations as it rarely affects management. **HVC**

Goals and Therapeutic Management

The management goals during an acute exacerbation are to relieve acute symptoms and to prevent future exacerbations. Supplemental oxygen should be used to maintain oxygen saturation between 89% and 92%. Noninvasive mechanical ventilation may be required if oxygenation or ventilation

CONT.

cannot be maintained. Patients may require mechanical intubation if they cannot tolerate noninvasive mechanical ventilation, have an altered mental status, or have worsening hypercapnic or hypoxemic respiratory failure despite the use of noninvasive mechanical ventilation. Short-acting β_2-agonists with or without anticholinergic agents should be used to relieve acute symptoms. The use of oral glucocorticoids during acute exacerbations has been shown to decrease the frequency of treatment failures, length of stay, and the time to subsequent exacerbations while improving FEV_1 and hypoxemia. Glucocorticoids have also been shown to decrease the need for hospitalization if used early. Recent randomized trials have demonstrated that short courses of lower-dose oral glucocorticoids, 40 mg for 5 days, are usually equivalent to longer courses, higher doses, and intravenous administration.

Antibiotics should be prescribed in cases of moderate or severe exacerbations or for patients with mild exacerbations who have noted an increase or change in sputum production. The most common infectious triggers are viruses, but bacterial causes include *Streptococcus pneumoniae*, *Haemophilus influenzae*, *Moraxella catarrhalis*, and *Mycoplasma pneumoniae*. If the patient is still smoking, treatment should also focus on smoking cessation because this can prevent future exacerbations. Because the prevalence of pulmonary embolism is higher in patients with COPD, a thromboembolic event should be considered as a potential trigger if patients do not improve with typical therapies for a COPD exacerbation, and appropriate testing should be performed.

Bronchiectasis

Definition

Bronchiectasis is a chronic suppurative lung disease associated with irreversible enlargement of the airways due to destruction of airway architecture. An injury to the lung typically results in prolonged airway inflammation, which leads to localized injury with subsequent mucus stasis, which can lead to further airway obstruction, chronic infection, and inflammation with worsening bronchiectasis.

Causes

In many cases of bronchiectasis, an underlying cause is not identified. The most common causes of bronchiectasis include cystic fibrosis, aspiration, immunodeficiencies, and connective tissue diseases (**Table 11**).

Presentation

Bronchiectasis should be considered in the differential diagnosis of any patient with a chronic cough, especially if the patient has a history of frequent respiratory infections or if the cough is productive. Other possible symptoms include hemoptysis, wheezing, and chest pain. Features that should alert the clinician to consider bronchiectasis include previous

TABLE 11. Common Causes of Bronchiectasis
Airway obstruction
Tumor
Foreign body
Aspiration
COPD
Congenital
Mounier-Kuhn syndrome
Young syndrome
Connective tissue diseases
Rheumatoid arthritis
Sjögren's syndrome
Cystic fibrosis
Hypersensitivity
Allergic bronchopulmonary aspergillosis
Immunodeficiency
Common variable immunodeficiency
HIV
Mucociliary dysfunction
Primary ciliary dyskinesia
Postinfection
Tuberculosis
Pneumonia, especially recurrent

sputum cultures growing uncommon pathogens such as *Pseudomonas aeruginosa*, *Aspergillus*, or nontuberculous mycobacteria; clubbing; and minimal or no smoking history.

Patients with bronchiectasis may also present with extrapulmonary symptoms, especially fatigue.

Diagnosis

Initial evaluation should include a comprehensive medical history, including childhood diseases, family history, and careful evaluation to exclude known causes of bronchiectasis. Bronchiectasis is diagnosed by high-resolution chest CT. Diagnostic criteria include airway diameter that is greater than that of its accompanying vessel and lack of distal airway tapering (**Figure 4**). Bronchial wall thickening or cysts are often present. For every diagnosed patient, it should be determined whether there is an underlying cause that can be treated. This may involve testing for chronic bacterial or mycobacterial infections. These tests can identify causes of disease progression and help determine targeted antimicrobial therapy for exacerbations. Patients should also be evaluated for the presence of connective tissue disease and immune function. In selected patients, testing for cystic fibrosis, ciliary dysfunction, or α_1-antitrypsin deficiency may be appropriate if suspected. However, even with rigorous evaluation, more than half of all cases are still considered idiopathic.

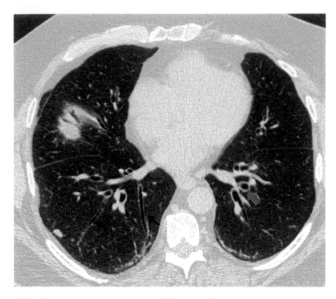

FIGURE 4. Bronchiectasis on chest CT. The airway is larger than its accompanying blood vessel (*thick arrow*), and the airway fails to taper distally (*thin arrows*).

Treatment

The presence of chronic symptoms of cough and sputum production typically indicates irreversible airway dilation. Therefore, treatment of the underlying cause may not lead to improvement in current symptoms but could prevent further progression. Otherwise, treatment of bronchiectasis focuses on airway clearance, treating infections, and preventing exacerbations. The goal of airway clearance is to improve mucous clearance and thereby prevent chronic or recurrent infections. Bronchodilators, inhaled glucocorticoids, and combination inhalers have been shown to decrease symptoms but have no effect on the decline of lung function or frequency of exacerbations. Studies suggest that long-term use of macrolide antibiotics may prevent future exacerbations due to their anti-inflammatory effects. When deciding whether to use macrolide antibiotics, the risk of future exacerbations should be weighed against the possibility of developing macrolide resistance. Antibiotics may also be used in the management of chronic non–cystic fibrosis bronchiectasis to eradicate organisms such as *Pseudomonas aeruginosa* or methicillin-resistant *Staphylococcus aureus*. If eradication of bacterial colonization is not successful, there may be some symptomatic benefit from suppressive therapy with inhaled antibiotics. Patients should also be encouraged to exercise, which can improve airway clearance and symptoms. Surgical resection should be considered in patients who have localized disease with persistent symptoms despite therapy.

Treatment of Exacerbations

Exacerbations of bronchiectasis may be difficult to differentiate from baseline symptoms. However, changes in sputum volume, viscosity, or purulence; increased cough; wheezing; shortness of breath; hemoptysis; or declines in lung function are considered evidence of an exacerbation. Therapy for an exacerbation is ideally guided by routine sputum and acid-fast bacilli culture results to identify a possible predominant organism for treatment. Empiric antibiotic therapy is recommended and may be based on previous culture data until the results of the current sputum culture become available. If previous data are not available, a fluoroquinolone can be started to ensure *Pseudomonas* coverage until sputum culture results are available.

Cystic Fibrosis

Cystic fibrosis (CF) is an autosomal recessive disease affecting the CF transmembrane conductance regulator (*CFTR*) gene. It is diagnosed in approximately 1 of 2000-3000 live births with a predilection for disease in those of European descent. The most common genetic variant resulting in disease is ΔF508, but there are at least 1500 other genetic mutations. The pathogenesis for clinical manifestations of CF remains incompletely understood; however, the abnormal homozygous *CFTR* genotype results in abnormally thick secretions that are difficult to clear. There is an increased concentration of chloride in sweat gland secretions, and sweat chloride testing is a primary diagnostic tool for CF. The changes in respiratory secretions lead to bacterial colonization of airways and chronic bacterial infection, resulting in chronic inflammation and, ultimately, bronchiectasis. Further tissue destruction results from insufficient lung antiproteases to counteract the effect of elastase released from neutrophils. This ongoing inflammatory process also results in large amounts of free DNA and matrix protein deposition within areas of tissue destruction, which further drives increased viscosity of lung secretions.

Thickened secretions in the gastrointestinal tract impair flow of bile and pancreatic secretions, leading to pancreatic exocrine and endocrine deficiency, liver disease, and the development of malabsorption and maldigestion. The secretions increase the risk for bowel obstruction (distal ileal obstructive syndrome, intussusception, and rectal prolapse). Consequently, individuals with CF often present with malnutrition and weight loss.

Diagnosis

Few patients with CF are diagnosed as adults. Adults diagnosed with CF most often present with pulmonary or gastrointestinal symptoms. Pulmonary manifestations often include chronic productive cough, recurrent sinusitis, and recurrent pulmonary infections requiring several courses of antibiotics. For those with gastrointestinal symptoms, loose and frequent stools with abdominal pain are the most common. Pancreatic insufficiency (either endocrine or exocrine) may occur but is less common. Chronic, persistent pulmonary or gastrointestinal symptoms requiring repetitive treatment should raise suspicion for CF. Radiographic findings of upper lobe–predominant with mucoid impaction may be present.

Often the greatest challenge to making the diagnosis is failing to include CF in the differential diagnosis. A family history of CF can be quite helpful in this regard. Sweat chloride testing is the initial test for CF, although it is less sensitive in adults. Abnormal results on repeat testing are diagnostic of CF. DNA testing confirms the diagnosis and helps with prognosis. A negative sweat chloride test in an adult patient does not rule out disease. Therefore, if the clinical suspicion remains high after negative repeat sweat chloride testing, consideration for referral to a center with expertise in CF or genetic testing is appropriate.

KEY POINTS

- Adults diagnosed with cystic fibrosis most often present with pulmonary or gastrointestinal symptoms; pulmonary manifestations often include chronic productive cough, recurrent sinusitis, and recurrent pulmonary infections requiring several courses of antibiotics.

- A negative sweat chloride test in a patient who presents as an adult should not rule out cystic fibrosis.

Treatment

The pillars of CF management are airway clearance, antibiotic therapy, nutritional support, and psychosocial support. The primary objectives of CF treatment are maintaining lung health and controlling/minimizing the impact of CF-affected organ disease. The Cystic Fibrosis Foundation practice guidelines recommend use of chronic medications to improve lung function and reduce exacerbations. These medications include mucolytics, hydrating agents, inhaled antibiotics, oral macrolide antibiotics, and *CFTR* potentiators. The treatment of CF lung disease is experiencing a period of rapid evolution, and management is suboptimal unless it involves a multidisciplinary approach best provided at a CF care center.

Diffuse Parenchymal Lung Disease

Diffuse parenchymal lung diseases (DPLDs) are a group of disorders based on similar clinical, radiographic, physiologic, and pathologic changes that affect the alveolar walls and often the related small airways and distal pulmonary vasculature. Like other lung diseases, these disorders present primarily with shortness of breath. Imaging studies will typically demonstrate bilateral rather than unilateral lung disease. Although COPD and pulmonary hypertension affect the distal airways and vasculature, these are excluded from the category of DPLD.

Classification and Epidemiology

Although there are hundreds of disorders that can present with diffuse parenchymal lung disease, they are typically divided into those with a known cause or those which are idiopathic (**Table 12**). The updated classification of idiopathic interstitial pneumonia will be discussed below. A thorough history that defines the time course is a critical first step in making the diagnosis.

DPLD is uncommon, compared to other pulmonary diseases such as asthma or COPD. The true prevalence of DPLDs is unknown; however, the literature estimates the prevalence at approximately 70 per 100,000 persons, with idiopathic cause accounting for 30% to 40% of disease in these patients.

Diagnostic Approach and Evaluation

Nonproductive cough and dyspnea are the most common presenting symptoms of a DPLD. Dyspnea that comes on suddenly and is of short duration is more likely due to respiratory infection, asthma, pulmonary embolism, or heart failure than DPLD. In contrast, patients presenting with subacute or chronic dyspnea lasting weeks to months without response to treatment should be evaluated for DPLD. As opposed to the typical nonproductive cough of DPLD, a long history of cough with sputum production can suggest an underlying chronic infection, airways inflammation such as chronic bronchitis, or bronchiectasis.

When DPLD is suspected, questions should focus on determining the onset of symptoms, the disease course (improving or worsening), medications, and exposures. The most common identifiable etiologies of DPLDs are those associated with exposures, and the history should include a thorough review of occupations, home environment, hobbies, and other activities. Medication review should include current medications as well as those taken before the onset of symptoms.

Connective tissue diseases can lead to the development of DPLD; therefore, the review of systems should assess for symptoms of arthralgia, myalgia, arthritis, tenosynovitis, dry eyes, dry mouth, dysphagia, gastroesophageal reflux, and unexplained rash. A family history of DPLD due to connective tissue disease should substantially increase clinical suspicion.

Physical examination findings differ depending on the underlying cause of DPLD. In patients with connective tissue disorders, findings may include Raynaud phenomenon, skin

TABLE 12. Classification and Distinguishing Features of Select Forms of Diffuse Parenchymal Lung Disease

Known Causes	
Drug-induced	Examples: amiodarone, methotrexate, nitrofurantoin, chemotherapeutic agents (see www.pneumotox.com for a complete listing).
Smoking-related	"Smokers'" respiratory bronchiolitis characterized by gradual onset of persistent cough and dyspnea. Radiograph shows ground-glass opacities and thickened interstitium. Smoking cessation improves prognosis.
	Desquamative interstitial pneumonitis and pulmonary Langerhans cell histiocytosis are other histopathologic patterns associated with smoking and DPLD.
Radiation	May occur 6 weeks to months following radiation therapy.
Chronic aspiration	Aspiration is often subclinical and may exacerbate other forms of DPLD.
Pneumoconioses	Asbestosis, silicosis, berylliosis.
Connective tissue diseases	
Rheumatoid arthritis	May affect the pleura (pleuritis and pleural effusion), parenchyma, airways (bronchitis, bronchiectasis), and vasculature. The parenchymal disease can range from nodules to organizing pneumonia to usual interstitial pneumonia.
Systemic sclerosis	Nonspecific interstitial pneumonia pathology is most common; may be exacerbated by aspiration due to esophageal involvement; antibody to Scl-70 or pulmonary hypertension portends a poor prognosis. Monitoring of diffusing capacity for early detection is warranted.
Polymyositis/dermatomyositis	Many different types of histology; poor prognosis.
Other connective tissue diseases	Varying degrees of lung involvement and pathology can be seen in other forms of connective tissue disease.
Hypersensitivity pneumonitis	Immune reaction to an inhaled antigen; may be acute, subacute, or chronic. Noncaseating granulomas are seen.
Unknown Causes	
Idiopathic interstitial pneumonias	
Idiopathic pulmonary fibrosis	Chronic, insidious onset of cough and dyspnea, usually in a patient aged >50 years. Usual interstitial pneumonia pathology (honeycombing, bibasilar infiltrates with fibrosis). Diagnosis of exclusion.
Acute interstitial pneumonia	Dense bilateral acute lung injury similar to acute respiratory distress syndrome; 50% mortality rate.
Cryptogenic organizing pneumonia	May be preceded by flu-like illness. Radiograph shows focal areas of consolidation that may mimic infectious pneumonia or may migrate from one location to another.
Sarcoidosis	Variable clinical presentation, ranging from asymptomatic to multiorgan involvement. Stage 1: hilar lymphadenopathy. Stage 2: hilar lymphadenopathy plus interstitial lung disease. Stage 3: interstitial lung disease. Stage 4: fibrosis. Noncaseating granulomas are hallmark.
Rare DPLD with Well-Defined Features	
Lymphangioleiomyomatosis	Affects women in their 30s and 40s. Associated with spontaneous pneumothorax and chylous effusions. Chest CT shows cystic disease.
Chronic eosinophilic pneumonia	Chest radiograph shows "radiographic negative" heart failure, with peripheral alveolar infiltrates predominating. Other findings may include peripheral blood eosinophilia and eosinophilia on bronchoalveolar lavage.
Pulmonary alveolar proteinosis	Median age of 39 years, and males predominate among smokers but not in nonsmokers. Diagnosed using bronchoalveolar lavage, which shows proteinaceous material in and around alveolar macrophages. Chest CT shows "crazy paving" pattern.

DPLD = diffuse parenchymal lung disease.

thickening, sclerodactyly, malar rash, inflammatory arthritis, or tenosynovitis. Lung examination findings are variable and may be normal. This is more likely early in disease or in those with imaging findings of ground-glass opacity or micronodules. Decreased breath sounds and dullness to percussion may suggest a pleural effusion, which is atypical for many DPLDs. Wheezes may suggest small airways disease, while inspiratory dry "Velcro" crackles are more suggestive of fibrosis. In more severe disease there may be right heart strain on electrocardiography or evidence of right-sided heart failure with findings of jugular venous distention, peripheral edema, a pronounced pulmonic second sound, and an S_3. These findings are also suggestive of more long-standing disease.

The physical examination should include resting and exertional pulse oximetry. It is common for patients with DPLD to have normal resting pulse oximetry. However, because of reductions in the functional pulmonary capillary bed, individuals with DPLD will often demonstrate desaturation when ambulating. The desaturation may not require supplemental oxygen; however, desaturation of greater than 4% while ambulating is consistent with a diffusion limitation, which is a hallmark of interstitial lung disease.

Patients with a clinical suspicion of DPLD should undergo full pulmonary function testing, including lung volumes and DLCO. The vast majority of DPLDs have restrictive physiology. However, there are a few diseases that have obstruction or exhibit a combined obstructive and restrictive deficit. Simple spirometry has a limited role because it can only identify obstruction and may be normal in the setting of restriction or reduced DLCO.

Plain chest radiography is an appropriate initial test for the evaluation of dyspnea and cough in patients suspected of having DPLD. Chest radiography may show various findings in patients with DPLD, including diffuse reticular and reticulonodular patterns, increased septal line thickening, consolidation, pleural effusions with or without pleural calcification, bronchiectasis, and hilar or mediastinal lymphadenopathy. The chest radiograph can be normal in patients with minimal disease, and a normal chest radiograph does not rule out DPLD.

KEY POINTS

- Patients presenting with subacute or chronic symptoms of dyspnea lasting weeks to months without response to treatments should be evaluated for diffuse parenchymal lung disease.
- Patients with a clinical suspicion of diffuse parenchymal lung disease should undergo full pulmonary function testing, including lung volumes and DLCO.
- A normal chest radiograph does not rule out diffuse parenchymal lung disease.

High-Resolution CT Scanning

High-resolution CT (HRCT) scan of the chest (slice thickness 1-2 mm) is the best imaging study to identify abnormalities that can help diagnose the underlying disease (**Table 13**). When disease of the small airways is suspected, HRCT imaging should be obtained both on inspiration and on expiration to accentuate air trapping. Prone images may be helpful if there is subtle septal thickening posteriorly that can be difficult to

TABLE 13. Patterns of Disease Associated with a Diagnosis of Diffuse Parenchymal Lung Disease

Lung Disease	Imaging	Comments
Acute interstitial pneumonia	Diffuse ground glass with consolidation	Indistinguishable from ARDS but without a risk factor for ARDS
Organizing pneumonia	Patchy ground glass, alveolar consolidation, peripheral and basal predominance	Connective tissue diseases, infections, drug-related, or idiopathic
Idiopathic pulmonary fibrosis/usual interstitial pneumonia	Basal-predominant and peripheral-predominant septal line thickening with traction bronchiectasis and honeycomb changes	The usual interstitial pneumonia pattern can be seen in connective tissue disease, asbestosis, and chronic hypersensitivity pneumonitis; idiopathic pulmonary fibrosis is a diagnosis of exclusion
Nonspecific interstitial pneumonia	Ground glass, basal predominance	Idiopathic and common finding in connective tissue disease
Respiratory bronchiolitis	Centrilobular nodules and ground-glass opacity in an upper-lung predominant distribution	May be an asymptomatic finding in an active smoker
Desquamative interstitial pneumonia	Basal-predominant and peripheral-predominant ground-glass opacity with occasional cysts	
Hypersensitivity pneumonitis	Acute: ground-glass opacification; centrilobular micronodules that are upper- and mid-lung predominant Chronic: mid- and upper-lung predominant septal lung thickening with traction bronchiectasis; usual interstitial pneumonia pattern may be seen	Acute: associated with flulike illness Chronic: often cannot identify a causative antigen
Sarcoidosis	Upper lobe–predominant; mediastinal and hilar lymphadenopathy; cystic changes including development of aspergilloma; small nodules oriented along bronchovascular bundles	Findings for sarcoidosis are often not specific; DPLD with diffuse mediastinal and hilar lymphadenopathy greater than 2 cm in size should raise suspicion

ARDS = acute respiratory distress syndrome; DPLD = diffuse parenchymal lung disease.

distinguish from dependent atelectasis. The findings on HRCT highly correlate with the histopathology identified on open lung biopsy. In fact, most of the time the diagnosis of idiopathic pulmonary fibrosis can be made without lung biopsy based on the results of HRCT.

Serologic Testing

Although the American Thoracic Society guidelines recommend screening all patients with DPLD with an antinuclear antibody (ANA), rheumatoid factor, and anti-cyclic citrullinated peptide antibodies, it is most appropriate in younger patients, in particular those younger than 40 years of age, patients with symptoms of an underlying rheumatologic disorder, and patients with a family history of autoimmune or rheumatologic disease. Standard serological testing for individuals who have no clinical evidence of autoimmune disease remains controversial. Additional serologic tests for connective tissue and vascular diseases should be based on history and physical examination. See MKSAP 18 Rheumatology for further discussion of testing for connective tissue disease.

Lung Biopsy

When pulmonary function tests and HRCT are insufficient for making the diagnosis, the physician must consider the risks and benefits of either a bronchoscopic or surgical lung biopsy, including the patient's general health and risk of intervention. Careful assessment of risk factors, alternate diagnostic strategies, and impact of the results of lung biopsy on treatment should be discussed within a multi-disciplinary team, including a thoracic radiologist, thoracic surgeon, and pulmonary specialist with expertise in DPLD. Although a bronchoscopic biopsy provides much less tissue than a surgical lung biopsy, it has a high yield for making a diagnosis of sarcoidosis and is typically performed as an outpatient procedure. Overall in-hospital mortality associated with a surgical lung biopsy (either thoracoscopic or open biopsy) for DPLD remains low for scheduled cases (1.7%), but is much higher for emergency cases (16%).

KEY POINTS

HVC
- The diagnosis of diffuse parenchymal lung disease can often be made based on high-resolution CT without a lung biopsy.
- Serologic testing for diffuse parenchymal lung disease is most appropriate in young patients, those with symptoms of rheumatologic disease, or those with a family history of rheumatologic conditions.

Diffuse Parenchymal Lung Diseases with a Known Cause

Smoking-Related Diffuse Parenchymal Lung Disease

There are several DPLDs that occur almost exclusively in individuals who are current smokers. Examples include respiratory bronchiolitis-associated interstitial lung disease (RB-ILD), desquamative interstitial pneumonia (DIP), and pulmonary Langerhans cell histiocytosis (PLCH). A history of smoking is also believed to be a risk factor for the development of idiopathic pulmonary fibrosis.

RB-ILD is the histopathologic diagnosis associated with the HRCT finding of centrilobular micronodular disease in current smokers. This diagnosis may incidentally be made in asymptomatic smokers undergoing low-dose CT lung cancer screening. DIP is characterized by alveolar filling with macrophages and is associated with ground-glass opacities on CT imaging, although this imaging finding is not specific for DIP. Patients with DIP typically are symptomatic with a dry cough and dyspnea.

PLCH, on the other hand, has diffuse thin walled cysts and several pulmonary nodules that are mid- and upper-lung zone predominant on HRCT. PLCH can also be associated with the development of pulmonary hypertension. Demonstrating the presence of Langerhans cells with S100 or CD1a staining of tissue obtained by either transbronchial or open lung biopsy confirms the diagnosis.

On physiologic testing, RB-ILD may have combined restriction and obstruction, whereas DIP typically is associated with pure restrictive disease. PLCH often produces restrictive disease, but may have preserved total lung capacity and evidence of obstruction when significant cystic disease is present. D_{LCO} is reduced in all of these conditions.

For all smoking-related DPLDs, the primary management is smoking cessation. The use of glucocorticoids for those with more severe smoking-related DPLD or who have quit smoking and have persistent symptoms is often attempted, but has uncertain treatment effect.

KEY POINTS

- Respiratory bronchiolitis-associated interstitial lung disease may be diagnosed in asymptomatic smokers based on high-resolution CT findings and pulmonary function testing.
- The primary management of all smoking-related diffuse parenchymal lung diseases is smoking cessation.

Connective Tissue Diseases

Individuals younger than 40 years of age who present with DPLD have a high prevalence of connective tissue disease (CTD). The review of systems should include a thorough review of rheumatologic symptoms. Signs and symptoms of CTD warrant serologic evaluation based on the most likely disorder. Ruling out this potential cause for DPLD is very important even in the older population, despite the lower prevalence of CTD, because of the implications for treatment with immunomodulating agents. Pulmonary abnormalities are extremely common in patients with rheumatoid arthritis and include bronchiolitis, organizing pneumonia, rheumatoid nodules, nonspecific interstitial pneumonia (NSIP), and usual interstitial pneumonia (the same pathology that is seen with idiopathic pulmonary fibrosis). Furthermore, patients with rheumatoid arthritis treated with methotrexate are also at risk for possible drug-induced DPLD.

Patients with systemic sclerosis are at high risk for the development of lung disease, which is the leading cause of death in these patients. NSIP is the most common histopathologic diagnosis on lung biopsy, and HRCT imaging typically demonstrates findings of bilateral lower lobe ground-glass opacities with or without septal line thickening and traction bronchiectasis. The pathologic pattern of NSIP can occasionally be diagnosed in a patient before the development of systemic disease. Although cyclophosphamide has been shown to be of modest benefit, it has high toxicity and has been replaced by mycophenolate mofetil, which has similar efficacy and is better tolerated with decreased side effects. As a result, mycophenolate mofetil is considered first-line therapy for those with progressive DPLD and systemic sclerosis. For patients thought to have idiopathic NSIP, rheumatology consultation and evaluation for immunosuppressive treatment is appropriate.

KEY POINTS

- Pulmonary abnormalities are extremely common in patients with rheumatoid arthritis and can include bronchiolitis, organizing pneumonia, rheumatoid nodules, nonspecific interstitial pneumonia, and usual interstitial pneumonia.
- Patients with systemic sclerosis are at high risk for the development of lung disease, which is the leading cause of death in these patients.

Hypersensitivity Pneumonitis

Repetitive inhalation of antigens in a sensitized patient can result in hypersensitivity pneumonitis (HP), an immunologic response that results in noncaseating granulomas and peribronchial mononuclear cell infiltration with giant cells. The antigens are typically complex proteins, which can come from several sources including agricultural dusts, thermophilic fungi, and bacteria, but can also be some small-molecular-weight chemical compounds. There are three forms of HP, and they each present differently. The acute form, which is most easily identified, results after a large exposure to an inciting antigen. The patient will develop fevers, cough, and fatigue, typically within 12 hours of exposure. Chest radiography can demonstrate diffuse micronodular disease but may be normal. Physical examination will reveal inspiratory crackles. If a HRCT scan is performed, it will demonstrate diffuse centrilobular micronodules and ground-glass opacities (**Figure 5**). After removal from the offending antigen, symptoms will resolve within approximately 48 hours. The recurrence of symptoms if the patient is rechallenged is the hallmark of the disease.

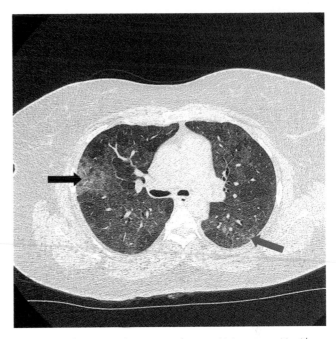

FIGURE 5. Chest CT scan demonstrating hypersensitivity pneumonitis with patchy, bilateral ground-glass opacities (*red arrow*) and centrilobular micronodules (*blue arrow*) in the mid-lung section.

Subacute and chronic forms of HP likely occur after more prolonged lower-level antigen exposure. Bird fanciers disease is an example of a chronic disorder. These patients have a chronic low-level exposure to avian antigens within the home and will ultimately experience cough, fatigue, weight loss, and shortness of breath. Similar to the acute form, the HRCT will show micronodules and ground-glass opacities, but there is also evidence of septal line thickening and fibrosis. In its most severe and chronic form, significant traction bronchiectasis and honeycomb changes will be evident. Evidence of severe fibrosis on CT imaging significantly increases the risk for progression of disease and death.

Removal of exposure to the offending antigen is essential in the treatment of HP. To identify potential antigens, careful history is vital, as serologic testing is often limited and may not include antibodies to the responsible antigen. Glucocorticoids are often used for those with more severe symptoms. Response to this therapy is variable. Prolonged glucocorticoid use is associated with significant side effects, and should be avoided without clear objective evidence of improved pulmonary function.

KEY POINTS

- The acute form of hypersensitivity pneumonitis is characterized by fever, cough, and fatigue within 12 hours of a major exposure to an inciting antigen; recurrence of symptoms with rechallenge is the hallmark of acute hypersensitivity pneumonitis.
- Removal of exposure to the offending antigen is essential in treatment of hypersensitivity pneumonitis.

Drug-Induced Diffuse Parenchymal Lung Disease

Many medications have been implicated in the development of DPLD (Table 14). A review of medications should include those that are new and those taken for prolonged periods because the duration of exposure to the development of disease can vary, even for the same agent. For instance, amiodarone lung toxicity has an acute form consistent with acute lung injury/acute respiratory distress syndrome, and a chronic indolent form with reticular abnormalities and subpleural nodules. Prompt treatment by removal of the offending agent is important for resolution of symptoms. For those with more severe symptoms, glucocorticoids may have some benefit, although data are anecdotal.

Radiation Pneumonitis

Radiation pneumonitis typically occurs 4 to 12 weeks after initial radiation exposure. Patients present with cough, shortness of breath, and a new radiographic infiltrate. Fever, pleuritic chest pain, fatigue, and weight loss are accompanying nonspecific symptoms. Differential diagnosis often includes infection and drug-induced lung injury. HRCT will demonstrate ground-glass opacities, usually within the field of

TABLE 14.	Select Drug-Induced Parenchymal Lung Diseases	
Drug	**Clinical Points**	**Radiographic Findings and Treatment**
Amiodarone	More common in: Older patients Increased dosage and higher cumulative dose First year of therapy (but can occur late)	Multiple radiographic presentations possible, including ground-glass opacities, subpleural nodules, and reticular abnormalities Very long half-life prevents clearance from the pulmonary parenchyma: Rare improvement with discontinuation of the drug alone High risk of recurrence with tapering of glucocorticoids
Methotrexate	Occurs in less than 5% of treated patients Unpredictable time to presentation No clear correlation between dose and disease severity	Diffuse reticular and ground-glass attenuation Patients generally do well after stopping medication. Glucocorticoids are often given and duration is based on response.
Nitrofurantoin	Acute (more common): Fevers, chills, cough, shortness of breath, chest pain; rash can occur in 10%-20% of patients. Peripheral eosinophilia common Chronic: Distinct from the acute form Onset months to years after prolonged exposure	Acute: Faint bilateral lower lobe septal lines; moderate pleural effusions may be present. Treatment: Often will resolve with discontinuation but will recur with repeat exposure. Chronic: Reticular opacities with subpleural lines and thickened peri-bronchovascular areas. Treatment: Possible benefit of glucocorticoids from anecdotal reports.
Busulfan	Occurs in less than 8% of treated patients. Currently used solely as a conditioning regimen for HSCT; often combined with other agents associated with pulmonary toxicity. Injury typically occurs 30 days to 1 year after exposure.	Multiple patterns including: ground glass opacities, reticulation, bibasilar septal lines, asymmetric peripheral and peribronchial consolidation, centrilobular nodules, and dependent consolidation Optimal treatment unknown and is often supportive. Glucocorticoids may be used for more progressive disease.
Bleomycin	Risk significantly increases with cumulative dose. Increased age, renal insufficiency, concomitant chemotherapy and/or radiation also increases risk of toxicity. Typically subacute presentation 1-6 months after exposure; may resemble hypersensitivity pneumonitis but with more rapid onset and progressive course.	Imaging patterns suggest the multiple possible pathologic findings seen: Consolidation with ground glass (diffuse alveolar damage) Septal line thickening, traction bronchiectasis, and honeycomb change (end-stage fibrosis) Patchy ground glass with subpleural consolidation or peribronchial consolidation (organizing pneumonia) Diffuse ground glass with centrilobular micronodules (hypersensitivity pneumonitis) Glucocorticoids are used for more severe disease and disease may recur with tapering of steroids.

HSCT = hematopoietic stem cell transplantation.

radiation exposure. A well-defined nonanatomic demarcation between normal and abnormal lung consistent with the radiation field is pathognomonic but not always present. Radiographic abnormalities, such as organizing pneumonia, may also be seen outside the field of exposure and can be nodular or alveolar. Treatment of radiation pneumonitis is typically glucocorticoids for severe disease with more extensive abnormalities on imaging, respiratory symptoms, or with hypoxemia. Observation may be appropriate for those with mild disease. From 6 to 12 months after radiation exposure, additional findings on HRCT may develop, including septal line thickening, traction bronchiectasis, and volume loss more consistent with chronic fibrosis. In addition, individuals exposed to radiation are at risk for the development of radiation-recall pneumonitis, which can occur when exposed to select chemotherapy agents including adriamycin, etoposide, gemcitabine, paclitaxel, and pemetrexed.

KEY POINTS
• Radiation pneumonitis typically presents 4 to 12 weeks after initial radiation exposure, with cough, shortness of breath, and a new radiographic infiltrate.
• Treatment of severe forms of radiation pneumonitis typically is glucocorticoids, whereas observation may be appropriate for those with mild disease.

Diffuse Parenchymal Lung Diseases with an Unknown Cause

Idiopathic Pulmonary Fibrosis

Idiopathic pulmonary fibrosis (IPF), which is associated with the histopathologic appearance of usual interstitial pneumonia (UIP), is the most common idiopathic form of DPLD. It typically presents in patients between 50 and 70 years of age who have a greater than 6-month duration of a dry cough and dyspnea on exertion. History will reveal no potential cause for the development of fibrosis, and lung examination is notable for Velcro inspiratory crackles that are predominant at the bases and may be subtle in early disease. Clubbing is present in up to 50% of patients and should raise suspicion for IPF. The diagnosis of IPF is challenging because it is uncommon and indolent. Because smoking is a risk factor, patients are often treated for COPD without significant improvement. Similarly, crackles on examination may lead to management for presumed heart failure. Chest radiographs may demonstrate bibasilar septal line thickening with reticular changes, and volume loss and bronchiectasis when the disease is more severe. The best diagnostic test is HRCT, which may show abnormalities, such as bilateral, peripheral, and basal predominant septal line thickening with honeycomb changes, when the chest radiograph is normal (**Figure 6**). When HRCT is consistent with UIP, lung biopsy may not be necessary for diagnosis.

IPF is progressive, with a median survival of 3 to 5 years after diagnosis. The progression of disease, however, is variable

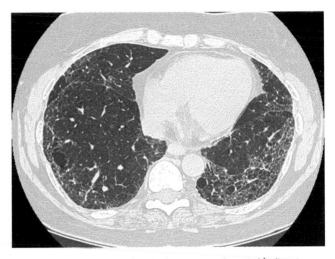

FIGURE 6. High-resolution chest CT demonstrating the typical findings in idiopathic pulmonary fibrosis, including increased reticular changes that are predominantly peripheral and basilar in distribution, honeycombing (at the left base), and absence of significant ground-glass opacification.

and may be associated with periods of stability with intermittent periods of acute decline. A subset of patients develop an acute exacerbation with a worsening of symptoms, typically of less than 1 month's duration, and associated new findings on chest CT of bilateral ground-glass opacities after having relatively stable disease over time. These events can be "triggered" by an inciting event such as an infection or may be "idiopathic." Heart failure and volume overload should be excluded as causes of the radiographic changes or clinical decompensation.

An important aspect of treatment of IPF includes optimum management of comorbidities such as obesity, heart failure, and deconditioning. Sleep-disordered breathing is common in this population due to nocturnal hypoxemia and increased prevalence of obstructive sleep apnea. Treatment of hypoxemia includes supplemental oxygen with exertion and at rest as needed based on pulse oximetry testing. For those with deconditioning, pulmonary rehabilitation has demonstrated benefits in exercise tolerance and quality of life in several small studies. In progressive and severe disease, pulmonary hypertension and right-sided heart failure are commonly observed. One preliminary study suggesting improvement in quality of life with sildenafil needs further study before recommending its use in this population.

In 2014, two FDA-approved therapies, nintedanib and pirfenidone, became available. Both therapies target the fibroblast, which is considered central in the progression of fibrosis. Although the mechanisms of these two medications differ, clinical response is quite similar, with both demonstrating a decline in the rate of progression of disease. Although these medications delay IPF progression, they are not curative. Referral to a pulmonologist or interstitial lung disease (ILD) center may be appropriate before initiating treatment with these medications.

Lung transplantation is a life-prolonging therapy for those without comorbidities that may otherwise limit life expectancy. Typically, transplant centers exclude those with untreatable end-organ damage outside the lungs. Early referral of eligible patients to a transplant center is appropriate given the unpredictability of disease progression.

The most common cause of death in patients with IPF is respiratory failure. In patients with respiratory failure, the need for mechanical ventilation portends an extremely poor prognosis. As a result, consensus-based guidelines recommend against mechanical ventilation for IPF patients if lung transplantation is not an option. Palliative care consultation to establish advanced care plans should be considered for patients with IPF who are not candidates for lung transplantation and who have a severe exacerbation and poor performance status. Ideally, advance care planning, including end-of-life goals of care and palliative strategies, should be decided before urgently facing the decision of whether to begin mechanical ventilation in the setting of respiratory failure. **H**

> **KEY POINTS**
> - FDA-approved therapy with nintedanib and pirfenidone decreases the rate of progression of idiopathic pulmonary fibrosis but is not curative.
> - Consensus-based guidelines recommend against mechanical ventilation for patients with idiopathic pulmonary fibrosis if lung transplantation is not an option.

Nonspecific Interstitial Pneumonia

Nonspecific interstitial pneumonia (NSIP) is the most common DLPD associated with autoimmune disorders, but it can occasionally be idiopathic and not associated with an underlying connective tissue disease. There are two forms of NSIP: cellular and fibrotic. The fibrotic form has a worse prognosis and is poorly responsive to treatment. The cellular form has a better prognosis and will typically respond to immunosuppressive treatments. Although the overall prognosis is better than for IPF, the 5-year mortality of idiopathic NSIP remains approximately 15% to 25%. Individuals with progressive decline in pulmonary function are at increased risk of death regardless of the underlying pathology. Similar to IPF, select patients may benefit from lung transplantation. NSIP affects a younger population than IPF. HRCT will demonstrate bilateral lower-lobe reticular changes and an absence of honeycombing, but can also demonstrate areas of ground-glass opacification. These findings on HRCT have been associated with systemic sclerosis, systemic lupus erythematosus, Sjögren's syndrome, dermatomyositis, and polymyositis, as well as undifferentiated connective tissue disease. Because idiopathic NSIP is rare, a thorough investigation for an underlying autoimmune disorder is essential. NSIP was common in patients with AIDS in the pre-antiretroviral therapy era; however, it is much less common since the advent of antiretroviral therapy.

> **KEY POINTS**
> - Nonspecific interstitial pneumonia is the most common diffuse parenchymal lung disease associated with autoimmune disorders.
> - Bilateral lower-lobe reticular changes and an absence of honeycombing on high-resolution CT scan, often accompanied by areas of ground-glass opacification, have been associated with systemic sclerosis, systemic lupus erythematosus, Sjögren's syndrome, dermatomyositis, and polymyositis, as well as undifferentiated connective tissue disease.

Cryptogenic Organizing Pneumonia

Organizing pneumonia is defined by histopathologic findings of patchy proliferation of granulation tissue that affects the terminal bronchiole, and alveolar ducts and spaces, and is associated with surrounding inflammation. This pattern often follows or is associated with various types of injury to the lung, including acute infection, radiation exposure, drug-induced pneumonitis, and autoimmune diseases. In patients in whom no cause is identified, the diagnosis is termed cryptogenic organizing pneumonia (COP).

Patients with COP typically present with cough, fever, and malaise for 6 to 8 weeks. Initial chest radiographs will demonstrate patchy opacities that mimic pneumonia and, as a result, patients are often initially misdiagnosed with community-acquired pneumonia and treated with standard antibiotics (**Figure 7**). However, nonresolving symptoms and failure to respond to antibiotics should raise suspicion for organizing pneumonia or COP. HRCT imaging will demonstrate ground-glass opacities or areas of alveolar consolidation resembling an infectious pneumonia, but findings can include peripheral nodules and nodules along the bronchovascular bundle. The diagnosis may not require lung biopsy if the clinical presentation and HRCT findings are consistent with COP. For cases with atypical presentation, lung biopsy may be necessary to make the diagnosis. **H**

Patients with COP typically respond to glucocorticoid therapy. In organizing pneumonia associated with an autoimmune disorder, treatment should focus on the autoimmune condition. Relapses of COP with tapering of glucocorticoids are common, and therefore a long taper of glucocorticoids or transition to alternate immunosuppressive therapy should be considered.

> **KEY POINT**
> - Patients with cryptogenic organizing pneumonia typically present with complaints of cough, fever, and malaise for 6 to 8 weeks, which may mimic community-acquired pneumonia.

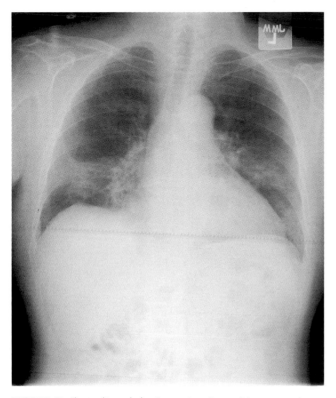

FIGURE 7. Chest radiograph showing cryptogenic organizing pneumonia, demonstrating multiple patchy bilateral alveolar opacities that are nonspecific and may be difficult to distinguish from more typical infectious pneumonia. Infiltrates may be migratory, with resolution of established opacities as new areas appear on serial imaging. Imaging may also be nonspecific, showing interstitial infiltrates and alveolar opacification or one or more rounded nodules that may be interpreted as malignancy.

Acute Interstitial Pneumonia

Acute interstitial pneumonia develops rapidly during days to weeks, resulting in acute respiratory failure with bilateral alveolar opacities on HRCT of the chest consistent with pulmonary edema. The pathologic findings on open lung biopsy are those of diffuse alveolar damage. This process is clinically, radiographically, and pathologically indistinguishable from acute respiratory distress syndrome. The differentiating factor is the lack of risk factors for the development of acute respiratory distress syndrome. The history should carefully assess any history of aspiration, sepsis, or inhalational exposure that could result in acute lung injury.

Management includes supportive care, as for other patients with acute lung injury or acute respiratory distress syndrome. This includes low tidal volume ventilation if required and critical care management to avoid complications of illness. Although glucocorticoids are often used, there is little evidence other than case reports of improvement with their use. Mortality remains high (approximately 50%), and those who recover from the initial illness often have complications, are at risk for the development of chronic lung disease, and may have a relapse. Long-term management of these patients includes consideration of immunosuppression; however, there are limited data to guide therapy.

KEY POINT

- Acute interstitial pneumonia is clinically, radiographically, and pathologically indistinguishable from acute respiratory distress syndrome; the differentiating point is the lack of risk factors for the development of acute respiratory distress syndrome.

Sarcoidosis

Sarcoidosis is a granulomatous disease of unknown cause that can affect several organ systems. Greater than 90% of patients with sarcoidosis have lung involvement. The prevalence of sarcoidosis is approximately 10 to 20 per 100,000 individuals. Sarcoidosis affects blacks more frequently than whites and typically occurs in younger patients. Many patients are asymptomatic, and lung involvement is incidentally found on chest radiography done for other reasons (**Figure 8**). Findings from chest radiography can help predict the probability of spontaneous resolution (**Table 15**). CT scanning can show pulmonary parenchymal disease or intrathoracic lymphadenopathy, either alone or in combination. Although there are various appearances of sarcoidosis on chest CT scanning, a particularly characteristic finding is the presence of small nodules alongside bronchovascular bundles.

Pulmonary function testing is typically abnormal and findings can be obstructive, restrictive, or both. Sarcoidosis is a diagnosis of exclusion. Diagnosis, with a few exceptions (**Table 16**), typically requires bronchoscopic biopsy, with tissue obtained from a lymph node or from the pulmonary

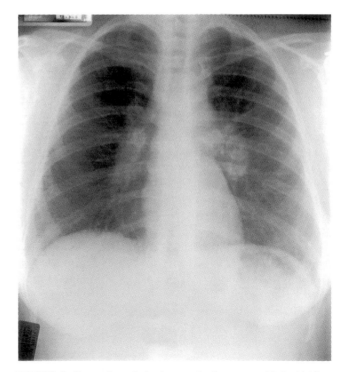

FIGURE 8. Chest radiograph showing stage I pulmonary sarcoidosis with hilar lymphadenopathy and normal lung parenchyma.

TABLE 15. Chest Radiograph Staging of Pulmonary Sarcoidosis

Stage	Radiographic Pattern	Clinical Course and Comments
0	Normal	
I	Hilar lymphadenopathy with normal lung parenchyma	>90% will have spontaneous resolution without treatment
II	Hilar lymphadenopathy with abnormal lung parenchyma	Approximately 50% rate of spontaneous improvement without treatment
III	No lymphadenopathy with abnormal lung parenchyma	Approximately 20% rate of spontaneous improvement without treatment
IV	Parenchymal changes with fibrosis and architectural distortion	

TABLE 16. Clinical Presentations of Sarcoidosis that Do Not Require a Biopsy

Syndrome	Additional Findings/Symptoms
Asymptomatic bilateral hilar lymphadenopathy	No evidence of fevers, malaise, or night sweats to suggest a malignancy
Löfgren syndrome	Bilateral hilar lymphadenopathy, migratory polyarthralgia, erythema nodosum, and fever
Heerfordt syndrome	Anterior uveitis, parotiditis, fever (uveoparotid fever), and facial nerve palsy

parenchyma. The diagnosis is made by the finding of noncaseating granulomas with exclusion of potential mimicking infections (mycobacteria, fungi), exclusion of other systemic granulomatous diseases, and ideally with involvement of more than one organ system.

Pulmonary hypertension may develop through several different mechanisms, including chronic hypoxemia, destruction of the capillary bed resulting in severely reduced capillary surface area, granulomatous inflammation of the pulmonary arteries, compression of pulmonary arteries secondary to contiguous lymphadenopathy, pulmonary veno-occlusion from granulomatous inflammation, and left ventricular dysfunction from cardiac involvement. Development of pulmonary arterial hypertension is a poor prognostic indicator, with a median survival of approximately 3 years.

The primary treatment of sarcoidosis is glucocorticoids, although many patients do not need to be treated. In addition, spontaneous resolution without treatment is common and related to the radiographic stage of disease (see Table 15). The decision to treat and assessment of response should be based on symptoms and organ dysfunction, not radiographic findings. For those without symptoms or organ dysfunction, observation is appropriate. If treatment is required, low- to medium-dose glucocorticoid therapy, often on alternate days, is appropriate. Short-term symptomatic benefit is clear from retrospective study data; however, long-term benefits remain less clear. For patients with more severe or prolonged symptoms, side effects from chronic glucocorticoids should be

considered. In this setting, adjunctive glucocorticoid-sparing therapies are often used. Pulmonary consultation should be considered for management of persistent disease. For patients with pulmonary hypertension or severe disease with significant activity limitation due to lung disease, evaluation for lung transplantation is appropriate. **H**

KEY POINTS

- Greater than 90% of patients with sarcoidosis have lung involvement; radiographic staging can predict the probability of spontaneous resolution.
- The primary treatment of symptomatic sarcoidosis is glucocorticoids.

Occupational Lung Disease

When to Suspect an Occupational Lung Disease

Occupational lung disease can affect any part of the respiratory tract, including sinuses, airways, the lung parenchyma, and the surrounding pleura. As a result, signs and symptoms associated with occupational exposure include rhinitis, reactive airways disease, COPD, pleural disease, diffuse parenchymal lung disease, and malignancy. Occupational lung diseases can present acutely, subacutely, or slowly after many years of exposure. As a result, these diseases require that clinicians maintain suspicion for and obtain a careful history of occupational exposures. Clinical presentations related to silica and asbestos exposures are well characterized and recognized. However, new agents that may lead to respiratory diseases are frequently introduced in industry. Factors suggesting an underlying occupational lung disease include patient concerns about an exposure, a temporal association with an exposure, unexplained signs or symptoms, and evidence of coworkers with similar symptoms (**Table 17**). In addition, patients may experience relief of symptoms when away from the work environment and recurrence of symptoms upon their return. For the patient with occupational lung disease, similar to diffuse parenchymal lung disease, cough and dyspnea on exertion are common.

TABLE 17. Occupational Lung Disease Screening Questionnaire

Occupation
What do you do every day at your job?
Have you always done these tasks at work?
Have you had other duties?
How long have you been working in this job? Have you had a similar job elsewhere?
What other types of work have you done?*

Type and Extent of Exposure
Describe your work area. Is there adequate ventilation? Is there visible dust in the air? Is visibility across the work area limited due to the extent of dust in the air?
Are you exposed to vapors, gases, dust, or fumes in your work?
Does your employer require you to wear personal protective equipment? If so, do you wear it for the full extent of your exposure?
Do you know the amount and type of chemicals used?
Do you have Material Safety Data Sheets (MSDSs) from your workplace?

Temporal Relationship of Symptoms to the Work Environment
Before symptoms began, were there any changes in the processes at work or new exposures?
When you are off work, do your symptoms improve?
Are there others at work who have developed similar symptoms?
Has a process change at work resulted in improved symptoms?

Other Relevant Exposures
Do you perform activities at home that may expose you to organic or inorganic dust (for example, refurbishing old cars or wood working)?
Do you have any pet birds at home? Do you have any pets?
Have you always lived in the area?
Have you traveled recently?

*Obtain a full accounting of other jobs as well.

Key Elements of the Exposure History

The time course from exposure to the development of signs and symptoms of occupational lung disease is highly variable. Therefore, it is essential to obtain a complete history, including employment history. Exposures within the same industry can vary based on use of best practices and on the type of workplace. For example, coal worker's pneumoconiosis in the United States has substantially decreased since the institution of federal safety standards. However, rates of coal worker's pneumoconiosis are higher for individuals who work for companies with fewer than 50 employees, and for those who work in thin-seam mines. Thin-seam mines appear to have higher crystalline silica exposure and pose greater risk. More than

95% of these mines are located in Kentucky, West Virginia, and Virginia. Adequate determination of exposure requires a clear description of job duties and determination of the extent of dust exposure. Clinicians should also obtain a history of additional exposures from hobbies or the home environment (see Table 17).

When an occupational lung disease is suspected, clinicians should request Material Safety Data Sheets (MSDSs) from the employer, which detail chemical properties and known health risks associated with substances within the workplace. The U.S. Occupational Safety and Health Administration (OSHA) requires that this information is available upon request for employees who work with potentially harmful materials.

For individuals who have undiagnosed disorders, persistent unexplained symptoms, or permanent impairment possibly due to an occupational lung disease, referral to an occupational and environmental lung disease specialist is appropriate.

KEY POINTS

- Presentations of occupational lung disease include rhinitis, reactive airways disease, COPD, pleural disease, diffuse parenchymal lung disease, or malignancy.
- When an occupational lung disease is suspected, it is essential to obtain a complete history, including occupation, type and extent of exposure, temporal relationship of exposure to symptoms and disease, and other exposures at home and from hobbies.

Management

The key to management of occupational lung disease is removal of the offending agent from the workplace or the worker from the offending agent. Because workers typically have colleagues in a similar environment, further investigation of the workplace to ensure identification of all affected individuals is essential. Beyond one specific patient, prevention through mitigation of further exposures in the workplace is best practice.

Workers' compensation often becomes an issue during medical management. It may be difficult to define the degree of impairment resulting from the exposure, and the determination of disability related to the impairment may require referral to a specialist with expertise in occupational lung disease.

KEY POINT

- The key to management of occupational lung disease is removal of the offending agent from the workplace or the worker from the offending agent; further investigation of the workplace to ensure identification of all affected individuals is essential.

Surveillance

For individuals at high risk for the development of pulmonary disease, the use of health questionnaires and pulmonary function screening is appropriate; such screening can also identify a new exposure and any associated risk of disease development. Surveillance systems that catalogue sentinel cases of disease can help identify clustering of cases. However, one major limitation of these databases is the failure of physicians to report events.

Asbestos-Related Lung Disease

Asbestos includes a group of minerals that, when crushed, will break into fibers. These fibers are chemically heterogeneous hydrated silicates that are used in industry because of their high tensile strength, heat resistance, and acid resistance. In the past, asbestos fibers were widely used in insulation, brake linings, flooring, cement paint, and textiles. Because of the known toxicities associated with asbestos, these compounds are used far less frequently today.

Asbestos-associated diseases have a prolonged latency period (15 to 35 years), resulting in continued identification of new cases despite the decreased use of asbestos in the United States. Continued exposures within the United States and the developed world occur through updating, demolition, and abatement of older construction. Asbestos exposure remains an occupational hazard for workers in developing nations.

Risk Factors

Duration and extent of exposure are key risk factors for the development of disease. Asbestos-related lung diseases are common in mine workers who procure the asbestos and in industries that make use of the products. In the United States, workers in construction, naval shipyards, and the automotive service industries are particularly at risk. Exposure is also possible in areas where manufacturing of asbestos leads to environmental contamination. Similarly, there are reports of people who develop asbestos-related lung diseases after exposure to asbestos dust from family members working in an asbestos-related industry.

KEY POINT

- Asbestos-related lung diseases are common in mine workers who procure the asbestos and in industries that make use of products containing asbestos; in the United States, workers in construction, naval shipyards, and the automotive service industries are particularly at risk.

Pathophysiology

Inhaled asbestos fibers deposit deep within the lung, reaching airway bifurcations; respiratory bronchioles; and the alveolus, where they promote alveolitis. Type I alveolar epithelial cells take up the fibers, which migrate to the interstitium. Lymphatic channels transport asbestos fibers to the pleural surface. Although activated macrophages phagocytose and remove fibers, remaining fibers stimulate the macrophage to produce inflammatory mediators. These and other cell mediators stimulate fibroblast proliferation and chemotaxis, resulting in collagen deposition and development of fibrosis.

Asbestos exposure increases the risk for development of lung cancer regardless of smoking status, but the risks are substantially higher in smokers. This risk of cancer is apparent when any form of asbestos-related lung disease is present; however, for those with a history of asbestosis (that is, diffuse parenchymal lung disease secondary to asbestos), the risk of lung cancer is 36 times higher than in those with no history of smoking. Smoking cessation is essential. Findings of parietal pleural calcifications or plaques on chest radiograph should alert the clinician to the possibility of asbestos exposure. Although most patients with pleural plaques are asymptomatic, the most common symptom is exertional dyspnea. Additional evaluation including evaluation for lung cancer or mesothelioma should be considered.

Silicosis

Silicosis is a fibrotic lung disease caused by the inhalation of silica dust. Silica exposure typically occurs in industries that grind, cut, or drill silica-containing materials such as concrete, tile, and masonry. Pottery making, foundry work, and sand blasting can also result in exposure. Sandblasting of denim jeans (stone washing) recently resulted in an outbreak of disease in Turkey. Hydraulic fracturing for natural gas and oil may expose workers to hazards, as this process involves fine sand and a wide variety of chemicals.

There are four main types of silicosis (**Table 18**), and they are associated with altered cell immunity and macrophage function. Patients with silicosis are at increased risk for the development of mycobacterial infection and connective tissue disease. Chronic silicosis is associated with the development of infection, including tuberculosis, and clinicians should have a high index of suspicion for this complication. Once fibrosis develops in silicosis, there is little evidence that any therapies alter disease course. If individuals have continued exposure, removal from the environment will prevent further lung injury. Silica exposure is associated with increased risk of lung cancer, particularly for smokers. As a result, smoking cessation remains an essential intervention.

KEY POINTS

- Silica exposure can occur in individuals who work with hydraulic fracturing, concrete, tile, masonry, pottery, sand blasting, or in those who do foundry work.
- Once fibrosis develops in patients with silicosis, no therapies alter the course of the disease.

Pleural Disease

The two main abnormalities affecting the pleura result from the presence of fluid (pleural effusion) or air (pneumothorax) in the pleural space.

TABLE 18. Key Features of Silica-Related Lung Diseases

Type	Latency	Exposure Level[a]	Imaging Findings	Clinical
Acute silicoproteinosis (acute silicosis)	A few weeks to 3 years	High level	Crazy-paving pattern (extensive ground-glass opacity and interlobular septal thickening)	Rapidly progressive dyspnea with constitutional symptoms. Typically fatal. BAL yields a thick, milky effluent
Chronic simple silicosis	10-20 years	Low to moderate	Upper-zone predominant with centrilobular or peri-lymphatic nodules 1-9 mm in diameter Hilar lymph nodes may have eggshell calcification.	Often asymptomatic Rarely will progress to PMF
Chronic complicated silicosis (PMF)[b]	10-20 years	Low to moderate for those who progress from simple silicosis	Coalescent fibrosis >1 cm in diameter, typically in the periphery, enlarging over time and progressing towards the hilum. May contain air bronchograms and calcifications	Debilitating disease marked by progressive dyspnea and functional impairment
Accelerated silicosis	3-10 years	Accelerated disease may occur with very high exposure for a shorter period of time	Similar to chronic disease other than more rapid development	As for chronic disease

BAL = bronchoalveolar lavage; PMF = progressive massive fibrosis.

[a]Exposure refers to both quantity of dust exposure and duration

[b]A form of chronic silicosis that may progress from simple silicosis

Pleural Effusion

Each year more than 1.5 million new cases of pleural effusion are diagnosed in the United States. Most effusions are benign; however, approximately 16% of them are secondary to malignancy. Heart failure, pneumonia, and malignancy are the most common etiologies in the United States. The pleurae are thin membranes that cover the surface of the lung (visceral pleura) and the chest wall (parietal pleura). Normally the pleural space contains only a small amount of fluid (less than 15 mL). Pleural effusions result from conditions that affect the rate of fluid entry from pleural capillaries and the ability of lymphatics to absorb the fluid.

KEY POINT

- Heart failure, pneumonia, and malignancy are the most common causes of pleural effusion in the United States.

Evaluation
History and Physical Examination
The cause of a pleural effusion is often suggested by patient history and physical exam. Symptoms typically include dyspnea, cough, and pleuritic chest pain. Key questions include severity and duration of symptoms; constitutional symptoms such as fevers, night sweats, and weight loss; occupation; recent illness, injury, or travel; exposures (for example, asbestos); and medical history such as heart failure, previous surgeries, and medications. The chest examination may reveal dullness to percussion and diminished or

absent fremitus and breath sounds if the effusion is larger than 300 mL. There are several other key physical examination findings that may suggest the cause of the effusion (**Table 19**).

Diagnostic Imaging
A chest radiograph should be performed as the first test in an evaluation of a possible pleural effusion. The radiographic findings are variable, but abnormalities may be seen with as little as 200 mL on the posterior-anterior (PA) chest radiograph or 50 mL on the lateral view (**Figure 9**).

TABLE 19. Key Physical Examination Findings in the Evaluation of a Pleural Effusion

Finding	Possible Cause of Pleural Effusion
Distended neck veins, S_3 gallop, pulmonary crackles	Heart failure
Bilateral peripheral edema	Heart failure, nephrotic syndrome, cirrhosis
Calf or thigh swelling, erythema, edema, tenderness, palpable cord	Pulmonary embolus
Accentuated cardiac pulmonic sound, right ventricular heave	Pulmonary embolus
Lymphadenopathy	Malignancy
Ascites	Cirrhosis

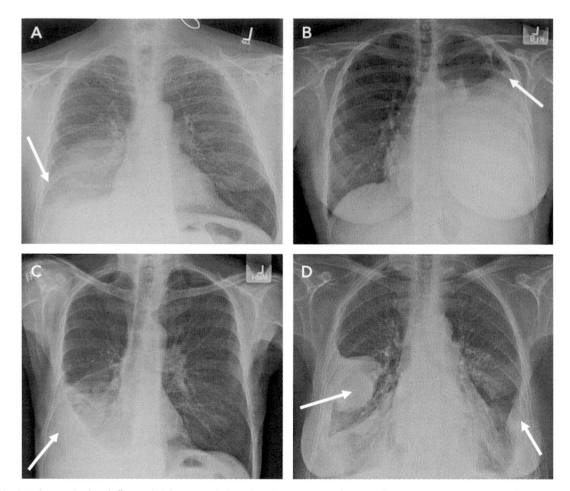

FIGURE 9. *A:* Moderate right pleural effusion which layers over the lower hemithorax; *B:* Large left pleural effusion with meniscus sign (a rim of fluid ascending the lateral chest wall); *C:* Loculated pleural effusion along the right lateral chest wall (presence of septations and separate compartments within the effusion); *D:* Bilateral multi-loculated pleural effusions.

CONT.

Thoracic ultrasound is a helpful addition to chest radiography for identification of small effusions, particularly in patients who are semirecumbent, such as those who are critically ill. This imaging allows estimation of the quantity of the fluid and determination of whether it is free-flowing or loculated (that is, with septations) (**Figure 10**). In addition, there is no radiation exposure with ultrasound.

Advantages of CT imaging include the ability to detect small amounts of pleural fluid; assessment of coexisting intrathoracic abnormalities, such as pulmonary masses and malignant pleural disease; and identification of an empyema, as enhancement of the pleura around the fluid creates a lenticular-shaped opacity (**Figure 11**).

KEY POINTS

- A chest radiograph should be performed in the initial evaluation of possible pleural effusion.

- In supine patients and in those with small effusions, thoracic ultrasound is more sensitive than chest radiography for diagnosis of pleural effusion.

Indications for Thoracentesis

Once a pleural effusion is identified, the next diagnostic test to consider is thoracentesis.

Indications include pleural effusion of unknown cause and greater than 1 cm of fluid thickness on ultrasound or lateral decubitus film. Fluid less than 1 cm thick is technically difficult to sample and less likely to be clinically meaningful, but still may be appropriate for thoracentesis based on clinical judgment. Thoracentesis should be done with ultrasound guidance, as it allows for both a greater success rate and a reduced risk of solid organ puncture and iatrogenic pneumothorax.

Pleural Fluid Analysis

The first step in pleural fluid evaluation is assessing the appearance of the pleural fluid (**Table 20**). The next step is to determine whether it is a transudate or exudate. Transudates are due to an imbalance between hydrostatic and oncotic pressures, as occurs with heart failure and cirrhosis. Exudates are due to inflammation causing increased capillary permeability, impaired drainage by lymphatics, or both.

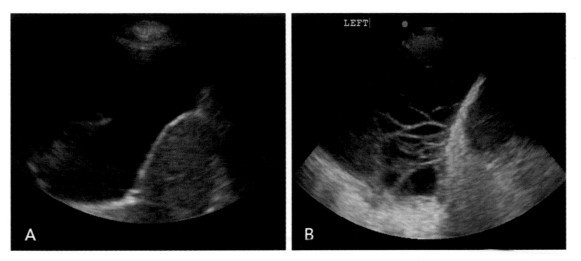

FIGURE 10. Comparison of a simple (*A*) and complicated (*B*) pleural effusion on thoracic ultrasound. A hypoechoic effusion (*A*) may be transudate or exudate. A multi-septated (loculated) effusion (*B*) is exudate.

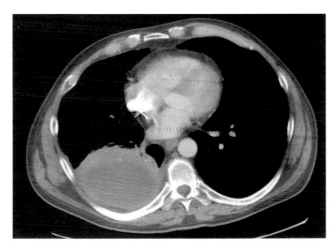

FIGURE 11. CT imaging reveals an empyema, as enhancement of the pleura around the fluid creates a lenticular-shaped opacity.

There are many causes of exudative effusions but the most common are infection and malignancy. Differentiation is commonly made using Light's criteria, based on the levels of lactate dehydrogenase and total protein in both serum and pleural fluid (**Table 21**). However, a recent review also found that checking pleural fluid cholesterol was an accurate method for classifying the effusion as an exudate. Exudative and transudative effusions have a wide range of causes (**Table 22**).

In addition to characterizing a pleural effusion as a transudate or exudate, other tests are often performed depending on clinical suspicion. If infection is suspected then pH, glucose, cell count, Gram stain, and aerobic and anaerobic cultures should also be performed. If malignancy is suspected, then cytological analysis of fluid should be performed.

TABLE 20. Pleural Fluid Characteristics and Diagnostic Considerations		
Appearance	**Possible Cause**	**Additional Tests to Perform**
Bloody	Malignancy, pulmonary embolus, trauma, pneumonia, benign asbestos pleural effusion	Hematocrit If >50% of the serum, it is a hemothorax; consider aortic rupture, myocardial rupture, and injuries to hilar structures, lung parenchyma, and intercostal vessels
Milky	Chylothorax or cholesterol effusion	Triglyceride level
Yellow-green	Rheumatoid pleurisy	Serum rheumatoid factor Pleural fluid glucose <60 mg/dL (3.33 mmol/L)
Dark green	Bilothorax	Bilirubin
Dark brown/black	Long-standing hemothorax, fungal infection, malignancy	Hematocrit, cytology, fungal cultures
Purulent	Empyema	Aerobic and anaerobic cultures

TABLE 21. Criteria for Exudative Pleural Effusion

Test	Sensitivity (%)	Specificity (%)
Combined Light's criteria (1 or more of the following 3):	97	85
Ratio of pleural-fluid protein to serum protein level >0.5	90	90
Ratio of pleural-fluid LDH level to serum LDH level >0.6	88	91
Pleural-fluid LDH level >2/3 the upper limit of normal for serum LDH	88-89	93-100
Pleural fluid cholesterol level >55 mg/dL	85-94	95-99
Ratio of pleural-fluid cholesterol to serum cholesterol >0.3	93	94

LDH = lactate dehydrogenase.

Data from Wilcox ME, Chong CA, Stanbrook MB, Tricco AC, Wong C, Straus SE. Does this patient have an exudative pleural effusion? The Rational Clinical Examination systematic review. JAMA. 2014;311:2422-31. [PMID: 24938565] doi:10.1001/jama.2014.5552

TABLE 22. Causes of Transudates and Exudates

Transudates	Exudates
Very Common	**Very Common**
Heart failure	Parapneumonic
Cirrhosis	Malignancy
Less Common	**Less Common**
Nephrotic syndrome	Pulmonary embolism
Hypoalbuminemia	Tuberculosis
Unexpandable (trapped) lung	Autoimmune diseases (RA, SLE)
Peritoneal dialysis	Benign asbestos effusion
Atelectasis	Post-coronary artery bypass
Urinothorax	Pancreatitis
Constrictive pericarditis	Post-myocardial infarction
Meigs syndrome (ovarian fibroma with ascites)	Yellow nail syndrome (lymphatic disorders)
	Drugs

RA = rheumatoid arthritis; SLE = systemic lupus erythematosus.

Cell Counts and Differential

CONT. Cell counts are useful for determining the cause of a pleural effusion; however, they are not disease-specific. Neutrophil-predominant effusions are secondary to an acute process such as pneumonia (parapneumonic effusion) or pulmonary embolus. Lymphocyte predominance (more than 50%) is common in chronic effusions. The most common causes worldwide of lymphocyte-predominant effusions are tuberculosis and cancer. An eosinophilic effusion of greater than 10% is most commonly due to current or recent air or blood in the pleural space and is a nonspecific finding (**Table 23**).

Chemical Analysis

Pleural fluid acidosis (pH less than 7.3) is nonspecific and occurs in malignant effusions, complicated parapneumonic effusions, esophageal rupture, and inflammatory conditions such as rheumatoid and lupus pleuritis. Clinically, pH is most useful if an infection is suspected. A pH less than 7.2 in a parapneumonic effusion indicates a complicated pleural effusion is present and tube thoracostomy drainage is needed. Glucose normally diffuses freely across the pleural membrane. A pleural glucose concentration of less than 60 mg/dL (3.33 mmol/L) narrows the differential significantly and suggests that the effusion is secondary to malignancy, empyema or complicated parapneumonic effusion, tuberculosis, esophageal rupture, or rheumatoid or lupus pleuritis.

Pleural fluid amylase concentration should be checked if there is concern that the effusion may be due to pancreatitis or esophageal rupture. Pleural fluid amylase greater than the upper limit of normal for serum amylase, or a pleural fluid to serum amylase ratio greater than 1.0, is indicative of pancreatitis or esophageal rupture.

Pleural fluid triglycerides elevated above 110 mg/dL (1.24 mmol/L) support the diagnosis of chylothorax. If the triglyceride level is between 50 and 110 mg/dL (0.56 and 1.24 mmol/L), chylomicrons should be checked. A true chylothorax results from a disruption of the thoracic duct and is usually the result of thoracic surgery or trauma. Other causes include malignancy (lymphoma), tuberculosis, and lymphatic malformations.

Tests for Tuberculous Effusions

The diagnosis of tuberculosis should be considered in a patient with a lymphocyte-predominant exudative effusion of unclear cause; however, confirming the diagnosis may be challenging. An acid-fast smear of pleural fluid has a sensitivity of less than 5%, and mycobacterial culture has a sensitivity of only 10% to 20% due to the low mycobacterial load. Adenosine deaminase (ADA) is an enzyme present in lymphocytes that is elevated in most tuberculous pleural effusions (sensitivity 90%). In countries with a low incidence of tuberculosis, testing for ADA can be useful, as a negative test helps exclude tuberculosis. Pleural biopsy is useful for histology and is also the most likely source to yield a positive mycobacterial culture (greater than 70%).

TABLE 23. Pleural Cell Counts and Clinical Conditions

Cell Type	Cell Count	Clinical Conditions
Erythrocyte	5000-10,000/μL (5-10 × 10⁹/L)	Hemothorax if pleural fluid hematocrit >50% peripheral hematocrit
Nucleated cells	>50,000/μL (50 × 10⁹/L)	Complicated parapneumonic effusions and empyema
	>10,000/μL (10 × 10⁹/L)	Simple parapneumonic effusion, acute pancreatitis and lupus pleuritis
	<5000/μL (5 × 10⁹/L)	Chronic exudates (TB pleuritis and malignancy)
Lymphocytes	>80%	TB, lymphoma, malignancy, RA pleuritis, sarcoidosis, late post-CABG effusions
Eosinophils	>10%	Air or blood in the pleural space. Also parapneumonic effusions, drug-induced pleuritis, eosinophilic granulomatosis with polyangiitis, benign asbestos effusions, malignancy (lymphoma), pulmonary infarction, parasitic disease

CABG = coronary artery bypass graft; RA = rheumatoid arthritis; TB = tuberculosis.

Tests for Pleural Malignancy

Cytologic examination of pleural fluid has an average sensitivity of 60%. This is slightly higher in adenocarcinoma and lower in mesothelioma, squamous cell carcinoma, and lymphoma. There is minimal benefit for obtaining and sending more than two fluid samples. If cytology is negative and malignancy is still suspected, thoracoscopy may be the next step in evaluation. This procedure allows for the direct visualization and biopsy of the pleural surface and has a diagnostic sensitivity for malignant disease of greater than 90%. Closed pleural biopsy provides only a random sample of pleural tissue without visualization of pleural abnormalities. It is less sensitive than fluid cytology and has been replaced by thoracoscopy in the diagnostic evaluation of pleural malignancy.

Management

Parapneumonic Effusions and Empyema

A pleural effusion associated with a bacterial pneumonia is called a parapneumonic effusion. It can be uncomplicated (sterile and free-flowing) or complicated (either infected or loculated). Uncomplicated effusions are typically small and resolve on their own with treatment of the pneumonia. Complicated parapneumonic effusions occur with significant inflammation or when bacteria invade the pleural space. An empyema is defined as a bacterial infection of the pleural space, which results in purulent fluid or a positive Gram stain. Pleural fluid cultures identify pathogens in only 60% of cases. If infection is suspected, culture bottles should be inoculated at the bedside to increase yield. Any pleural effusion greater than 10 mm in depth on lateral decubitus radiograph and associated with a pneumonic illness should be sampled with a diagnostic thoracentesis. Drainage is required if there is a positive Gram stain or culture, or when the pH is less than 7.2. The bacteriology of pleural space infection differs depending on if it is community-acquired or hospital-acquired. In the community, *Streptococcus pneumoniae*, *Streptococcus pyogenes*, *Staphylococcus aureus*, and *Streptococcus anginosus* group are the organisms typically associated with pleural infection. Methicillin-resistant *Staphylococcus aureus* and *Enterobacteriaceae* are more prevalent in nosocomial empyema. Anaerobic bacteria are cultured in greater than 20% of pleural-space infections and may be due to the common association with aspiration or the anaerobic environment of the pleural space. Polymicrobial infections are common, and empiric antibiotic regimens before obtaining culture results should include coverage for anaerobes.

Complicated parapneumonic effusions and empyema require drainage. The combined use of intrapleural fibrinolytics (streptokinase, urokinase, tissue plasminogen activator) and a mucolytic agent (deoxyribonuclease, or DNase) has demonstrated utility in decreasing the size of the effusion and lowering the rate of surgical referral for definitive treatment. The size of drainage tube needed to best manage pleural-space infection remains controversial, but several studies have demonstrated equal efficacy and improved patient comfort with the use of smaller (10 to 14 Fr) thoracostomy tubes. Effusions due to infection refractory to antibiotics and drainage require surgical debridement.

Malignant Pleural Effusion

The diagnosis of a malignant pleural effusion signifies advanced disease and overall poor prognosis. As a result the goal of management is the relief of symptoms. Several therapeutic options exist, and treatment decisions should be based on symptoms, prognosis, degree of anticipated lung re-expansion, and patient performance status. Repeat therapeutic thoracentesis is appropriate for patients with poor prognosis (less than 3 months) and slow re-accumulation of fluid. Patients with rapid re-accumulation of fluid and dyspnea should be offered more definitive management. Indwelling pleural catheters with intermittent outpatient drainage provide significant symptom relief, and 50% to 70% of patients achieve spontaneous pleurodesis after 2 to 6 weeks. Chemical pleurodesis refers to obliteration of the pleural space with a sclerosing agent (typically talc). Talc can be introduced through a thoracostomy tube (talc slurry) or during a thoracoscopy (talc poudrage). Talc pleurodesis is very effective, with a success rate of 60% to 90% depending on the degree of lung re-expansion. Pleurectomy and pleuro-peritoneal shunt are other management options but are rarely performed.

Pneumothorax

Evaluation

Air in the pleural space is defined as a pneumothorax, which can occur spontaneously or as a result of trauma or a procedural complication. A primary spontaneous pneumothorax (PSP) occurs in someone without known underlying lung disease. A secondary spontaneous pneumothorax (SSP) occurs in someone with known underlying lung disease, such as COPD. Risk of recurrence for PSP is 23% to 50% over 1 to 5 years, and greater than 50% over 1 to 3 years in those with SSP. Risk factors for pneumothorax are listed in **Table 24**.

Symptoms include the sudden onset of dyspnea and sharp pleuritic chest pain. The symptoms are typically more severe with SSP, as patients have less respiratory reserve. Physical examination findings can be subtle but usually reveal reduced lung expansion, hyperresonance to percussion, and diminished breath sounds on the side of the pneumothorax. Tension pneumothorax should be suspected in patients presenting with significant cardiorespiratory distress (worsening dyspnea, hypotension, absent breath sounds on one side, tracheal deviation, and distended neck veins).

A chest radiograph is an appropriate initial test and can confirm the diagnosis and determine the size of the pneumothorax. If the lung margin is greater than 2 cm away from the chest wall at the level of the hilum, it is considered a large pneumothorax. A CT scan is the most sensitive imaging modality for small pneumothoraces and is particularly useful in patients with bullous emphysema.

Management

Management of pneumothorax is driven by clinical symptoms. A tension pneumothorax (large and hemodynamically significant) should be managed by emergent needle thoracostomy followed by thoracostomy tube placement and hospitalization. Observation alone has been shown to be safe for small pneumothoraces in patients with minimal symptoms (**Table 25**).

Recurrence prevention is recommended after the second episode of pneumothorax on the ipsilateral side in PSP and after the first occurrence in SSP. Patients should be encouraged to stop smoking, as the lifetime incidence rates for PSP are much higher in men who are lifelong heavy smokers than men who have never smoked (12% vs 0.1%). Intervention to prevent recurrence includes both chemical and mechanical pleurodesis. Air travel should be avoided until complete resolution of the pneumothorax, and scuba diving is not recommended unless definitive therapy, such as surgical pleurectomy, has been applied. **H**

Pulmonary Vascular Disease

Pulmonary Hypertension

Pulmonary hypertension (PH) is defined as a resting mean pulmonary artery pressure of 25 mm Hg or greater measured during right heart catheterization. The normal mean pulmonary artery pressure is less than 20 mm Hg. Untreated PH eventually leads to right ventricular failure and may directly contribute to death; however, the rate of progression is highly variable and dependent upon the origin of disease and comorbidities.

The current classification system subdivides PH into five groups, which are based on similarities in mechanisms, hemodynamics, clinical presentation, and approach to treatment (**Table 26**).

TABLE 24. Risk Factors for Pneumothorax
Risk Factors for PSP
Smoking
Family history
Thoracic endometriosis
Tall stature
Risk Factors for SSP
COPD
Interstitial lung disease
Tuberculosis
Cystic fibrosis
Malignancy
Necrotizing pneumonia
Marfan syndrome
PSP = primary spontaneous pneumothorax; SSP = secondary spontaneous pneumothorax.

TABLE 25. Management of Pneumothorax	
Size[a] and Clinical Symptoms	**Management**
<2 cm on chest radiograph, minimal symptoms	Admit to hospital for observation and supplemental oxygen (PSP may be managed as an outpatient if good access to medical care)
>2 cm on chest radiograph, breathlessness, and chest pain	Insertion of a small-bore (<14 Fr) thoracostomy tube with connection to a high-volume low-pressure suction system
Cardiovascular compromise (hypotension, increasing breathlessness) regardless of size	Emergent needle decompression followed by thoracostomy tube insertion Note: If persistent air leak (>48 hours) refer to a thoracic surgeon
[a]Measured between lung and chest wall PSP = primary spontaneous pneumothorax.	

TABLE 26. Classification of Pulmonary Hypertension

1	Pulmonary arterial hypertension (includes idiopathic and heritable, and disease related to drugs and toxins, connective tissue diseases, HIV infection, schistosomiasis, and portal hypertension)
2	Pulmonary hypertension due to left-sided heart disease
3	Pulmonary hypertension due to lung diseases and/or hypoxia
4	Chronic thromboembolic pulmonary hypertension and other pulmonary artery obstructions
5	Pulmonary hypertension with unclear or multifactorial causes

Data from Simonneau G, Gatzoulis MA, Adatia I, Celermajer D, Denton C, Ghofrani A, et al. Updated clinical classification of pulmonary hypertension. J Am Coll Cardiol. 2013;62:D34-41. [PMID: 24355639] doi:10.1016/j.jacc.2013.10.029

KEY POINT

- Pulmonary hypertension is defined as a resting mean pulmonary artery pressure of 25 mm Hg or greater measured during right heart catheterization.

Pathophysiology

Most cases of PH are caused by left-sided heart disease (group 2) and hypoxic respiratory disorders (group 3). Left-sided heart disease (heart failure with reduced or preserved ejection fraction, valvular disease) results in elevations in left atrial and pulmonary venous pressures. Chronic hypoxia is probably the primary contributor to PH in advanced respiratory disorders such as COPD, interstitial lung disease, and sleep hypoventilation syndromes; obliteration of the vascular bed in emphysema also contributes. Regardless of the underlying causes or disease associations, untreated PH is usually progressive, eventually leading to vascular remodeling and right ventricular hypertrophy and dilatation. PH is often a risk factor for death in patients with group 2 and 3 disease, and may be directly contributory in death due to right ventricular ischemia, arrhythmias, or heart failure.

KEY POINT

- Most cases of pulmonary hypertension are secondary and caused by left-sided heart disease and hypoxic respiratory disorders.

Diagnosis

Because early symptoms of PH (exertional dyspnea and fatigue) are nonspecific and may be attributed to an underlying disorder such as heart failure or lung disease, a high index of suspicion can help identify PH in its earlier stages. Progressive disease, eventually resulting in right ventricular impairment, is associated with symptoms of exertional chest pain, syncope, and edema. Findings on physical examination depend on the severity of disease. An early sign is a prominent S_2; an audible split eventually widens. A prominent jugular venous a wave and a parasternal heave reflect right ventricular hypertrophy. As the right ventricle dilates, a holosystolic

tricuspid regurgitant murmur may be detected. Right ventricular failure leads to jugular venous distention, hepatomegaly, ascites, and peripheral edema. Pulmonary findings reflect underlying lung disease.

Enlarged central pulmonary arteries with peripheral pruning, along with a prominent right ventricle detectable on the lateral view on chest radiograph, are suggestive of PH (**Figure 12**). If PH is suspected, transthoracic echocardiography should be performed, as it allows an estimation of pulmonary arterial systolic pressure and assessment of both right and left heart size and function. However, echocardiography does not confirm the diagnosis because the estimation of true pulmonary artery pressure may be inaccurate. Right heart catheterization confirms the diagnosis of PH and is typically an essential component of the diagnostic evaluation, although it may be deferred in certain situations, such as in patients whose PH is attributable to advanced lung disease such as COPD.

Once PH is confirmed, further testing, guided by clinical history, helps determine underlying causes and important comorbid conditions. Left heart catheterization can assess the coronary arteries if ischemic cardiomyopathy is suspected. Additional diagnostics may include pulmonary function tests, high-resolution CT if interstitial lung disease is a consideration, and tests for nocturnal hypoxemia. Abnormal overnight pulse oximetry to detect nocturnal hypoxemia followed by polysomnography to characterize the cause can identify sleep-related breathing disorders as a cause of PH. Assessment of functional status with the 6-minute walk test should be performed to provide prognostic information and to determine a baseline for assessment of therapeutic response.

KEY POINTS

- If pulmonary hypertension is suspected, echocardiography should be performed, as it allows an estimation of pulmonary arterial systolic pressure and assessment of both right and left heart size and function.

- Right heart catheterization confirms the diagnosis of pulmonary hypertension and is an essential component of the diagnostic evaluation.

Treatment of Pulmonary Hypertension

Therapy for patients with groups 2, 3, and 5 PH is directed at the underlying condition. Optimization of treatment of underlying left ventricular systolic and diastolic function and valvular disease is appropriate. COPD should be managed in a stepwise fashion. For a discussion of treatment of COPD, see Airways Disease. Supplemental oxygen for hypoxemia due to underlying lung disease causing PH may provide mortality benefit. Positive airway pressure therapy may be indicated for sleep-disordered breathing and hypoventilation syndromes. The use of advanced vasodilator therapy in groups 2 through 5 PH can be considered on a patient-by-patient basis. Treatment with such pulmonary vasodilators, however, may be harmful in patients with PH due to left ventricular dysfunction (group 2)

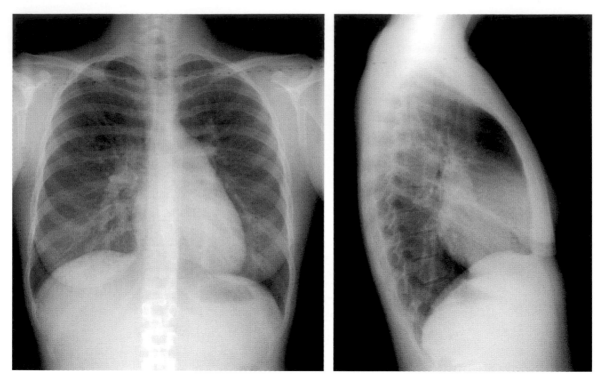

FIGURE 12. Posteroanterior chest radiograph (*left*) of a woman with pulmonary arterial hypertension showing right atrial dilatation (straightening of the right heart border), pulmonary artery enlargement, attenuation ("pruning") of the peripheral vessels, and oligemic lung fields. The lateral chest radiograph (*right*) demonstrates diminished retrosternal airspace, a sign of right ventricular hypertrophy.

or lung disease (group 3) because of the potential to overload a compromised left ventricle and to worsen ventilation-perfusion ($\dot{V}/\dot{Q}$) mismatching, respectively.

KEY POINTS

- Therapy for patients with pulmonary hypertension caused by left-sided heart disease, lung diseases, or hypoxia, is typically directed at the underlying condition.

- Treatment with pulmonary vasodilators may be harmful in patients with pulmonary hypertension due to left ventricular dysfunction or lung disease because of the potential to overload a compromised left ventricle and to worsen ventilation-perfusion mismatching, respectively.

Chronic Thromboembolic Pulmonary Hypertension (Group 4)

Progressive exertional dyspnea is the most common symptom of chronic thromboembolic pulmonary hypertension (CTEPH). Less than 5% of patients who experience an acute pulmonary embolism (PE) develop CTEPH. Greater than 25% of patients diagnosed with CTEPH do not have a documented history of PE. For further discussion of pulmonary embolism, see MKSAP 18 Hematology and Oncology. In patients with CTEPH, the organized thrombus is incorporated into the pulmonary arterial endothelium, increasing pulmonary vascular resistance and pressures, eventually leading to right-sided heart failure. Such patients are only occasionally diagnosed with an underlying hypercoagulable state.

Diagnosis

Because PE (acute or previous) isn't always evident, CTEPH remains an underrecognized cause of PH and requires a high index of suspicion. The diagnosis is made in the setting of PH in the absence of left heart pressure overload accompanied by imaging evidence of chronic thromboembolism.

Ventilation/perfusion scanning is the most sensitive indicator of CTEPH and should be performed in all patients in whom the diagnosis is suspected. CT pulmonary angiography (CT-PA), which is often performed in the evaluation of a dyspneic patient, may demonstrate proximally located vascular abnormalities such as webs, intimal irregularities, and luminal narrowing, but may be less sensitive for more distal lesions. Conventional pulmonary angiography is used to best characterize the extent and distribution of organized thrombus to determine suitability for surgical intervention.

KEY POINTS

- The diagnosis of chronic thromboembolic pulmonary hypertension is made in the setting of pulmonary hypertension in the absence of left heart pressure overload accompanied by imaging evidence of chronic thromboembolism.

(Continued)

- Ventilation/perfusion scanning is the most sensitive indicator of chronic thromboembolic pulmonary hypertension and should be performed in all patients in whom the diagnosis is suspected.

Management

Anticoagulation and consideration of thromboendarterectomy are indicated for CTEPH. Lifelong anticoagulant therapy is indicated in all patients to help prevent further thromboembolism. The only potentially curative therapy for CTEPH is pulmonary thromboendarterectomy. Because the disease usually irreversibly progresses, surgical evaluation at an experienced center is warranted in all patients with CTEPH regardless of disease severity. About half of patients with CTEPH will be eligible for surgery; a proportion will opt for the operation. Pulmonary thromboendarterectomy can result in normalization of pulmonary hemodynamics in about one-third of patients who undergo surgery. Riociguat, an advanced therapy vasodilator, may be used in those who are not candidates for surgery or have persistent PH following surgery. The role of inferior vena cava filters in patients with a coexisting clot in the lower extremities is controversial, and its effect on long-term outcomes is not known.

KEY POINT

- Lifelong anticoagulation and consideration of thromboendarterectomy are indicated for chronic thromboembolic pulmonary hypertension.

Pulmonary Arterial Hypertension

Pulmonary arterial hypertension (PAH) is caused by changes in the small pulmonary arterioles resulting in high pulmonary vascular resistance. PAH is defined by a proliferative vasculopathy originating in the pulmonary arteriolar bed, with pathophysiologic contributions from endothelial cell proliferation, vasoconstriction, and in-situ thrombosis. Imbalances in nitric oxide, prostacyclin, and endothelin that affect vascular tone and endothelial and smooth muscle cellular growth drive the process and are targets for currently available therapy. PAH is classified as idiopathic (previously referred to as primary pulmonary hypertension), heritable, or associated with drugs, toxins, or other conditions.

Idiopathic PAH is typically seen in younger adults, particularly women. Heritable forms account for less than 10% of cases of PAH, with the majority due to mutations in bone morphogenetic protein receptor type 2 (*BMPR2*). Mutations in *BMPR2*, a gene related to the apoptotic process, might explain the propensity for cellular proliferation in PAH. Although otherwise clinically indistinguishable from sporadic disease, those with heritable PAH may have a worse prognosis.

PAH is most commonly associated with connective tissue diseases, portal hypertension, HIV infection, drug use, and toxin exposure.

In connective tissue disease, PAH is classically seen in systemic sclerosis, where it is a leading cause of death. Patients with limited cutaneous disease in association with CREST syndrome (calcinosis cutis, Raynaud phenomenon, esophageal dysmotility, sclerodactyly, and telangiectasia) may be at highest risk. PAH can also be seen in rheumatoid arthritis and systemic lupus erythematosus.

Portopulmonary hypertension affects some patients who have chronic liver disease (see MKSAP 18 Gastroenterology and Hepatology). The mechanism may relate to the diseased liver's inability to clear vasoactive substances.

PAH in patients with HIV infection is not common, but HIV-infected patients have an approximately 10-fold higher risk of PAH compared with patients without HIV infection. Both viral and host factors have been implicated, and disease can occur in the absence of AIDS-related complications.

The drugs most strongly associated with PAH are the anorectics, including fenfluramine, phentermine, and dexfenfluramine. The tyrosine kinase inhibitors dasatinib and imatinib have been implicated, as well as interferon alfa. There is an increasing association between PAH and illicit drugs such as methamphetamine and cocaine. H

KEY POINT

- Pulmonary arterial hypertension is most commonly associated with connective tissue diseases, portal hypertension, HIV infection, drug use, and toxin exposure.

Diagnosis

The diagnosis of PAH requires confirmation of high pulmonary vascular resistance as well as a normal pulmonary capillary wedge pressure to exclude left-sided heart disease. During right heart catheterization, vasoreactivity testing can help guide subsequent therapy (see below). Lung biopsy poses a significant risk in PAH and is not indicated in the diagnostic evaluation. The role of genetic testing is yet to be defined. Laboratory studies to investigate underlying cause of PAH depend on the clinical situation and may include HIV serologies, tests of liver function, and autoantibody titers. H

KEY POINT

- The diagnosis of pulmonary arterial hypertension requires confirmation of high pulmonary vascular resistance as well as a normal pulmonary capillary wedge pressure to exclude left-sided heart disease.

Treatment

Therapy for PAH is directed at PH itself, referred to as "advanced therapy." These vascular-targeted treatments are directed at reducing vasoconstriction and interrupting the pathways mediating cellular proliferation. Use of advanced agents may be guided by disease severity (**Table 27**). Before administering advanced therapy for patients with PAH, vasoreactivity testing with nitric oxide is performed to identify those who may respond to calcium channel blockers. Calcium channel

TABLE 27. Pharmacologic Therapy for Pulmonary Arterial Hypertension

Class	Comments
Calcium channel blockers	Only for patients with acute vasodilator response at catheterization; acute response does not assure chronic response; side effects such as hypotension can occur.
Prostanoids (epoprostenol, treprostinil, iloprost)	Parenteral prostacyclin analogues such as epoprostenol, administered by a continuous central venous infusion, are first-line therapy for severe disease and for those in whom disease progresses despite oral therapy; inhaled iloprost requires frequent administration; prostanoids supplement endogenous levels of prostacyclin (PGI_2), a vasodilator with antismooth muscle proliferative properties.
Endothelin-1 receptor antagonists (bosentan, ambrisentan)	Reasonable initial oral therapies for mild to moderate disease. Blocks action of endogenous vasoconstrictor and smooth muscle mitogen endothelin; class-wide risk of liver injury and teratogenicity; liver chemistry testing and pregnancy testing for reproductive-aged women are required[a].
Phosphodiesterase-5 inhibitors (sildenafil, tadalafil)	Reasonable initial oral therapies for mild to moderate disease. Prolongs effect of intrinsic vasodilator cyclic GMP by inhibiting hydrolysis by phosphodiesterase-5.

GMP = guanosine monophosphate.

[a]Although not required for ambrisentan, some experts suggest that it is prudent to perform liver chemistry tests at the outset of treatment for pulmonary arterial hypertension and at periodic intervals thereafter at the discretion of the managing physician.

blockers are desirable therapy because they are less expensive and have fewer side effects than other forms of advanced therapy. Failure to achieve a favorable hemodynamic response with nitric oxide predicts unresponsiveness to calcium channel blockers and the need for other advanced therapy. Given the complexity of management, the increasing number of drugs available to treat PAH, and cost, these patients are best managed by specialists at a center experienced with PAH management.

Additional treatments include diuretic therapy to combat volume overload and supplemental oxygen for hypoxemia at rest or with exercise. Women of reproductive age who have PAH should be counseled on the risks of pregnancy; most specialists would advise against pregnancy. Because PAH predisposes patients to in-situ pulmonary vascular thrombosis and embolism, anticoagulation is often prescribed. Experience with direct oral anticoagulants in this setting is limited; therefore, warfarin remains the agent of choice. Digoxin might be used to improve right ventricular function or as a rate-control adjunct for supraventricular dysrhythmias or atrial fibrillation. Supervised exercise training has been shown to improve functional capacity.

Lung or heart-lung transplantation should be considered for patients in whom drug treatment is unsuccessful.

KEY POINTS

- Therapy for pulmonary arterial hypertension is directed at pulmonary hypertension itself, referred to as *advanced therapy*, and is best managed by specialists at a center experienced with pulmonary arterial hypertension management.

- Before administering advanced therapy for patients with pulmonary arterial hypertension, vasoreactivity testing with nitric oxide is performed to identify those who may respond to calcium channel blockers.

Lung Tumors
Pulmonary Nodule Evaluation

Pulmonary nodules are small rounded radiographic opacities that are less than 3 cm in size. A solitary pulmonary nodule is a nodule completely surrounded by aerated lung and not associated with atelectasis, hilar enlargement, or pleural effusion. These nodules are usually asymptomatic and found either incidentally or on screening. In contrast, a focal pulmonary opacity larger than 3 cm is considered a lung mass and is presumed malignant until proved otherwise.

The finding of a pulmonary nodule is increasingly common because of the frequency of CT scans done for other reasons, as well as lung cancer screening programs. Management of these lesions can be complicated and often requires subspecialty referral. Principles of pulmonary nodule evaluation include the review of imaging history, estimating the probability of malignancy, performing functional imaging tests (PET scan) to further characterize the nodule, and discussing management preferences with the patient. Guidelines recommend management based on nodule size and characteristics. When more than one nodule is present, follow-up is dictated by the size and characteristics of the largest lesion. Shared decision making is an integral part of the evaluation and management of pulmonary nodules.

KEY POINTS

- Principles of pulmonary nodule evaluation include the review of imaging history, estimating the probability of malignancy, performing functional imaging tests to further characterize the nodule, and discussing management preferences with the patient.

- A focal pulmonary opacity larger than 3 cm are presumed malignant until proved otherwise.

Solid Indeterminate Nodule Larger Than 8 mm

The first step in evaluating a solid nodule that is larger than 8 mm in size is to estimate the probability of malignancy. Criteria included in the calculation include age, smoking history, nodule size, location within the lung, and presence of spiculated or lobular border (https://brocku.ca/lung-cancer-screening-and-risk-prediction/risk-calculators/). Solid nodules with low to moderate probability of malignancy should be characterized further with a PET scan. If the PET scan is negative for metabolic activity, continued surveillance is warranted (**Table 28**). A nodule with moderate or intense uptake is suggestive of malignancy and requires further evaluation, including complete staging followed by surgical resection or chemotherapy and radiation, for definitive management.

If the probability of malignancy is initially high, the next step is staging with a PET scan followed by definitive management with surgical resection or chemotherapy and radiation.

TABLE 28. Fleischner Society Recommendations for Single Pulmonary Nodule Follow-Up

Risk Factors for Lung Cancer?	Size	Recommended Follow-Up
No (Low-risk patient)	<6 mm	No follow-up
	6-8 mm	CT at 6-12 months then consider CT at 18-24 months
	>8 mm	Consider CT at 3 months, PET/CT, or tissue sampling
Yes (High-risk patient)	<6 mm	Optional CT at 12 months
	6-8 mm	CT at 6-12 months then CT at 18-24 months
	>8 mm	Consider CT at 3 months, PET/CT, or tissue sampling

Data from MacMahon H, Naidich DP, Goo JM, Lee KS, Leung ANC, Mayo JR, et al. Guidelines for management of incidental pulmonary nodules detected on CT images: From the Fleischner Society 2017. Radiology. 2017;284:228-243. [PMID: 28240562] doi:10.1148/radiol.2017161659

- The first step in evaluating a solid pulmonary nodule larger than 8 mm in size is to estimate the probability of malignancy.

Solid Indeterminate Nodule of 8 mm or Smaller

Solid indeterminate nodules of 8 mm or smaller are usually detected incidentally. The first step as with larger nodules is an estimation of the likelihood of malignancy (https://brocku.ca/lung-cancer-screening-and-risk-prediction/risk-calculators/). Nodules of 8 mm or smaller have a lower probability of being malignant, are difficult to biopsy, and are not reliably characterized by PET scan. As a result, these small nodules are usually followed by serial CT scans. The frequency and duration of follow-up is based on the recommendations of the Fleischner Society and endorsed by other professional societies (see Table 28).

Subsolid Nodule

A subsolid nodule is a focal rounded opacity that is either pure ground glass in appearance (focal density with underlying lung architecture still preserved) or has a solid component (part solid) but is still more than 50% ground glass (**Figure 13**). These nodules often represent premalignant disease, such as adenocarcinoma in situ, and can be very slow growing. Observed growth rates for subsolid nodules can range between 400 to 800 days. This has implications for both the frequency and duration of follow-up. Subsolid nodules are not reliably characterized by PET scans and nonsurgical biopsies also have limited sensitivity. Development of a solid component in a pure ground-glass nodule or enlargement of the solid component suggests malignancy (see Figure 13). Recommendations for nonsolid and part-solid nodule follow-up are in **Table 29**.

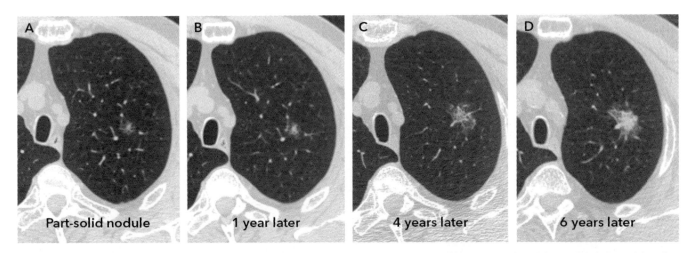

FIGURE 13. Radiographs show the evolution of a part-solid nodule from adenocarcinoma in situ to invasive adenocarcinoma: part-solid, part-ground-glass nodule in the left upper lobe (*A*); growth in the solid component of the nodule 1 year after initial imaging (*B*); an increase in size in the ground-glass component 4 years after initial imaging (*C*); and further increase in the solid component of the nodule 6 years after initial imaging (*D*). This growth rate is characteristic of a part-solid, part-ground-glass nodule and demonstrates why patients with this finding must be followed for at least 5 years.

TABLE 29. Fleischner Society Recommendations for Follow-Up of Solitary Subsolid Lung Nodule

Imaging Findings	Size	Recommended Follow-Up
Pure ground glass	<6 mm	No follow-up
	≥6 mm	CT at 6-12 months to confirm persistence, then CT every 2 years until 5 years
Part solid nodule	<6 mm	No follow-up
	≥6 mm	CT at 3-6 months to confirm persistence. If unchanged and solid component remains <6 mm, annual CT should be performed for 5 years

Data from MacMahon H, Naidich DP, Goo JM, Lee KS, Leung ANC, Mayo JR, et al. Guidelines for Management of Incidental Pulmonary Nodules Detected on CT Images: From the Fleischner Society 2017. Radiology. 2017;284:228-243. [PMID: 28240562] doi:10.1148/radiol.2017161659

Lung Cancer

Lung cancer is the leading cause of cancer death worldwide. In the United States, it is estimated that 225,000 new cases will be diagnosed and more than 160,000 deaths occur each year. The overall 5-year survival rate remains low at 17.7%. However, much progress has been made recently regarding screening, diagnosis, and treatment.

KEY POINT

- Lung cancer is the leading cause of cancer death worldwide, with an estimated 225,000 new cases and more than 160,000 deaths each year.

Lung Cancer Types

There are two major classes of lung cancer: non–small cell lung cancer (NSCLC) and small cell lung cancer (SCLC). NSCLC accounts for most lung cancer cases (80%) and is divided into adenocarcinoma, squamous cell carcinoma, and large cell carcinoma. Adenocarcinoma is the most common NSCLC and accounts for almost all lung cancer diagnoses in nonsmokers. The most frequent location of adenocarcinoma is in the peripheral aspects of the lung parenchyma as a solitary nodule or mass.

Squamous cell carcinoma is the second most common subtype of NSCLC. It correlates highly with smoking history and usually originates in the central airways (trachea, main stem bronchi, lobar and segmental bronchi) (**Figure 14**). Individuals with squamous cell carcinoma often have symptoms of cough and hemoptysis due to central airway involvement. Radiographically, squamous cell carcinoma may present with postobstructive pneumonia or lobar collapse. Large cell carcinoma is an undifferentiated carcinoma and characteristically presents as a peripheral mass with prominent necrosis (**Figure 15**).

In the past decade the development of targeted therapy for specific gene mutations has revolutionized the treatment of lung cancer. The separation of adenocarcinoma and squamous cell carcinoma is important for determining the optimal therapy. Testing for epidermal growth factor receptor (*EGFR*) mutation, anaplastic lymphoma kinase receptor tyrosine kinase (*ALK*) translocation, and ROS proto-oncogene 1 receptor tyrosine kinase (*ROS1*) translocation is recommended in advanced-stage adenocarcinoma or mixed cancers. Targeted treatment has resulted in better responses than standard chemotherapy.

SCLC accounts for about 15% of all lung cancers. It is the most strongly associated with cigarette smoking and typically occurs adjacent to the central airways with extensive lymphadenopathy and distant metastasis at diagnosis. Imaging commonly shows a large mediastinal mass that encompasses lymph nodes with an uncertain primary site of origin (**Figure 16**). Paraneoplastic syndromes are most commonly associated with SCLC, including hyponatremia due to the syndrome of inappropriate antidiuretic hormone secretion (rare in other lung tumors), hypertrophic pulmonary osteoarthropathy, inflammatory myopathies, Cushing syndrome caused by ectopic adrenocorticotropic hormone secretion, and other hematologic and neurologic syndromes. **H**

KEY POINTS

- There are two major classes of lung cancer: non–small cell lung cancer and small cell lung cancer; non–small cell lung cancer accounts for 80% of lung cancers and is divided into adenocarcinoma, squamous cell carcinoma, and large cell carcinoma.

(Continued)

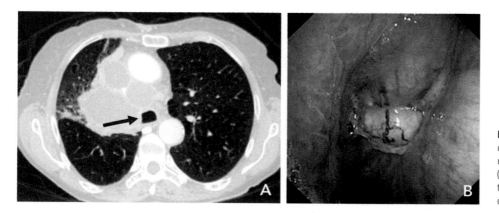

FIGURE 14. Metastatic squamous cell carcinoma can be seen as an 8-cm right hilar mass with invasion into the trachea on CT scan (*A*), and as tumor invasion into the distal trachea and occlusion of the right main stem on bronchoscopy (*B*).

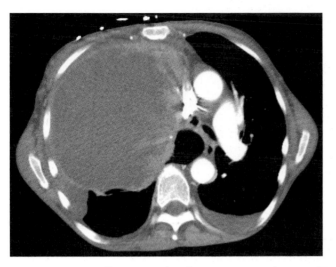

FIGURE 15. Large cell carcinoma with predominant necrosis can be seen on CT scan as a large necrotic tumor that has completely replaced the right upper and middle lobes, with deviation of the central airway structures to the left. Necrosis is noted by the mixed attenuation of the mass as noted on CT.

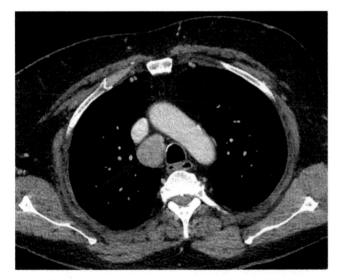

FIGURE 16. Small cell lung cancer can be seen on chest CT with a right paratracheal mass (*arrow*). This patient initially presented with encephalitis (paraneoplastic syndrome).

KEY POINTS *(continued)*

- Testing for epidermal growth factor receptor (*EGFR*) mutation, anaplastic lymphoma kinase receptor tyrosine kinase (*ALK*) translocation, and ROS proto-oncogene 1 receptor tyrosine kinase (*ROS1*) translocation is recommended in advanced-stage adenocarcinoma or mixed cancers.

Risk Factors

The main risk factor for lung cancer is smoking tobacco (voluntary or secondhand). This risk increases based on the number of pack-years of smoking and other carcinogenic exposures. Any reduction in lung cancer mortality will be linked to an overall reduction of cigarette smoking. Other risk factors that have been associated with lung cancer include previous radiation therapy, exposure to environmental toxins (asbestos, radon, metals, and diesel fumes), pulmonary fibrosis, HIV infection, family history of lung cancer, and alcohol abuse.

Screening

Until recently, screening for lung cancer was not widely done, as previous studies had not shown early detection resulted in any mortality benefit for lung cancer. The National Lung Screening Trial (NLST) was a randomized trial comparing CT screening to chest radiograph for detecting lung cancer in current or heavy smokers. The trial demonstrated a 20% reduction in lung cancer mortality in heavy smokers who were screened annually for 3 years. As a result, the U.S. Preventive Services Task Force has recommended annual lung cancer screening using low-dose CT scan for high-risk current and former smokers. The criteria for screening are based on the inclusion criteria for the NLST and include those who are age 55 to 80 years (other guidelines offer different ages to discontinue screening, ranging from 74 to 77 years), have at least a 30-pack-year smoking history, and are current smokers or have quit within the last 15 years. Cessation of screening should be considered in those with limited life expectancy or those who would not be candidates for or willing to undergo surgery.

KEY POINT

- The U.S. Preventive Services Task Force recommends annual lung cancer screening using low-dose CT scan for those who are age 55 to 80 years, have at least a 30-pack-year smoking history, and are either current smokers or have quit smoking within the last 15 years.

Diagnosis and Staging

When evaluating a patient who has a lung nodule or mass for possible lung cancer, two questions must be answered: first, what is the cell type?; and second, what is the stage? The radiographic abnormality should first be compared to any previous chest imaging studies the patient has undergone in order to determine the age and growth pattern of the lesion. A solid lung nodule that has been stable for 2 years or longer is unlikely to represent malignancy. However, ground-glass or part-solid lesions usually grow at a much slower rate (400 to 800 days) and need a longer period of time (5 years) to exclude cancer based on radiographic stability.

Initial evaluation should start with a full history, physical exam, complete blood count, serum chemistries, and CT scan of the chest. Most lung cancers present at a late stage. Symptoms result from the local effects of the tumor, metastatic spread involving other organs, or paraneoplastic syndromes. The most common symptoms at presentation include cough, dyspnea, chest pain, weight loss, and hemoptysis. NSCLC and SCLC present with similar symptoms. Similarly, the presence of findings on physical examination (consolidation, effusion, bone tenderness, neurological findings) will indicate advanced disease. CT scan findings that are suggestive of malignancy are listed in **Table 30**. A CT scan provides an accurate assessment of the location and size of the tumor within the chest and helps to direct tissue biopsy for diagnosis and staging. PET scans can be very helpful in the initial evaluation of potential lung cancer, as several studies have demonstrated that PET identifies unsuspected mediastinal involvement, distant disease, or both, which informs staging biopsies and reduces futile (noncurative) surgery. The sensitivity of a PET scan to detect lung cancer is affected by the mass of the nodule and its metabolic rate, with increased potential for false negative results for cancers smaller than 1 cm and slow-growing cancers, such as carcinoid tumors.

The definitive diagnosis of lung cancer requires tissue histopathology. If the nodule has a high probability for malignancy and the PET scan shows uptake only in the lesion, it is reasonable to offer surgical resection to diagnose and treat in a single procedure. In patients with radiographic evidence of advanced stage disease, diagnosis and staging are best accomplished with a single invasive test at a location that will establish both the diagnosis and the stage. Because there are many techniques available for tissue diagnosis, the strategy will depend on size and location of the tumor, patient characteristics, and surgical expertise. In general, mediastinal and central lesions are best approached with bronchoscopy, and smaller peripheral lesions are best approached with a transthoracic needle aspiration.

Definitive staging of lung cancer is essential, allows for accurate prognostication, and serves as a guide for treatment decision making. NSCLC is staged based on the TNM staging system, taking into account the characteristics of the primary tumor (T), regional lymph node involvement (N), and metastatic disease (M).

SCLC is generally staged as either "limited" or "extensive" disease. Limited disease is defined as disease limited to one hemithorax and ipsilateral supraclavicular lymph nodes. The presence of disease outside these locations defines extensive stage disease.

Treatment of lung cancer is discussed in MKSAP 18 Hematology and Oncology. **H**

KEY POINTS

- The definitive diagnosis of lung cancer requires tissue histopathology.
- In patients with radiographic evidence of advanced-stage lung cancer, diagnosis and staging are best accomplished with a single invasive test at a location that will establish both the diagnosis and the stage of disease.

TABLE 30. CT Findings Suggestive of Lung Malignancy
Irregular or Spiculated Borders
Upper-lobe location
Thick-walled cavitation
Solid component within a ground-glass lesion
Detection of growth on follow-up imaging

Other Pulmonary Neoplasms

Carcinoid tumors are low-grade neoplasms comprised of neuroendocrine cells and are uncommon, accounting for 1% to 2% of all lung cancers. Unlike the case for NSCLC and SCLC, smoking is not a risk factor. Most lung carcinoid tumors arise in the proximal airways, and the predominant symptoms or signs are those of an obstructing tumor mass (cough, dyspnea, monophonic wheezing) or bleeding. Bronchial obstruction may be responsible for lobar atelectasis and recurrent episodes of pneumonia in the same pulmonary segment, but may be asymptomatic (**Figure 17**). Misdiagnosing carcinoid tumors as asthma or pneumonia is responsible for delayed diagnosis. It is rare for lung carcinoid tumors to produce and release serotonin and other vasoactive substances into the systemic circulation and be associated with carcinoid syndrome. Surgical resection is often curative, and 10-year survival rates are higher than 90%.

Adenoid cystic carcinoma is a salivary gland tumor that occurs in the lower respiratory tract and accounts for less than 1% of all lung cancers. Surgical resection is the preferred treatment. Hamartomas are the most common benign lung neoplasm. These rare lesions are a combination of cartilage, connective tissue, smooth muscle, fat, and respiratory epithelium. On imaging they tend to be smooth-bordered nodules, which may contain fat. Additionally, they may be recognized by their classic appearance on CT of "popcorn" calcification; however, this only occurs 25% of the time.

The lung is a frequent site for metastatic disease from primary malignancies, which include head and neck, colon, kidney, breast, thyroid, and melanoma. Metastatic disease can present as solitary or multiple nodules; lymphangitic spread; and endobronchial, pleural, or embolic lesions. Surgical resection may be appropriate when a solitary pulmonary metastasis is identified without evidence of other metastatic disease.

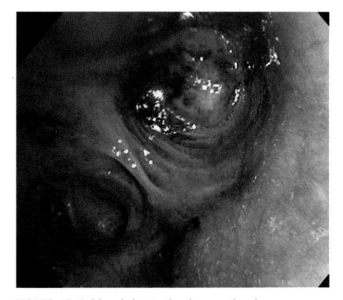

FIGURE 17. Endobronchial carcinoid can be seen on bronchoscopy as a smooth, polypoid, vascular-appearing mass that completely occludes a subsegmental airway of the right lower lobe.

- Surgical resection of carcinoid tumors is often curative, and 10-year survival rates are higher than 90%.

Mesothelioma

Malignant pleural mesothelioma is a rare neoplasm that originates from the cells that line the pleural cavity (mesothelium). It can present as small nodules, plaque-like masses, or confluent sheets that can encase the lung. It is associated with inhalational exposure to asbestos fibers and has a latency of 20 to 40 years. Asbestos is a naturally occurring silicate mineral that is found in soil and rock as long fibers. It is valued for its resistance to heat and combustion and has been used in cement, ceiling tiles, pool tiles, automobile brake linings, and shipbuilding. In addition to malignant pleural mesothelioma and lung cancer, asbestos exposure has been linked to a spectrum of nonmalignant pleuropulmonary diseases (**Table 31**); for further discussion of asbestos-related disease, see Occupational Lung Disease. Because of environmental control of asbestos, the rate of mesothelioma in the United States has been declining since 2000.

Patients with malignant pleural mesothelioma usually present with advanced disease. Symptoms include chest pain, dyspnea, cough, hoarseness, night sweats, or dysphagia. Clinical suspicion for malignant pleural mesothelioma should arise in the setting of pleural thickening or exudative pleural effusion and a history of asbestos exposure. Pleural fluid cytology is typically negative in this scenario and the diagnosis requires a pleural biopsy. Medical or surgical thoracoscopy allows for direct visualization of the pleural surface and has a greater than 90% sensitivity for malignancy. Treatment options depend on the extent of disease and patient factors and preferences, and may include surgery, radiation therapy, and systemic chemotherapy. The overall prognosis of malignant pleural mesothelioma remains poor, with a median survival of 6 to 8 months.

- Mesothelioma is associated with inhalational exposure to asbestos fibers and has a latency of 20 to 40 years.

- Clinical suspicion for malignant pleural mesothelioma should arise in the setting of pleural thickening or exudative pleural effusion and a history of asbestos exposure.

TABLE 31. Nonmalignant Asbestos-Related Pleural and Pulmonary Diseases

Disease	Characteristics
Asbestosis	Slowly progressive diffuse pulmonary fibrosis caused by inhalation of asbestos fibers
Benign asbestos pleural effusion	Small unilateral pleural effusion, may be associated with concomitant pleural plaques
Pleural plaques	Benign circumscribed areas of pleural thickening with linear or nodular appearance

Mediastinal Masses

The mediastinum is anatomically near the center of the thoracic cavity and is bound by the sternum anteriorly, the lungs and pleura laterally, and the vertebral column posteriorly. Tumors in the mediastinum can be either benign or malignant, and symptoms vary depending on size (mass effect) and systemic effects of the tumor. Dividing the mediastinum into compartments can be useful in developing a differential diagnosis when a mediastinal mass is discovered (**Figure 18**).

Anterior Mediastinum

The anterior mediastinal compartment lies between the posterior sternum and the great vessels and heart. It is the most common mediastinal location where malignant tumors occur. Masses in this location are usually remembered as the "terrible T's": thymoma, teratoma/germ cell tumor, "terrible" lymphoma, and thyroid. Thymic lesions are the most common and are associated with various paraneoplastic syndromes, such as myasthenia gravis. Myasthenia gravis is an autoimmune disorder of the neuromuscular junction that commonly presents with muscular weakness, fatigability, ptosis, diplopia, and bulbar symptoms. Diagnosis can be confirmed with an acetylcholine receptor antibody test. **H**

- Thymic lesions are the most common tumor in the anterior mediastinum and are associated with various paraneoplastic syndromes, such as myasthenia gravis.

Middle Mediastinum

Masses in the middle mediastinum are common and are attributed to lymphadenopathy, cysts, esophageal disorders, or vascular lesions (aneurysm). Lymphadenopathy is most common and can be secondary to lymphoma, sarcoid, or metastatic disease. **H**

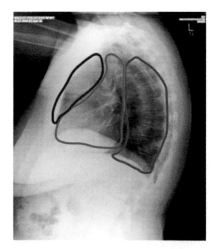

FIGURE 18. A lateral chest radiograph demonstrates the anterior (*red*), middle (*yellow*), and posterior (*blue*) mediastinal compartments.

KEY POINT

- Lymphadenopathy is the most common mass in the middle mediastinum and can be secondary to lymphoma, sarcoid, or metastatic disease.

Posterior Mediastinum

Masses in the posterior mediastinum include neurogenic tumors, meningoceles, and spine lesions. Neurogenic neoplasms are most common and are classified based on their neural origin. **H**

KEY POINT

- Neurogenic neoplasms are the most common tumors in the posterior mediastinum and are classified based on their neural origin.

Sleep Medicine
Classification of Sleep Disorders

Sleep disorders are broadly grouped into six classifications: insomnia, sleep-related breathing disorders, central disorders of hypersomnolence, circadian rhythm sleep-wake disorders, parasomnias, and sleep-related movement disorders (which includes restless leg syndrome).

Excessive Daytime Sleepiness

Excessive daytime sleepiness refers to difficulty staying awake and alert during daytime hours. Sleepiness is most prominent during passive situations such as reading or watching television. Lack of self-recognition is common and can pose a safety hazard if sleepiness occurs while driving or operating machinery. When obtaining a history from the patient, it is important to distinguish sleepiness, a cardinal symptom of many sleep disorders, from fatigue, which refers to a lack of energy or sense of exhaustion that prevents mental or physical activity at the intensity or pace desired. Fatigue is unlikely to be explained solely by a sleep disorder, and is more likely to occur in the setting of certain medical conditions (malignancies, autoimmune disorders, anemia, endocrinopathies, infections), neurologic disorders (myasthenia gravis, multiple sclerosis, Parkinson disease), psychiatric conditions (mood disorders), and chronic fatigue syndrome.

Causes of excessive daytime sleepiness can be categorized as extrinsic (circumstantial) or intrinsic (disease-related) processes (**Table 32**).

Sleepiness can occur acutely when a person is deprived of the 7 to 8 hours of sleep most adults require. Functional impairment resulting from chronic sleep debt due to inadequate amount of sleep is termed insufficient sleep syndrome. It likely is the most common cause of excessive daytime sleepiness and has been associated with cardiovascular

TABLE 32. Extrinsic and Intrinsic Causes of Excessive Daytime Sleepiness

Extrinsic Causes
Insufficient sleep duration (or inadequate opportunity for sleep)
Circadian rhythm disturbance (shift work sleep disorder, jet lag)
Drug-, substance-, or medical condition–related hypersomnia
Environmental sleep disorder (ambient noise, pets)

Intrinsic Causes
Sleep-disordered breathing syndromes, such as obstructive sleep apnea and central sleep apnea
Narcolepsy
Idiopathic hypersomnia
Restless leg syndrome and periodic limb movement disorder
Circadian rhythm sleep disorders (misalignment of the intrinsic circadian timing with the desired sleep schedule; for example, dementia and blindness)

disease and metabolic disorders such as glucose intolerance and obesity.

The initial evaluation of excessive daytime sleepiness should include a thorough history to assess the time available for and spent sleeping before pursuing additional testing. A 1- or 2-week diary of the sleep-wake schedule is a simple tool that promotes self-realization of suboptimal sleep habits. A more objective assessment of sleep and wakefulness can be obtained with a wrist actigraph, a device that measures movement and ambient light during a period of 1 or 2 weeks. Wrist-worn consumer fitness products using similar technology may provide useful feedback. Questionnaires such as the Epworth Sleepiness Scale can quantify sleepiness and help gauge the response to treatment.

Objective sleep testing, either in-lab or at-home multi-channel recordings, is often indicated when a primary sleep disorder (such as obstructive sleep apnea) is suggested by the history and physical examination. In certain cases a multiple sleep latency test, a sleep laboratory–based study that measures the time to sleep during a series of daytime nap opportunities following a normal night of sleep, provides an objective measure of sleepiness and is key to establishing the diagnoses of narcolepsy and idiopathic hypersomnia. A mean sleep latency of more than 15 minutes is considered normal and less than 5 minutes is indicative of pathologic sleepiness.

All patients with excessive daytime sleepiness should be counseled about the dangers of drowsy driving and the need to maintain a routine sleep-wake schedule that allows for 7 to 8 hours of sleep per night. Specific treatment depends on the underlying condition (positive airway pressure for obstructive sleep apnea or stimulant medications for narcolepsy). Short-term management of the occasional bout of acute sleepiness may include strategically timed naps or caffeinated beverages.

- The initial evaluation of excessive daytime sleepiness should include a thorough history to assess the time available for and spent sleeping before pursuing additional testing.
- All patients with excessive daytime sleepiness should be counseled about the dangers of drowsy driving and the need to maintain a routine sleep-wake schedule that allows for 7 to 8 hours of sleep per night.
- Functional impairment resulting from chronic sleep debt due to inadequate amount of sleep is termed insufficient sleep syndrome; it likely is the most common cause of excessive daytime sleepiness and has been associated with cardiovascular disease and metabolic disorders such as glucose intolerance and obesity.
- When obtaining a history from the patient, it is important to distinguish sleepiness, a cardinal symptom of many sleep disorders, from fatigue, which refers to a lack of energy or sense of exhaustion that prevents mental or physical activity at the intensity or pace desired.

Conditions that Disrupt Circadian Rhythm

Jet Lag

Jet lag results when the internal circadian clock is out of phase with the local time following air travel across multiple (typically more than five) time zones. Symptoms occur within one to two days following travel and may include insomnia, daytime sleepiness, and neuropsychiatric impairment. For short trips (one to two days), remaining on origin time might be preferable, if feasible. For longer trips, adjusting to the destination time may alleviate jet lag. Ways to promote adjustment include pretravel measures (avoidance of sleep deprivation and dehydration and, for the highly motivated, bright light therapy starting up to 3 days before travel with the intention to advance the circadian phase). In-flight hypnotic medications are popular, though they pose a risk of parasomnias, particularly if alcohol is consumed. Postarrival measures include timed bright light exposure and melatonin, depending upon the direction traveled, caffeine intake, and naps.

Shift Work Sleep Disorder

As much as one fifth of the American work force maintains a job schedule outside the usual day shift hours. Although some people acclimate well to this schedule (and may even prefer it), many do not and suffer daytime symptoms such as excessive sleepiness, mood perturbations, and neurocognitive dysfunction. Such symptoms can render the next-morning drive home from work dangerous. Symptoms persisting at least 3 months meet criteria for shift work sleep disorder. Management should first include consideration of eliminating shift work by a change in work schedule. If this isn't feasible, interventions to improve daytime sleep may include bright light avoidance in the morning (wearing sunglasses if necessary), maintaining a structured sleep-wake pattern, and melatonin, which is of modest benefit in shifting the physiologic sleep cycle. Hypnotic medications have been used to promote daytime sleep but are of varying effectiveness and pose the risk of carryover effects into the nighttime work period. Interventions to promote nighttime wakefulness include bright light treatment in the evening before the night shift, caffeinated beverages or wake-promoting stimulants (such as modafinil) during work hours, and planned napping during work breaks.

Obstructive Sleep Apnea

Obstructive sleep apnea (OSA) is an increasingly common disorder defined by sleep interruption due to repetitive upper airway narrowing or collapse. These disordered breathing events, captured during sleep testing, are classified as *apneas* (complete cessation of airflow) or *hypopneas* (reductions in airflow), and when these events are divided by total sleep time (in hours) collectively comprise the apnea-hypopnea index (AHI). Although, this frequency-based measure doesn't incorporate every important OSA outcome (for example, it does not capture the degree of oxyhemoglobin desaturations), the AHI is probably the best composite metric of disease severity. An AHI of 5/hour to 15/hour indicates mild OSA, 15/hour to 30/hour indicates moderate OSA, and more than 30/hour indicates severe OSA.

- Obstructive sleep apnea is an increasingly common disorder defined by sleep interruption due to repetitive upper airway narrowing or collapse.
- The apnea-hypopnea index (AHI) is the total number of apnea and hypopnea events divided by total sleep time (in hours) and can classify obstructive sleep apnea as mild (5/hour to 15/hour), moderate (15/hour to 30/hour), or severe (more than 30/hour).

Pathophysiology

With sleep onset, pharyngeal muscles acting to maintain upper airway patency relax, resulting in redundancy of the soft tissues that line the airway. Snoring is often (though not universally) a result of this process, as inspired air collides with these tissues. In OSA, airflow is further compromised by forces (see Risk Factors) that overwhelm the neuromuscular mechanisms promoting upper airway patency. Posture and sleep stage are also important factors. The supine position promotes posterior displacement of the tongue, further narrowing the airway lumen. Disordered breathing events are most prominent during rapid eye movement (REM), a stage of sleep characterized by atonia of nearly all muscles, with the exception of the extraocular muscles and respiratory diaphragm. Efforts to breathe persist against the airway occlusion, resulting in intrathoracic pressure swings. The process is terminated with a brief awakening from sleep (called a microarousal), during which upper airway patency is restored and ventilation resumes, typically followed by resumption of sleep and continual repetition of the process.

Repetitive arousals and disruption of sleep architecture contribute to the development of excessive daytime sleepiness and neurocognitive symptoms of OSA. Oxyhemoglobin desaturations can be profound, particularly in those with underlying cardiopulmonary disease. This hypoxic stress, along with a host of other intermediary mechanisms including inflammation and high adrenergic tone, raise the question of whether OSA may directly contribute to commonly comorbid systemic disorders such as metabolic and cardiovascular disease. Current evidence, based in part on results of randomized controlled trials of positive airway pressure therapy, suggest a causal link between OSA and systemic hypertension. However, relationships with other disorders such as heart failure, cardiac arrhythmias, diabetes mellitus, and mortality are merely associative; causation remains unproven.

Risk Factors

The most important risk factor for OSA is obesity, particularly in those with prominence of adipose tissue in the trunk and neck. Partially on account of gender-specific distribution of fat tissue, men are at higher risk than women, though rates equalize following menopause. The prevalence of OSA increases with age. Blacks and Asians are at higher risk. Alcohol and sedative drugs can exacerbate OSA. Tonsillar hypertrophy, macroglossia, retrognathia/micrognathia, and upper airway mass lesions can contribute to upper airway narrowing.

KEY POINT

- The most important risk factor for obstructive sleep apnea is obesity, particularly in those with prominence of adipose tissue in the trunk and neck.

Clinical Features and Diagnosis

Patients are commonly brought to medical attention by the concerns of a bed partner who observes loud snoring, gasping, and breathing pauses. Nocturnal choking or gasping is probably the most sensitive pretest indicator of OSA. Other symptoms include overnight awakenings, nocturia, and feeling unrested after a night of sleep.

The most important established consequence of OSA is excessive daytime sleepiness. Although it is not a universal symptom, the lack of self-report may not reflect the true degree of impairment. Collateral history from a family member as well as questionnaires such as the Epworth Sleepiness Scale can help identify excessive daytime sleepiness. Neuropsychiatric symptoms are common, including mood alterations, difficulty in concentrating, and problems completing tasks at school or the workplace.

With increasing use of screening tools such as the STOP-BANG questionnaire and perioperative care pathways, unexpected patient events due to undiagnosed OSA following a surgical procedure involving general anesthesia or narcotic analgesics are less common than in the past.

Objective testing is required for a diagnosis of OSA. Physical examination findings (crowded oropharynx) and questionnaires might enhance pretest probability and guide decision-making about whether to pursue testing, but alone are insufficiently sensitive or specific. Overnight pulse oximetry is also poorly discriminative to diagnose OSA, but in those who are asymptomatic with a low pretest probability, normal overnight oximetry might be reassuring and support the decision to avoid further testing. The historic gold standard—in-laboratory polysomnography—which is costly and resource-intensive, is being replaced in many regions by home sleep testing. Home sleep testing doesn't measure electroencephalographic sleep like polysomnography. Yet, it is diagnostically similar in otherwise uncomplicated patients (without underlying cardiopulmonary or neuromuscular disease) who are felt to have at least moderate to severe OSA (to minimize false negatives that may occur in milder disease).

KEY POINTS

- Normal overnight pulse oximetry in those who are asymptomatic with a low pretest probability can be reassuring and supports the decision to avoid further testing for obstructive sleep apnea.

- Home sleep testing may be most appropriate in patients without underlying cardiopulmonary or neuromuscular disease who are felt to have at least moderate to severe obstructive sleep apnea.

Treatment

There are several treatment options for OSA, the efficacy of which are generally based upon the ability to reduce, if not abolish, apneas and hypopneas. Positive airway pressure therapy, which typically reduces the AHI toward zero, is the most reliable means to accomplish this, though because the AHI doesn't always correlate with important outcomes in OSA, other treatments may adequately manage OSA for a given patient, even in the face of residual sleep apnea.

Based upon clinical trial results, the strongest indication for treatment of OSA is excessive daytime sleepiness, which generally improves with effective therapy. Although they are not as easily measured as excessive daytime sleepiness, other associated symptoms such as choking or gasping would also be expected to respond to treatment. Neurocognitive and mood symptoms are probably indications for treatment. In patients who perform mission-critical work (truck drivers, pilots), the threshold for treatment may be lower than for others. The role of treatment in otherwise healthy or asymptomatic individuals is a matter of debate. Device therapy (positive airway pressure and oral appliances) has been shown to modestly reduce blood pressure in hypertensive patients with

OSA, but the effect of treatment to manage comorbid cardiovascular disease or to prevent major cardiovascular events is unproven.

Weight Loss, Behavioral Modifications

OSA severity improves with weight loss, so all overweight or obese patients with OSA should be counseled accordingly. In minimally symptomatic patients with mild OSA, weight loss might be preferred therapy. Weight loss associated with dieting programs or bariatric surgery generally improves but may not eradicate OSA, so close follow-up is required. Additional measures that may help manage mild OSA include reducing alcohol intake before bedtime and avoiding a supine posture if OSA is position-dependent. **H**

> **KEY POINT**
> - Obstructive sleep apnea severity improves with weight loss, so all overweight or obese patients with obstructive sleep apnea should be counseled accordingly.

H ## Positive Airway Pressure

Positive airway pressure remains the most effective therapy for preventing disordered breathing events and alleviating symptoms in patients who have OSA. It acts by pressurizing the upper airway to maintain lumenal patency, thereby eliminating snoring and airflow limitation.

As home sleep testing becomes more widespread in uncomplicated OSA, the traditional paradigm of in-lab polysomnography titration performed by a sleep technologist to arrive at an optimal fixed and constant value referred to as continuous positive airway pressure will be less common. The diagnosis by home sleep testing is coupled to treatment with auto-adjusting positive airway pressure, which uses a computer algorithm to detect and overcome upper airway resistance in real time. Auto-adjusting positive airway pressure and continuous positive airway pressure are considered therapeutic equivalents in terms of reducing the AHI and adherence to treatment. Bilevel positive airway pressure, which delivers separate inspiratory and expiratory pressures (the gradient is referred to as pressure support) to augment alveolar ventilation, has no proved role in OSA without a hypoventilation syndrome (see below).

The effectiveness of positive airway pressure therapy hinges upon patient adherence. Symptom burden probably drives adherence but for those who lack motivation, educational programs can help, as can direct-to-patient reports wirelessly transmitted from the device directly to smartphones or computers. Side effects such as xerostomia and nasal dryness and congestion can be ameliorated by in-line humidification. Intranasal glucocorticoids or anticholinergics may be useful for recalcitrant nasal congestion or rhinitis. Modified pressure profiles that slightly reduce pressure on exhalation may enhance comfort. Proper mask fit enhances comfort and mitigates air leak. Positive airway pressure interfaces, ranging from nasal pillows that sit at the nasal openings to nasal masks that cover the nose to oronasal (full face) masks that cover the nose and mouth, are frequently updated and improved. **H**

> **KEY POINTS**
> - Positive airway pressure remains the most effective therapy for preventing disordered breathing events and alleviating symptoms in patients who have obstructive sleep apnea.
> - Auto-adjusting positive airway pressure and continuous positive airway pressure are considered therapeutic equivalents for reducing the apnea-hypopnea index and increasing adherence to treatment.

Oral Appliances

Oral appliances increase upper airway caliber primarily by exerting traction to advance the mandible. They do not reduce the AHI or increase oxygen levels as reliably as positive airway pressure, and are, therefore, generally avoided in more severe cases of OSA. Oral appliances have some potential advantages over positive airway pressure, however, including a reduced incidence of side effects and a potentially higher rate of adherence. The most common side effects are morning occlusal changes, which are generally reversible, and sialorrhea.

Upper Airway Surgery

Although surgical procedures are generally not first-line therapy for OSA, maxillomandibular advancement (MMA) significantly improves the AHI, even in severe disease, and can be considered for patients who do not benefit from or refuse positive airway pressure therapy. Factors that predict surgical success are not fully known, though younger patients who are less obese probably fare better. Traditional soft palatal procedures such as uvulopalatopharyngoplasty (UPPP) are ineffective; tonsillectomy in adults may or may not be effective. Tracheotomy, which bypasses the entire upper airway, is an effective though uncommonly used treatment of OSA, limited by patient acceptance and aesthetics.

If surgery is performed, reassessment by objective testing should be performed within 3 to 6 months to assess effect.

> **KEY POINT**
> - Traditional soft palatal procedures such as uvulopalatopharyngoplasty are ineffective for treatment of obstructive sleep apnea.

HVC

Other Devices

A hypoglossal nerve stimulator approved for use in OSA has been shown to improve the AHI in some patients. Implanted in the chest wall, it synchronizes with the respiratory cycle to contract the tongue muscles during inspiration. It is expensive, and those patients most likely to benefit from this treatment are yet to be determined.

A nasal end-expiratory positive airway pressure device applied to the nasal openings by way of an adhesive has also been shown to reduce the AHI in some but not all patients. No drug therapy is effective for OSA. Supplemental oxygen is not recommended as primary therapy for OSA. A direct comparison of supplemental oxygen versus positive airway pressure therapy found that blood pressure was reduced in the positive airway pressure group but not in the supplemental oxygen group.

Central Sleep Apnea Syndromes
Classification and Pathophysiology

Central sleep apnea (CSA) syndromes are defined by pauses in airflow due to loss of output from the central respiratory generators in the brainstem, resulting in lack of respiratory effort. Ventilation during sleep is primarily determined by the arterial P_{CO_2}, particularly during non-REM sleep, which comprises about 75% of total sleep time. Under normal circumstances, a steady state exists where ventilation maintains the arterial P_{CO_2} in the normal range (approximately 40 mm Hg [5.3 kPa]). In CSA, the response to arterial P_{CO_2} is exaggerated, resulting in ventilatory overshoot, hyperventilation, and reduction of the arterial P_{CO_2} to a level near the apneic threshold, the level at which respiratory efforts cease. This central apnea further destabilizes ventilation and perpetuates the process. On polysomnography, a central apnea is identified by the absence of respiratory effort associated with loss of airflow for at least 10 seconds.

> **KEY POINT**
> - Central sleep apnea syndromes are defined by pauses in airflow due to loss of output from the central respiratory generators in the brainstem, resulting in lack of respiratory effort.

Risk Factors

Comorbid illnesses that predispose to instability of the ventilatory control system are the most common risk factors for CSA. The most important and prevalent association is between CSA and heart failure, which classically manifests as Cheyne-Stokes breathing, characterized by a crescendo-decrescendo pattern of ventilation. Atrial fibrillation, both in the setting of heart failure and also in those with normal left ventricular systolic function, is a risk factor for CSA.

Known for their respiratory depressant effects in high doses, opioid analgesics are also associated with CSA. Opioids have destabilizing effects on ventilation, resulting in CSA and a chaotic breathing rhythm.

Approximately 10% percent of OSA patients treated with positive airway pressure exhibit "treatment-emergent CSA," the significance of which is a matter of debate. In many, the central apneas dissipate as patients acclimate to positive airway pressure therapy.

Other risk factors for CSA include stroke, brainstem lesions, and possibly kidney failure. Men may be at higher risk than woman. High-altitude periodic breathing is a form of CSA. Primary or idiopathic CSA, in which no risk factors are identified, is uncommon.

Symptoms and Diagnosis

It can be difficult to determine which symptoms are specific to CSA and which are associated with the comorbid condition(s). Some symptoms may be indistinguishable from OSA, such as frequent awakenings from sleep and nocturnal dyspnea, although daytime sleepiness is uncommon in those with CSA and heart failure. In-lab polysomnography is required to accurately diagnose CSA, though the Cheyne-Stokes breathing pattern is sometimes recognizable on home sleep testing. It should also be noted that although the AHI is traditionally used to describe the severity of CSA, it hasn't been validated as a predictor of important clinical outcomes as it has been in OSA. Finally, abnormal oximetry does not reliably discriminate between OSA and CSA.

Treatment

There are few clinical trials proving a role for specific treatment of CSA, so initial management should target modifiable risk factors. For example, reduction or elimination of opioids improves CSA. Medical optimization of heart failure (with drugs or devices, optimizing fluid balance in the setting of volume overload, or surgery such as valve repair or cardiac transplantation) has been shown to improve CSA and Cheyne-Stokes breathing, though it remains controversial as to whether CSA is an independent risk factor for worsened prognosis in those with heart failure.

Sleep-related symptoms probably represent an indication for treatment. Continuous positive airway pressure may occasionally be useful, especially in patients with overlapping OSA, though "treatment-emergent CSA" may persist. Adaptive servo-ventilation is a form of positive airway pressure therapy that effectively suppresses CSA. Its role in treatment, however, was called into question by the results of a recent large trial showing an unexpected increase in mortality in patients with CSA and heart failure with reduced ejection fraction.

> **KEY POINT**
> - Initial management of central sleep apnea should target modifiable risk factors such as heart failure and elimination of opioids.

Sleep-Related Hypoventilation Syndromes

Sleep-related hypoventilation syndromes are associated with advanced COPD, obesity hypoventilation syndrome, and restrictive lung diseases related to kyphoscoliosis or neuromuscular disorders and others diseases (**Table 33**). These conditions are defined by impaired gas exchange during wakefulness that is further compromised with sleep, especially during the muscle atonia of REM. Capnometry (measurement of either transcutaneous or end-tidal carbon dioxide levels) are increasingly used to confirm hypoventilation during sleep, although oxygenation criteria are also used to diagnose

TABLE 33. Causes of Sleep-Related Hypoventilation Syndromes

COPD
Obesity hypoventilation syndrome
Myxedema
Neuromuscular disease
Muscular dystrophy
Amyotrophic lateral sclerosis
Myasthenia gravis
Guillain-Barré syndrome
Phrenic nerve injury
Poliomyelitis, post-polio syndrome
Cervical spine injury
Kyphoscoliosis

sleep-related hypoventilation syndromes. Sustained reductions in oxyhemoglobin saturation (less than 90% for at least 5 minutes or more than 30% total sleep time by oximetry or polysomnography) in the setting of a compatible medical condition signify a hypoventilation syndrome. Obstructive sleep apnea may or may not be an associated feature.

KEY POINT

- Sleep-related hypoventilation syndromes are defined by impaired gas exchange during wakefulness that is further compromised with sleep; common associated conditions include advanced COPD, obesity hypoventilation syndrome, and restrictive lung diseases related to kyphoscoliosis or neuromuscular disorders.

Chronic Obstructive Pulmonary Disease

Patients with severe airflow obstruction due to COPD often exhibit sleep-related hypoventilation. In addition to optimization of COPD therapy, supplemental oxygen is often used. The noninvasive pressure support of bilevel positive airway pressure can be used if hypercapnia is confirmed. In the overlap syndrome where OSA is superimposed on COPD, continuous positive airway pressure therapy has been shown to decrease mortality rates.

Obesity Hypoventilation Syndrome

The obesity hypoventilation syndrome (OHS) results from a combination of the mechanical load on the respiratory pump and blunting of the chemoreflex (ventilatory response to carbon dioxide) in those with marked obesity. The hallmark of OHS is daytime hypercapnia, defined as a P_{CO_2} greater than 45 mm Hg (5.9 kPa). OSA is usually but not always superimposed. Biventricular heart failure, pulmonary hypertension, and volume overload are common.

Weight loss is essential and consideration can be given to bariatric surgery. Positive airway pressure therapy is indicated.

Although comparative trials are lacking, most would consider bilevel positive airway pressure the mode of choice to augment ventilation. Supplemental oxygen may need to be added and its continued need reassessed at a later date. See Principles of Critical Care for a discussion of acute respiratory failure associated with OHS.

KEY POINT

- The hallmark of obesity hypoventilation syndrome is daytime hypercapnia, defined as an arterial P_{CO_2} greater than 45 mm Hg (5.9 kPa).

Neuromuscular Diseases

Noninvasive positive pressure ventilation devices are often prescribed to alleviate sleep-related symptoms and support blood oxygen levels in patients with neuromuscular disorders (**Table 34**). Bilevel positive airway pressure or volume-assured devices (average volume-assured pressure support, or AVAPS), with or without supplemental oxygen, are indicated once there is evidence of daytime hypercapnia indicative of chronic respiratory failure. Polysomnography may aid in optimizing machine and oxygen settings and in assessing concomitant sleep disorders, but is not always needed. Tracheostomy and home mechanical ventilation are effective and may be appropriate for some patients. Supplemental oxygen may further depress ventilation in patients with respiratory muscle weakness and should generally not be prescribed without

TABLE 34. Positive Airway Pressure Modes

Mode	Description	Indication
CPAP	Fixed pressure derived from an in-lab titration attended by a technician	OSA Occasionally CSA
APAP	Range of pressure delivered to maintain upper airway patency, determined by a proprietary computer algorithm	OSA
BPAP	Inspiratory pressure support delivered over and above a minimum expiratory pressure, derived from an in-lab titration	Hypoventilation syndromes OSA when CPAP fails (including patient intolerance)
Auto-BPAP	Range of bilevel pressures determined by a proprietary computer algorithm	Same as BPAP
ASV	Breath-by-breath adjustment of inspiratory pressure support and back-up rate determined by a proprietary computer algorithm; expiratory pressure set by a technician	CSA (including mixed CSA and OSA)
Auto-ASV	Inspiratory and expiratory pressures determined by a proprietary algorithm	Same as ASV

APAP = auto-adjusting positive airway pressure; ASV = adaptive servo ventilation; BPAP = bilevel positive airway pressure; CPAP = continuous positive airway pressure; CSA = central sleep apnea; OSA = obstructive sleep apnea.

adjunctive ventilatory support, either by noninvasive means or by tracheostomy.

- Noninvasive positive pressure ventilation devices are often prescribed to alleviate sleep-related symptoms and support blood oxygen levels in patients with neuro-muscular disorders.

High-Altitude–Related Illnesses

Sleep Disturbances and Periodic Breathing

Diminishing barometric pressure associated with an ascent to altitude reduces the amount of ambient oxygen available for gas exchange, a condition known as hypobaric hypoxia. Physiologic responses to hypobaric hypoxia mechanistically underlie many disorders collectively referred to as high-altitude illness. In general, high-altitude illnesses occur at elevations of 2500 meters (approximately 8200 feet) and higher but have been reported below this elevation. Susceptibility to high-altitude illness is individualized and difficult to predict. Although high-altitude illnesses can occur at all ages and in the fittest of sojourners, patients who have a history of high-altitude–related illness are at risk for recurrence. Higher altitudes and a rapid rate of ascent are two key risk factors. Prevention is the best method of management. Because high-altitude illnesses are likely to recur, prophylactic measures are indicated on subsequent trips to elevation.

With the onset of hypoxic stress associated with hypobaric hypoxia, there is stimulation of peripheral chemoreceptors that are sensitive to hypoxia, leading to an attendant increase in ventilation, which is a key pathophysiologic mechanism in the sleep disorder termed high-altitude periodic breathing. In high-altitude periodic breathing, arterial P_{CO_2} is driven toward the apneic threshold, which, when crossed, results in a pause in breathing (central apnea). With this pause, arterial P_{CO_2} eventually rises sufficiently to again stimulate breathing. The cycle of ventilatory overshoot, hypocapnia, and central apneas repeats, at night and at high altitude. Patients complain of interrupted sleep and insomnia and may experience paroxysms of dyspnea that awaken them. Alcohol ingestion, which promotes dehydration, can intensify the sequelae of high-altitude periodic breathing.

Gradual ascent of less than 1000 feet per day, especially at higher altitudes, is suggested to prevent high-altitude periodic breathing and other high-altitude illnesses. Spending one night at an intermediate altitude to allow acclimatization often suffices. Acetazolamide, a carbonic anhydrase inhibitor and weak diuretic, induces a slight metabolic acidosis, is used to stabilize ventilation and enhance gas exchange, and can be used prophylactically in patients who have previously suffered

high-altitude illness. Supplemental oxygen can relieve symptoms of disrupted sleep and paroxysmal nocturnal dyspnea, but because most cases of high-altitude periodic breathing are self-limited after a few nights, this is generally not indicated in otherwise healthy individuals.

- Gradual ascent of less than 1000 feet per day, especially at higher altitudes, is suggested to prevent high-altitude periodic breathing and other high-altitude illnesses.
- Acetazolamide is used to stabilize ventilation and enhance gas exchange at high altitude, and can be used prophylactically in patients who have previously suffered high-altitude illness.

Acute Mountain Sickness

Cerebral blood flow and oxygen delivery to the brain are altered by the hypoxia and hypocapnia associated with the ascent to altitude. Cerebral autoregulatory mechanisms can dampen the stress on blood flow, and symptoms can be mild in acute mountain sickness (AMS), but when the compensatory pathways are overwhelmed, severe, life-threatening cerebral edema can ensue. In AMS, the most common high-altitude illness, symptoms are nonspecific and include headache, fatigue, nausea, and vomiting; disturbed sleep related to high-altitude periodic breathing is also common. AMS is probably more common than what comes to medical attention, with estimates of as many as 25% of visitors to an altitude of 2000 meters (approximately 6500 feet), the elevation at most major U.S. ski areas. Heavy exertion and dehydration tend to amplify symptoms, which, provided there is no further ascent, typically resolve within 24 to 48 hours. As in high-altitude periodic breathing, slow ascent helps prevent the syndrome. For mild symptoms, conservative treatment may include rest, fluid replacement, aspirin, NSAIDs, or antiemetics. Acetazolamide is best used as a prophylactic but has been used as a treatment as it is believed to accelerate acclimatization. Dexamethasone is equally effective to reduce symptoms of AMS and can be used as an alternative to acetazolamide, which is a sulfonamide, for either prophylaxis or treatment in patients with sulfonamide allergy. Supplemental oxygen or portable hyperbaric therapies to simulate descent, when available, are also used to treat more symptomatic cases of AMS. Descent should also be considered when feasible.

- Symptoms of acute mountain sickness are nonspecific and include headache, fatigue, nausea, and vomiting; disturbed sleep related to high-altitude periodic breathing is common.

High-Altitude Cerebral Edema

High-altitude cerebral edema is a feared manifestation of acute mountain sickness that tends to occur at higher elevations (above 3000 to 4000 meters, or approximately 9800 to 13,000 feet). Vascular leak leads to brain swelling, resulting in a range of manifestations from confusion and irritability, to ataxic gait, to coma and death. Prophylactic acetazolamide should be considered in individuals planning to ascend to these elevations. Recognition of cerebral edema mandates immediate intervention. Definitive treatment is immediate descent from altitude, particularly when the patient is still ambulatory, because incapacitation at high altitude exponentially complicates evacuation. Dexamethasone, supplemental oxygen, and hyperbaric therapy may be used in addition to descent in altitude.

KEY POINT

- Definitive treatment of high-altitude cerebral edema is immediate descent from altitude, particularly when the patient is still ambulatory, because incapacitation at high altitude exponentially complicates evacuation.

High-Altitude Pulmonary Edema

Vascular leak resulting from hypoxia-induced high pulmonary vascular pressures is felt to be mechanistically important in the development of high-altitude pulmonary edema. Within 2 to 4 days of ascent (typically to at least 2500 meters, approximately 8200 feet), pulmonary artery pressures begin to rise in response to hypoxic stress. Cough, dyspnea, and exertional intolerance are usually insidious but may occur abruptly and awaken a patient from sleep. Other features of acute mountain sickness may or may not be present. A key feature of high-altitude pulmonary edema is dyspnea at rest. Patients are often tachypneic and tachycardic; crackles or wheezing can be heard on chest examination. Pink, frothy sputum or frank hemoptysis may occur, which heralds worsening gas exchange and respiratory failure. The treatment of choice is supplemental oxygen along with rest, both of which will acutely reduce pulmonary artery pressures. Descent from altitude should be considered. Salvage therapies in the absence of supplemental oxygen and descent include vasodilators such as nifedipine or phosphodiesterase-5 inhibitors (sildenafil or tadalafil). Conventional treatments for pulmonary edema in the setting of heart failure, such as diuretics and nitrates, are not recommended in this setting. Rarely, climbers may require assisted ventilation, including intubation.

Air Travel in Pulmonary Disease

The principles of hypobaric hypoxia also apply to commercial airline travel. Cabins are pressurized to the equivalent of 1500 to 2500 meters (approximately 5000 to 8000 feet) in altitude, resulting in an inspired oxygen tension between 110 and 120 mm Hg (about 70% of the levels encountered at sea level). The resultant arterial P_{O_2} of approximately 60 mm Hg (8.0 kPa) is adequate for healthy individuals, but those with underlying pulmonary disease are at risk for significant hypoxemia during flight. Patients most at risk include those with advanced COPD complicated by chronic hypercapnic respiratory failure, patients with pulmonary hypertension, and those with restrictive lung disease. Patients with a recent exacerbation of their chronic lung condition should be fully compensated back to baseline before air travel. Patients who have had previous in-flight symptoms are likely to have recurrent issues and warrant closer assessment. Pulse oximetry is a useful screening tool, where an oxyhemoglobin saturation less than 92% at sea level indicates a likely need for in-flight supplemental oxygen. In most cases, 2 to 3 liters per minute of supplemental oxygen by nasal cannula is adequate. In those with sea-level oxygen saturation between 92% and 95%, hypoxia altitude simulation testing, available at some centers, can be used to determine the need for oxygen supplementation. In patients who are already on long-term supplemental oxygen, doubling of the flow rate during flight is typically adequate.

Patients with advanced lung disease over time may develop air-filled bullae, blebs, or cysts. These noncommunicating cavities will expand under hypobaric conditions; however, because airline cabins are pressurized, the risk of in-flight rupture and subsequent pneumothorax is believed to be low. The risk of pneumothorax is probably higher in those who have had a recent exacerbation of obstructive airways disease (asthma or COPD), during which air trapping can be pronounced, and such patients should delay air travel until the acute phase resolves. Signs or symptoms indicative of a pneumothorax (acute chest pain, dyspnea) should prompt the in-flight administration of supplemental oxygen, which promotes resorption of pleural air.

Following cardiothoracic surgery, a delay of 3 to 4 weeks before air travel is reasonable. An existing pneumothorax has traditionally been considered a contraindication to flight owing to the potential risk of expansion and tension physiology. Air travel may be safe in the presence of a small postoperative pneumothorax that has been radiographically stable.

KEY POINTS

- Pulse oximetry is a useful screening tool for patients who have had previous in-flight symptoms of pulmonary disease, where an oxyhemoglobin saturation of less than 92% at sea level indicates a likely need for in-flight supplemental oxygen.

- In patients who are already on long-term supplemental oxygen, doubling of the flow rate during flight is typically adequate.

Critical Care Medicine: ICU Ⓗ Utilization

Recognizing the Critically Ill Patient

There are no commonly accepted criteria for admission to an ICU. Signs and symptoms of clinical instability including hypotension, hypoxemia, arrhythmias, and mental status changes may be useful to identify patients who require intense resources or may be at risk of deterioration. Several scoring systems (APACHE, SOFA, SAP) have been designed to help classify the severity of disease of patients admitted to the ICU. These scoring systems use vital signs and risk factors such as chronic disease, emergent surgery, and immunosuppression to calculate risk of mortality. Although they are rarely, if ever, used as ICU admission criteria, they are used to objectively compare severity and progression of disease and expected and observed mortality. Disease-specific scoring systems can also be used to triage patients based on risk of deterioration or death. Examples are the simplified Pulmonary Embolism Severity Index (sPESI), the Pneumonia Severity Index (PSI), or CURB 65 for predicting mortality in community-acquired pneumonia. Electronic early warning systems based on vital signs, age, and current or trending clinical information have also been developed to identify at-risk patients. These systems, which utilize telemedicine, have been available for some time, but data supporting their effectiveness are lacking.

Organization of Critical Care

To improve early management and resuscitation of patients at risk or deteriorating, many health care systems have developed rapid response teams (RRT) or medical emergency response teams, with the aim of recognizing patients promptly, triggering early evaluation and management, and moving the patient to a higher level of care. A key element of this system is the ability for any member of the health care team to trigger the RRT. Systematic reviews and meta-analyses of the effectiveness of these teams have demonstrated a decrease in cardiac and respiratory arrests and unexpected deterioration but not decreased mortality in adults.

Determining the admission to a critical care bed is more complicated than simply assessing the level of patient illness. This is determined in a significant way by hospital and unit policies and resources unique to each institution. No standard admission model exists, although international societies have published guidelines. Hospitals have developed institution-specific protocols to better manage patients who require life support technology.

An ICU is equipped with technology that allows continuous monitoring and delivery of life-sustaining interventions, such as mechanical ventilation or extracorporeal circulation. Hospital units designated as ICUs typically have the sickest patients and require nurse-to-patient ratios of 1:1 or 1:2, whereas a progressive care unit (also called intermediate, transitional, or step-down unit) may have a nurse-to-patient ratio as high as 1:5, reflecting patients with less acuity.

Critical care is generally defined as open-unit versus closed-unit, and low-intensity versus high-intensity. In an open unit, patients are managed by their primary team, which may include, but does not require a critical care consultant. Patients in a closed unit are managed primarily by the critical care team. Low-intensity units are open units. Although high-intensity units can be open or closed units, the critical care team is present throughout the day providing consultation. High-intensity and closed models with continuous staffing of ICUs by intensivists have been controversial; recent systematic reviews and meta-analyses show no differences in mortality between the staffing models, and minimal differences in length of stay.

KEY POINTS

- Rapid response teams have been shown to decrease the incidence of cardiac and respiratory arrests but not change hospital mortality in adults.
- Recent evidence shows no differences in mortality between open and closed ICUs, and minimal differences in length of stay.
- High-intensity and closed models of critical care with continuous staffing of ICUs by intensivists have been controversial; recent systematic reviews and meta-analyses show no differences in mortality between the staffing models, and minimal differences in length of stay.

HVC

Principles of Critical Care
Comprehensive Management of Critically Ill Patients

The care of patients in an ICU must be multidisciplinary and team-based. Critical care teams often include pharmacists, respiratory therapists, physical therapists, occupational therapists, case managers, and social workers in addition to nurses and physicians. The goal of care is to restore health and allow the patient to return home while minimizing time in the hospital, medical complications, and long-term effects of critical illness.

Patients in the ICU are at risk for developing many hospital-acquired conditions. The most common are health care-associated infections (central line-associated bloodstream infection, ventilator-associated pneumonia, catheter-associated urinary tract infection, *Clostridium difficile* colitis), skin and soft tissue pressure injury (including ulceration), malnutrition, gastrointestinal bleeding, delirium, and neuromuscular weakness (see MKSAP 18 Infectious Disease). Protocolized care can improve safety and decrease the incidence of these conditions. Hospital-acquired infections are considered avoidable and unacceptable events. Infections have become quality metrics and the focus of protocols standardizing care, for example to reduce central line infections. Other interventions include the use of a checklist during rounding on patients to improve compliance with ICU prophylaxis measures.

Protocols used in the ICU should be evidence-based and periodically reviewed to ensure accuracy. For instance, although stress ulcer prophylaxis with acid suppression has been standard practice, recent recognition of its association with increased risk of ventilator-associated pneumonia, *C. difficile* colitis, respiratory failure, and coagulopathy has raised concerns about the risk versus benefit for acid suppression. Coupled with data suggesting that the incidence of stress ulcers is decreasing, which may be due to early low-volume enteral feeding in critically ill patients, this emphasizes the importance of critical review of protocols as new evidence becomes available.

Skin and soft tissue pressure injuries are a key quality metric in the performance of an ICU. Scoring systems such as the Braden scale use clinical criteria to define risk of pressure injury in an objective manner. This helps establish specific care to prevent development of such injuries. Essential nursing care includes skin integrity monitoring and avoidance of high-risk situations, such as ongoing contact on pressure points and excessive skin moisture (see MKSAP 18 General Internal Medicine).

The complexity of disease and interventions in a critically ill patient requires a methodical approach to daily care. Many ICUs use an organ system–based approach, which allows caregivers to review the main disease process, its effects on organs and systems, and prophylactic and maintenance interventions that are essential to patient well-being.

Mechanical Ventilatory Support: General Ventilator Principles

Admission to the ICU for respiratory insufficiency is prompted by three basic conditions: (1) hypoxemic respiratory failure; (2) ventilatory (hypercapnic) respiratory failure; and (3) upper airway impairment. Acute hypoxemic respiratory failure is caused by ongoing perfusion of lung units that are no longer ventilating because of alveolar collapse or flooding with pus, edema fluid, or blood. Hypoxemia is reversed by application of positive end-expiratory pressure to the lung, which opens up flooded or collapsed alveoli. Adequate ventilation requires the generation of sufficient pressure by the respiratory muscles to create a pressure gradient that moves air from the mouth to the alveoli. The pressure generated has to overcome both elastic (chest wall and lung) and resistive (airway) forces. Ventilatory failure can result from elastic and resistive forces that are too high or respiratory muscles that are too weak to generate the necessary pressure gradient. Mechanical ventilator support for ventilatory failure can be accomplished by one of two methods: noninvasive, using a nasal or full face mask; or invasive, with an endotracheal tube or tracheostomy. Selection of noninvasive or invasive ventilation is dependent on the clinical situation and the goals of treatment. Initiation of any form of mechanical ventilatory support should be done in a monitored unit (for example, emergency department, ICU).

Noninvasive Mechanical Ventilation
Fundamental Concepts
Noninvasive positive pressure ventilation is administered through a facial or nasal mask. Higher pressures usually require a full face mask to achieve the desired level of positive pressure.

There are two types of noninvasive mechanical ventilation (NIV): continuous positive airway pressure (CPAP) and bilevel positive airway pressure (BPAP). CPAP delivers a constant airway pressure during inspiration and expiration. BPAP delivers a higher level of positive airway pressure during inspiration than during expiration, thus providing additional inspiratory support. This additional inspiratory support with BPAP increases tidal volume and maintains an appropriate level of gas exchange while requiring less respiratory effort by the patient. **Table 35** highlights the physiological effects and indications for these different modes of ventilatory support.

TABLE 35.	Modes of Noninvasive Ventilation		
Mode	**Function**	**Physiologic Effects**	**Indications**
CPAP	Applies and maintains a constant airway pressure throughout the respiratory cycle	Maintains patent airway in setting of obstructive sleep apnea, increases functional residual capacity, increases mean airway pressure	Obstructive sleep apnea Pulmonary edema Excessive dynamic airway collapse Pre-intubation Post-extubation
BPAP	Applies two different levels of airway pressure: inspiratory (IPAP) and expiratory (EPAP) positive airway pressure	Same as CPAP, but also decreases work of breathing and augments tidal volume	COPD exacerbation Obesity hypoventilation syndrome Neuromuscular diseases Time-limited trial in selected "do not intubate" patients with clear goals of care
BPAP with S/T mode	BPAP with a minimum set respiration rate	In case of apnea it will continue to deliver breaths	Hypoventilation, central apneas

BPAP = bilevel positive airway pressure; CPAP = continuous positive airway pressure; EPAP = expiratory positive airway pressure; IPAP = inspiratory positive airway pressure; S/T = spontaneous/timed.

Indications and Patient Selection

Evidence favors the use of NIV in the critical care setting in patients with COPD exacerbations, cardiogenic pulmonary edema, neuromuscular disease, obesity hypoventilation syndrome, and in patients who have been extubated, which places them at high risk of morbidity. However, NIV also increases the risk of mortality in some patients, such as those with COPD who require subsequent intubation. All patients placed on NIV need to be monitored and reevaluated within 2 hours to determine if the therapy is effective or if adjustments or more invasive therapy is needed.

The use of NIV has not been shown to benefit patients with asthma exacerbations, although the data are limited because of small numbers of patients and methodological design flaws. NIV is often used for patients who are not candidates for invasive mechanical ventilation, in part to decrease or palliate respiratory distress. NIV was thought to be beneficial for immunosuppressed patients, but recent trials have cast doubt about its effectiveness. Finally, the use of NIV in patients with hypoxemic respiratory failure remains controversial. Studies have not demonstrated benefit, and there is some evidence of harm.

Contraindications to the use of NIV include altered mental status, increased airway secretions, emesis, gastric distention, airway obstruction, recent esophageal surgery, cardiac arrest, inability to protect the airway, facial trauma/surgery (including oral, nasal, or sinus), and patient intolerance of the mask.

Application

NIV can be delivered with a critical care ventilator, a portable ventilator, or a home device. Initiation of NIV for patients with acute respiratory failure should always be done in a monitored unit by trained providers. Proper mask sizing and patient adaptation to the device are essential; these require time and coaching of the patient. The timing of instituting NIV is essential, as late application (impending respiratory failure) is related to the need for subsequent intubation and to worse outcomes. After initiation, patients should be closely monitored for tolerance and adverse effects (patient comfort, skin integrity, gastric distention, and eye irritation), effectiveness of the ventilatory settings (measured using tidal volumes and respiration rate), and clinical improvement (blood pH, respiration rate, oxygen saturation as measured by pulse oximetry, and mental status). Failure to improve on NIV is associated with increased mortality.

High-Flow Humidified Nasal Cannula Devices

High-flow humidified nasal cannula has surged as a new modality for oxygenation support in the critically ill. It consists of a device that mixes and humidifies high-flow air and oxygen (30 L/min or more) to deliver a reliable FIO_2 (0.21 to 1.0) through a nasal cannula. The high flow creates positive airway pressure; the amount of pressure depends on the flow rate and cannot be measured or monitored consistently. Delivery of inspired gas through high-flow humidified nasal cannula decreases the work of breathing, provides heated and humidified gas at a reliable FIO_2, and decreases dead space. High-flow humidified nasal cannula is effective for preoxygenating critically ill patients before intubation, as support for postoperative hypoxemic respiratory failure, and as support for acute hypoxemic respiratory failure. Its initial application should occur in the critical care setting with close monitoring for tolerance and effectiveness.

Invasive Mechanical Ventilation

Fundamental Concepts

Invasive mechanical ventilation involves the use of an endotracheal tube or tracheostomy to deliver positive pressure ventilation. Invasive mechanical ventilation allows the use of higher inspiratory pressures and addresses limitations of NIV, such as the ability to protect the airway. The indications for invasive mechanical ventilation are hypoxemic and ventilatory respiratory failure, contraindication to NIV, and inability to protect the airway. The timing, the ventilation mode, and the settings depend on the disease and the patient (**Table 36**).

The appropriate mode of invasive mechanical ventilation is chosen based on its ability to achieve safety, comfort, and ultimate liberation from the ventilator, as well as on the patient's disease and physiological status. Safe mechanical ventilation requires adequate minute ventilation and oxygenation while maintaining an appropriate tidal volume to prevent ventilator-induced lung injury (see Common ICU Conditions). Ventilator-induced lung injury can occur early or late in the course of inappropriate ventilation. Appropriate tidal volume is especially important for patients who cannot independently sustain minute ventilation because of paralysis or sedation, as well as for patients who require limited tidal volume, such as those with early acute respiratory distress syndrome.

When patients are awake and the risk of lung injury has decreased, patient-ventilator interaction should be optimized to provide comfort through adequate breath support. Important considerations include the patient's level of respiratory muscle weakness or fatigue, the presence of acidosis, and the patient's level of anesthesia.

Weaning

Patients should be liberated from mechanical ventilation as soon as possible. The concurrent use of daily awakening or targeted light sedation protocols and spontaneous breathing trials reduces mechanical ventilation time and mortality (**Table 37**). Weaning strategies have shifted from gradual reduction of support to intermittent testing for readiness to breathe, with trials of minimal or no ventilator assistance. Spontaneous breathing trials of 30 minutes to 2 hours using low levels of pressure support (8 cm H_2O or less) or T-piece can identify patients who will be successfully extubated. Recent guidelines suggest pressure support is the preferred method.

TABLE 36. Most Frequently Used Ventilator Modes

Common Name	Mode Classification	Breath Control Variable	Breath Sequence	Targeting Scheme
Volume control and assist/control	VC-CMVs	VC: The ventilator controls the flow (volume) during the mandatory breath. If the patient's effort, lung compliance, or resistance changes, the ventilator will still deliver the set tidal volume (but the pressure will change).	CMV: All breaths are mandatory. The patient may or may not trigger the breath, but the ventilator always ends the breath when the tidal volume is delivered. The name "assist/control" is a misnomer from the past.	Set-point, s: The operator sets all the parameters of the breath (flow waveform, flow rate, and volume). The ventilator only delivers the breath and does not adjust to the patient's effort or change in lung characteristics.
Pressure control and assist/control	PC-CMVs	PC: The ventilator controls the pressure during the mandatory breath. If the patient's effort, lung compliance, or resistance changes, the ventilator will still deliver the set inspiratory pressure (but the tidal volume delivered will change).	CMV: All breaths are mandatory. The patient may or may not trigger the breath, but the ventilator always ends the breath when the preset inspiratory time elapses.	Set-point, s: The operator sets all the parameters of the breath (inspiratory pressure and inspiratory time). The ventilator only delivers the breath and does not adjust to the patient's effort or change in lung characteristics.
Pressure support, continuous positive airway pressure	PC-CSVs	PC: The ventilator controls the pressure during the breath.	CSV: All breaths are spontaneous. The patient triggers and cycles the breath.	Set-point, s: The operator sets all the parameters of the breath (inspiratory pressure). The ventilator delivers the breath and does not adjust to the patient's effort or change in lung characteristics.
Synchronized intermittent mandatory ventilation	PC-IMVs,s or VC-IMVs,s	PC or VC: The mandatory breaths can be set to be volume or pressure controlled, not both.	IMV: Preset mandatory breaths are delivered by the ventilator at a minimum set rate. Spontaneous breaths are permitted in between mandatory breaths. The triggering of the mandatory breath will be coordinated with the patient if the inspiratory effort occurs close to the scheduled time trigger (determined by the set frequency).	Set-point, s: One "s" refers to the mandatory breath and the other to the spontaneous breath. Generally, all spontaneous breaths in IMV are pressure supported (PC-CSVs).

CMV = continuous mandatory ventilation; CSV = continuous spontaneous ventilation; IMV = intermittent mandatory ventilation; PC = pressure controlled; s = set-point; VC = volume controlled.

CONT.

Synchronized intermittent mechanical ventilation is a mode of ventilation that combines mandatory and spontaneous breaths. Some newer technologies are being marketed that use intermittent mandatory ventilation (IMV) sequences and different targeting algorithms, but evidence regarding their performance is scant, and synchronized IMV should not be used to wean patients from mechanical ventilation.

The use of NIV immediately (preemptive) after extubation prevents extubation failure in patients at high risk, such as those with heart failure, COPD, or hypercapnia. The delayed use of noninvasive ventilation after extubation, that is, when the patient develops features of respiratory failure, should be avoided as it is associated with increased mortality.

Ventilator-Associated Pneumonia
Ventilator-associated pneumonia develops 48 hours or more after endotracheal intubation. Preventive strategies include minimizing sedation, early mobilization, minimizing pooling of supraglottic secretions, scheduled oral care with chlorhexidine, head of bed elevation, minimization of changes of the ventilator circuit, and proper hand hygiene. For further discussion of pneumonia see MKSAP 18 Infectious Disease.

KEY POINTS

- Spontaneous breathing trials of 30 minutes to 2 hours using low levels of pressure support (8 cm H_2O or less) can identify patients who will be successfully extubated.

- The use of noninvasive mechanical ventilation immediately after extubation prevents extubation failure in patients at high risk, such as those with heart failure, COPD, or hypercapnia.

Invasive Monitoring

Patients in the ICU often require intensive monitoring of vital signs or vascular pressures, which necessitates the use of invasive methods. Monitoring devices increase the risk of adverse

TABLE 37. Common Criteria for Spontaneous Breathing Trials (SBT) and Extubation[a]

Criteria to Perform SBT
Cause of respiratory failure improved
FIO_2 ≤40% and PEEP ≤5-8 cm H_2O
pH >7.25
Hemodynamic stability
Able to spontaneously breathe

Criteria to Pass SBT: At Least 30 Minutes Without
Clinical evidence of respiratory distress
SpO_2 <90%
Respiration rate >35/min
New arrhythmias
Tachycardia
Hypotension or hypertension

Additional Considerations Before Extubation
Quantity of secretions
Adequacy of cough
Altered mental status

[a]These criteria may differ between institutions.

PEEP = positive end-expiratory pressure; SpO_2 = peripheral arterial oxygen saturation.

Intravenous Access

There are different types of devices for central intravenous (IV) access. The determination of the type of access depends on many factors including urgency of access, expected duration, and reason for access (**Table 38**). Removal of intraosseus devices must be done as soon as IV access is obtained. Peripheral venous access with a short, wide-bore catheter is the route of choice for rapid volume resuscitation. In general, all IV access should be removed as soon as possible to decrease the risk of complications, mainly infection and thrombosis. Procedure-related complications, such as arterial injury, nerve injury, or pneumothorax can be minimized with the use of ultrasound-guided placement. Devices with lower risk of complications (for example, peripheral IV access) should be used whenever possible. **H**

KEY POINTS

- All intravenous access should be removed as soon as possible to decrease the risk for complications.
- Peripheral intravenous access with a short, wide-bore catheter is the route of choice for volume resuscitation.

Blood Pressure Support

Systemic arterial pressure is determined by cardiac output and systemic vascular resistance. Maintenance of arterial blood pressure requires compensatory adjustments when there is either a decrease in cardiac output or inappropriate reduction in systemic vascular resistance (vasodilation). A mean arterial pressure of 65 mm Hg is considered to be the threshold at which there is sufficient pressure for organ perfusion. A study comparing a lower (65-70 mm Hg) vs a higher (80-85 mm Hg) mean arterial pressures strategy in patients

CONT. effects, so they should be used only when required to obtain information that cannot be obtained with noninvasive methods. For example, the routine use of pulmonary artery catheters does not lead to improved outcomes, is associated with increased side effects, and may increase mortality.

TABLE 38. Types of Central Venous Access

Type	Indications	Duration	Potential Complications	Contraindications
Peripherally inserted central venous catheter	Delivery of potentially caustic medications such as vasoactive agents, sedatives or antibiotics; central venous access	Few days up to 1 year	Low risk overall, avoiding pneumothorax and reducing infectious risk; clot formation or occlusion due to smaller vessel diameter	Current or pending dialysis
Temporary non-tunneled	Same as peripherally inserted central venous catheter; short-term dialysis; central venous pressure monitoring	Usually not more than 6 weeks	Infection; site-specific complications such as pneumothorax for subclavian or low intrajugular approach	
Long-term tunneled (valved tip and nonvalved tip)	Long-term TPN; chemotherapy; long-term antibiotics; dialysis	More than 6 weeks	Infection; valves prevent back bleeding but have an increased risk of catheter malfunction	
Ports or totally implanted	Long-term intermittent access such as chemotherapy	More than 6 weeks	Lowest risk of infection but more difficult to implant with more costs; hidden extravasation beneath skin	
Intraosseous (tibia or humeral head [adults])	When IV access otherwise not obtained but need emergency fluids and/or medications	About 24 hours	Low risk of infection; flow rates may be slower; if pain with infusion can use 2% preservative-free lidocaine injected slowly to control it	Do not place in a bone with a fracture, diagnosis of osteoporosis, or recent (24-48 h) intraosseous access attempt

IV = intravenous; TPN = total parenteral nutrition.

with septic shock demonstrated no difference in mortality. Blood pressure is usually monitored noninvasively with a blood pressure cuff. An arterial line for continuous monitoring is useful when the systolic blood pressure is less than 90 mm Hg, when frequent measurements are needed (particularly for patients requiring IV medication for blood pressure management), or when the cuff readings are unreliable. Assessment of tissue perfusion includes physical examination (skin temperature, mottling, jugular venous distention), ultrasound assessment of inferior vena cava diameter and other dynamic indices, and cardiac examination (echocardiogram, invasive and noninvasive cardiac output monitors). However, in a patient with several physical examination findings suggestive of decreased intravascular volume, the physical examination, including basic vital signs, is sufficient. Management should focus on the underlying cause of blood pressure derangement. For instance, hypotension due to deceased preload should be initially treated with volume resuscitation. Support of blood pressure may require the use of vasopressors (**Table 39**). Norepinephrine is the most commonly used agent and has been shown to reduce mortality. However, other agents are available and may be used in specific situations. **H**

KEY POINT

HVC
• A study comparing a lower (65-70 mm Hg) vs a higher (80-85 mm Hg) mean arterial pressures strategy in patients with septic shock demonstrated no difference in mortality.

Sedation and Analgesia

ICU patients often require sedation and analgesia. The need for analgesia should be monitored frequently, at least every 4 hours, and assessed using an objective scale such as the Behavioral Pain Scale or Critical Care Pain observation tool. Analgesics should be titrated to a goal and the patient should be monitored for side effects. Analgesia should include non-pharmacologic methods, such as relaxation techniques, non-narcotic and narcotic medication for general pain, and gabapentin or carbamazepine for neuropathic pain. Intravenous opioids are the drug of choice for treating non-neuropathic pain in critically ill patients, and all have similar efficacy and clinical outcomes when titrated to similar pain intensity endpoints. Additional analgesia should be given before painful procedures, such as thoracostomy tube placement. Most if not all patients requiring invasive mechanical ventilation will need some level of sedation. Sedation in the ICU requires monitoring and should be objectively assessed using a scale such as the Richmond Agitation Sedation Scale (RASS). Agents such as propofol or dexmedetomidine are preferred rather than benzodiazepines. If oversedation occurs, the drug should be stopped until the appropriate level of sedation is achieved, then restarted at half the previous dose.

Interruption of Sedation and Analgesia

Daily interruption of sedation and analgesia is appropriate in critically ill patients and is associated with decreased length of mechanical ventilation, length of ICU stay, and incidence of

TABLE 39.	Selection of Vasopressors			
Medication	**Type of Shock**	**Receptor Target**	**Primary Impact**	**Comments**
Dobutamine	Cardiogenic Distributive	β_1, β_2	↑Inotropy	First choice for cardiogenic shock without hypotension Add-on therapy for distributive shock with depressed cardiac function
Dopamine (high-dose)	Cardiogenic	D, α_1, β_1	↑SVR, ↑inotropy	Alternative to norepinephrine in (distributive) shock associated with absolute or relative bradycardia
Dopamine (low-dose)	Cardiogenic Distributive	D, β_1	↑Inotropy, ↑HR	Not recommended to augment renal blood flow
Epinephrine	Cardiogenic Distributive Hypovolemic	α_1, α_2, β_1, β_2	↑SVR, ↑inotropy	First choice anaphylactic (distributive) shock May be added to norepinephrine in distributive shock
Norepinephrine	Cardiogenic Distributive Hypovolemic	α_1, α_2, β_1	↑SVR, ↑inotropy	First choice in cardiogenic, distributive, and hypovolemic shock
Phenylephrine	Distributive	α_1	↑SVR	May be used when norepinephrine contraindicated (tachyarrhythmias) or failure of first-line drugs
Vasopressin	Distributive Hypovolemic	V	↑SVR	May be added to norepinephrine in septic shock

HR = heart rate; SVR = systemic vascular resistance.

CONT.

delirium. Protocolized light sedation has shown similar patient outcomes to daily sedation interruption.

Delirium

Delirium is characterized by an acute change in cognitive functioning occurring over hours to days, with fluctuations during the course of the day. Features of delirium include inattention, disorganized thinking, executive dysfunction, altered level of consciousness (lethargy or hypervigilance), perceptual disturbances (such as hallucinations or delusions), altered psychomotor activity (hyperactivity, hypoactivity, or alternating periods of hyperactivity and hypoactivity), sleep-wake disturbances, and labile mood. It is extremely common in ICU patients and is associated with increased length of ICU stay, morbidity, mortality, and post-intensive care cognitive impairment. Risk factors for delirium include preexisting dementia, hypertension, alcoholism, and high severity of illness on ICU admission. Patients should be monitored regularly and assessed using scales such as the Confusion Assessment Method-ICU (CAM-ICU) or Intensive Care Delirium Screening Checklist (ICDSC). Measures to decrease the risk of delirium include early mobilization, preservation of nocturnal sleep, adequate pain management, orientation of the patient, provision of visual and hearing aids, and minimization of nonessential medications. Early mobilization, consisting of interruption of sedation and physical and occupational therapy in the earliest days of critical illness, can be effective for treating and preventing delirium. In general, benzodiazepines should not be used for treating delirium in the ICU, unless needed in patients with alcohol withdrawal or seizures. Data do not support the routine use of haloperidol or atypical antipsychotics for the prevention of delirium. Treatment involves identification and correction of the underlying cause, maintaining adequate nutrition and hydration, and preventing complications. For further discussion of delirium see MKSAP 18 Neurology. **H**

KEY POINTS

- Sedation and analgesia should be monitored using objective standardized scales.

HVC - In general, benzodiazepines should not be used for treating delirium in the ICU, unless needed in patients with alcohol withdrawal or seizures; data do not support the routine use of haloperidol or atypical antipsychotics for the prevention of delirium.

Nutrition

Malnutrition in critically ill patients leads to increased morbidity and mortality, and all patients admitted to the ICU should have a nutritional evaluation. Enteral nutrition is preferred unless a contraindication is present (perforation, hemorrhage, or surgery). Guidelines recommend that enteral nutrition should be started within 24 to 48 hours of admission in critically ill patients. There is evidence that early enteral nutrition is associated with decreases in mortality and

infections, yet the level of evidence remains low. Critically ill patients who cannot maintain volitional nutritional intake may be fed using a gastric tube, large-bore tube, small-bore tube, or post-pyloric tube; there is no evidence of increased incidence of ventilator-associated pneumonia or aspiration among these methods. Routine measurement of gastric residuals is discouraged because it delays achievement of feeding goals, increases the risk of clogging the enteral access, and may increase the risk of aspiration.

Guidelines recommend that in patients at either low or high risk of problems with nutrition, use of supplemental parenteral nutrition should be considered only after 7 to 10 days of not meeting more than 60% of energy and protein requirements by the enteral route alone. Administration of parenteral nutrition to supplement enteral nutrition may lead to harm and should be avoided. In contrast, parenteral nutrition should be started as soon as possible for severely malnourished patients, those at high risk of malnutrition, and those for whom enteral nutrition is not possible. **H**

KEY POINTS

- Enteral nutrition is preferred unless a contraindication is present and should be started within 24 to 48 hours of admission in patients anticipated to have prolonged critical illness.

- Parenteral nutrition should be started as soon as possible for severely malnourished patients, those at high risk of malnutrition, and those for whom enteral nutrition is not possible.

- Routine measurement of gastric residuals is discouraged **HVC** in malnourished patients who are critically ill because it delays achievement of feeding goals, increases the risk of clogging the enteral access, and may increase the risk of aspiration.

- Administration of parenteral nutrition to supplement **HVC** enteral nutrition may lead to harm and should be avoided.

Early Mobilization

Many factors contribute to neuromuscular weakness in critically ill patients, including immobility, disease, medications, and medical interventions in the ICU. Immobility may result in muscular weakness, joint stiffness, ankylosis, pressure ulcers, osteoporosis, gastrointestinal dysmotility, and dysautonomia. Even a few days of immobility can have a prolonged effect on muscular strength; long-term follow-up of patients with critical illness demonstrates persistent muscular weakness at 1 and 5 years. The use of early mobilization strategies consisting of interruption of sedation and physical and occupational therapy in the earliest days of critical illness decreases length of time in the ICU and hospital stay, improves functional status, and decreases mortality. Despite the evidence favoring early mobilization and physical therapy, implementation remains low overall. **H**

- The use of early mobilization strategies decreases length of time in the ICU and hospital stay, improves functional status, and decreases mortality.

ICU Care Bundles

An ICU care bundle is a series of evidenced-based interventions that have been shown to improve patient outcomes when used together. Bundles can help clinicians monitor patients and guide appropriate interventions. The Institute for Healthcare Improvement has defined three bundles that apply to critical care (**Table 40**).

High Value Care in the ICU

The cost of health care in the United States is the highest per capita in the world. Critical care is responsible for a large proportion of health care costs. However, the survival and quality-of-life outcomes are not that different from those in other top-economy countries. Societal, organizational, and payment pressures have encouraged a focus on providing high value care, which is defined as care that maximizes benefit relative to harms and cost. The ICU is an environment in which high value care can have major effects, as the resources are expensive and the culture favors aggressive resource use. Internal medicine and critical care medical societies have joined the American Board of Internal Medicine (ABIM) Foundation's *Choosing Wisely®* campaign to promote cost-effective strategies that improve patient care (**Table 41**). The focus on resource utilization and cost will remain a central point of health care for the foreseeable future.

KEY POINTS

- Don't order diagnostic tests at regular intervals (such as every day), but rather in response to specific clinical questions. **HVC**
- Don't transfuse erythrocytes in hemodynamically stable, nonbleeding patients in the ICU who have a hemoglobin concentration greater than 7 g/dL (70 g/L). **HVC**
- Don't use parenteral nutrition in adequately nourished critically ill patients within the first 7 days of an ICU stay. **HVC**
- Don't deeply sedate mechanically ventilated patients without a specific indication and without daily attempts to lighten sedation. **HVC**
- Don't continue life support for patients at high risk for death or severely impaired functional recovery without offering patients and their families the alternative of care focused entirely on comfort. **HVC**

ICU Complications

Critical care illness is no longer viewed as an acute event that ends at the time of discharge from the ICU. ICU complications may be classified as early, which occur during the hospitalization, or late, which persist after the critical care illness. During the last decade, there has been increased recognition of

TABLE 40.   ICU Care Bundles
Prevention of Ventilator-Associated Pneumonia
Head of bed elevation at least 30 degrees
Daily sedation interruption and assessment of readiness to extubate
Stress ulcer prophylaxis
Deep vein thrombosis prophylaxis
Daily oral care with chlorhexidine
Central Line-Associated Bloodstream Infections
Hand hygiene
Maximal barrier precautions
Chlorhexidine skin antisepsis
Avoid femoral access
Daily review of line necessity
Sepsis
3-hour bundle
Measure lactate level
Obtain blood cultures before antibiotics
Administer broad-spectrum antibiotics
Administer 30 mL/kg crystalloids for hypotension or lactate ≥4 mEq/L (4 mmol/L)
6-hour bundle
Use vasopressors if no response to fluids; keep MAP above 65 mm Hg
Repeat volume status and tissue perfusion assessment
MAP = mean arterial blood pressure, calculated as [(2 × diastolic) + systolic]/3.

TABLE 41.   ICU *Choosing Wisely®* Top Five
Don't order diagnostic tests at regular intervals (such as every day), but rather in response to specific clinical questions.
Don't transfuse erythrocytes in hemodynamically stable, nonbleeding patients in the ICU who have a hemoglobin concentration greater than 7 g/dL (70 g/L).
Don't use parenteral nutrition in adequately nourished critically ill patients within the first 7 days of an ICU stay.
Don't deeply sedate mechanically ventilated patients without a specific indication and without daily attempts to lighten sedation.
Don't continue life support for patients at high risk for death or severely impaired functional recovery without offering patients and their families the alternative of care focused entirely on comfort.

CONT.

persistent disability and a focus on treatment to prevent late consequences of critical illness.

ICU-Acquired Weakness

Between 50% and 100% of critically ill patients develop muscle weakness. Muscle weakness may result from complications involving the nervous system (critical illness polyneuropathy), the muscles themselves (critical illness myopathy), or some combination thereof, or may be nonspecific (ICU-acquired weakness). It may also be related to prolonged neuromuscular blockade (**Table 42**). Identified risk factors include sepsis, multisystem organ failure, severe illness, prolonged immobility, and hyperglycemia. Evaluation for ICU-acquired weakness can initially be done at the bedside using the Medical Research Council muscle scale. ICU-acquired weakness generally improves over weeks to months, but may persist in a small percentage of patients for up to 2 years. Strategies to minimize ICU-acquired weakness include aggressive management of critical illness, early mobilization, and management of hyperglycemia. **H**

TABLE 42. Definitions and Characteristics of ICU-Acquired Weakness

ICU-Acquired Weakness

Clinically detected weakness with no other explanation other than the critical illness

Proximal and distal symmetrical flaccid weakness with sparing of cranial nerves

Often failure to wean from mechanical ventilation is first indication of weakness

Diagnosis of exclusion

Critical Illness Polyneuropathy

ICU-acquired weakness with electrophysiological evidence of axonal polyneuropathy

Quadriparesis or quadriplegia, decreased muscle tone, sparing of facial muscles. Deep tendon reflexes decreased

Critical Illness Myopathy

ICU-acquired weakness with electrophysiological and/or histological evidence of myopathy

Examination is similar to critical illness polyneuropathy. New sensory loss is suggestive, CK may be elevated

Critical Illness Neuromyopathy

Coexistence of critical Illness polyneuropathy and critical Illness myopathy

Mixed features, perhaps most prevalent form

Prolonged Neuromuscular Blockade

Prolonged effects in patients with renal failure, liver failure, hypermagnesemia

Flaccid areflexic quadriplegia with cranial nerve involvement

Repetitive nerve stimulation shows decremental response

CK = creatine kinase.

KEY POINT

- Strategies to minimize ICU-acquired weakness include aggressive management of critical illness, early mobilization, and management of hyperglycemia.

Long-Term Cognitive Impairment

As many as 30% to 80% of patients with critical care illness develop long-term impairment in cognition, which manifests clinically as cognitive impairment with similarities to acquired dementia. Observations have demonstrated that the level of impairment 1 year after critical illness is similar to mild Alzheimer disease. Although the specific risk factors and interventions related to developing cognitive impairment are not well defined, the development and duration of delirium during the ICU stay appear to be major predictors.

Post-Intensive Care Syndrome

Post-intensive care syndrome describes a group of symptoms that present in patients after an episode of critical care. The symptoms have been grouped according to the area that they affect (physical impairment, mental health, and cognitive impairments). Patients with post-intensive care syndrome have increased health care use, increased morbidity and mortality, and impaired quality of life. Post-intensive care syndrome also affects the caregivers and family of the critically ill patient; it has been reported that family members experience anxiety, depression, and post-traumatic stress disorder. Current research and interventions are focusing on how to improve recognition, prevention, diagnosis, and management. **H**

Common ICU Conditions **H**

Acute Respiratory Failure

Acute respiratory failure occurs when a patient cannot adequately oxygenate blood (hypoxemia) or remove carbon dioxide (hypercarbia or hypercapnia) from the blood. It is essential to quickly stabilize the patient and identify the cause of respiratory failure. History and physical examination are essential, but tests such as chest radiograph (**Table 43**), CT scan, arterial blood gas, and pulse oximetry are also useful. A structured approach allows clinicians to both identify and treat factors leading to respiratory failure. This approach includes evaluation for airway compromise, inadequate oxygenation, and inadequate ventilation. (**Figure 19**)

Acute Upper Airway Management

In patients who cannot maintain a patent airway or protect their airway against aspiration, a secure airway should be established by inserting a cuffed endotracheal or tracheostomy tube. High-flow oxygen; bag-valve mask ventilation; or oropharyngeal, nasopharyngeal, or laryngeal mask airway can aid oxygenation and ventilation when immediate intubation is not feasible and should be used until the airway can be secured. **H**

TABLE 43. Radiographic Findings and Differential Diagnosis in Acute Respiratory Failure

Finding	Differential Diagnosis
No infiltrate	Asthma/COPD exacerbation
	Drug overdose
	Intracardiac shunt
	Neuromuscular weakness
	Pulmonary embolus
Diffuse infiltrates	Acute respiratory distress syndrome
	Cardiogenic pulmonary edema
	Acute exacerbation of idiopathic pulmonary fibrosis
	Pneumonia
	Other (for example, acute hypersensitivity pneumonitis, acute eosinophilic pneumonia)
Focal infiltrate	Airway obstruction
	Atelectasis
	Pneumonia
	Pulmonary infarction

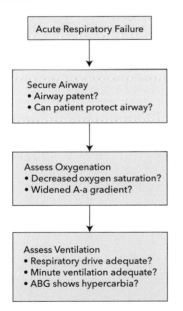

FIGURE 19. Key components to the assessment of acute respiratory failure. A-a = alveolar-arterial; ABG = arterial blood gas.

KEY POINT

- In patients who cannot maintain a patent airway or protect their airway against aspiration, a secure airway should be established by inserting a cuffed endotracheal or tracheostomy tube.

Airway Obstruction

Respiratory failure can result from intraluminal obstruction or extraluminal compression of the upper airways. Patients with partial airway obstruction may have tachypnea, increased respiratory effort, or an upright (tripod) posture with use of accessory muscles. Absent air movement, inability to talk, or cyanosis suggests complete obstruction and signifies a medical emergency. Inspiratory stridor suggests an obstruction above the level of the vocal cords, whereas expiratory stridor and wheezing suggest an intrathoracic process. Pulse oximetry in the setting of partial upper airway obstruction and stridor is usually normal. Patients with potential upper airway obstruction should be cautiously examined to prevent exacerbation of the condition. In patients with respiratory distress or for whom the risk of respiratory deterioration is high, early intubation is indicated.

Acute Inhalational Injuries

Smoke Inhalation

Pulmonary complications are a leading cause of morbidity and mortality in patients who have been burned or experienced significant smoke exposure from fires. Direct thermal injury due to smoke inhalation is usually limited to the upper airways. However, steam inhalation causes direct thermal injury throughout the tracheobronchial tree due to its ability to carry heat more efficiently than dry, hot gas. Following smoke inhalation, one-third of patients develop airway edema or mucosal sloughing from epithelial necrosis. Chest physiotherapy and serial bronchoscopic suctioning are frequently necessary to facilitate continued airway clearance. Injury to the distal tracheobronchial tree and lung parenchyma is caused by chemicals in smoke that generate a complex cascade of bronchoconstriction, pulmonary edema, ventilation-perfusion ($\dot{V}/\dot{Q}$) mismatch, and bronchial cast formation. Treatment is largely supportive.

Secondary respiratory infections are common and are a major cause of morbidity and mortality. Pneumonia is the most common complication following smoke inhalation injury, especially from *Staphylococcus* and *Pseudomonas* specie. Systemic toxicity from substances like carbon monoxide (CO) and hydrogen cyanide (HCN) are common following smoke inhalation. Clinicians should suspect CO and HCN poisoning in all patients with smoke exposure. Both can cause a reduction in the oxygen-carrying capacity of hemoglobin. Unfortunately this may not be apparent, as CO and HCN are not detected by standard pulse oximetry, and oxygen saturation measurement may be falsely normal. Additional details of CO and HCN poisoning are reviewed in Toxicology.

Other Forms of Inhalational Injury

Inhalational injuries related to chemical vapors are uncommon. War, industrial, or farming operations and exposure to home cleaning or pesticide agents constitute most chemical inhalational injuries. Water-soluble agents usually affect mucosal structures of the upper airway and have rapid onset of symptoms. Water insoluble agents affect deeper structures including lung parenchyma and distal airways, and symptoms are often delayed. Edema, bronchospasm, asphyxiation, and direct systemic toxicity are common. Key features of

CONT.

inhalational agents are listed in **Table 44**. Treatment is supportive, with a specific antidote, atropine, indicated only in cholinesterase inhibitor exposure.

Hypoxemic Respiratory Failure

Hypoxemic respiratory failure is caused by inadequate oxygenation of hemoglobin. The most common causes of hypoxemic respiratory failure in the ICU are $\dot{V}/\dot{Q}$ mismatch and shunt ($\dot{V}/\dot{Q}$ = 0), which occur when perfused areas of the lung are not ventilated, whether because of alveolar collapse (atelectasis) or filling of alveoli with blood, pus, protein, or water. An increased alveolar-arterial oxygen difference (gradient) is the key feature of $\dot{V}/\dot{Q}$ mismatch and shunt. The gradient is derived by subtracting the measured arterial P_{O_2} from the calculated alveolar P_{O_2}.

The alveolar P_{O_2} is calculated using the alveolar gas equation:

$$Alveolar\ P_{O_2} = (F_{IO_2} \times [P_{atm} - 47]) - (1.25 \times P_{CO_2})$$

F_{IO_2} is the fraction of inspired oxygen (0.21 in ambient air), P_{atm} is the atmospheric pressure (760 mm Hg at sea level), and 47 represents the partial pressure of water in mm Hg at 37°C (98.6°F). The alveolar-arterial gradient increases with age, and normal gradients in individuals breathing ambient air (but not applicable in patients on supplemental oxygen) can be estimated with the equation:

$$Expected\ alveolar\text{-}arterial\ oxygen\ gradient = 2.5 + 0.21 \times age\ in\ years$$

TABLE 44.	Key Features of Inhaled Agents	
Agent	**Characteristics**	**Clinical Features Following Exposure**
Ammonia	Colorless, ammonia odor	Cough, upper airway burns, pulmonary edema, asphyxiation in poorly vented areas
Chlorine	Yellow-green, chlorine odor	Upper airway irritation and burns, bronchospasm, pulmonary edema
Phosgene	Colorless, musty odor like fresh cut grass	Systemic toxicity including elevated methemoglobin level, cyanosis and metabolic acidosis. Pulmonary edema
Mustard gas	Yellow-brown vapor, odor like garlic or onions	Upper airways burns and obstruction can occur
Organophosphates and other cholinesterase inhibitors	Colorless, fruity odor	Systemic toxicity causing acetylcholine toxicity (rhinorrhea, bronchorrhea, diarrhea, bronchospasm, flaccid paralysis, apnea)

Scenarios of acute and chronic hypoxemia are difficult to distinguish using arterial blood gases alone. A helpful distinguishing feature is the time course of development of symptoms; in addition, the presence of polycythemia suggests chronic hypoxemia. Findings on chest imaging studies may be helpful, as diffuse alveolar filling is more suggestive of acute hypoxemic respiratory failure, whereas interstitial lung disease is more suggestive of a chronic process.

Signs of acute hypoxemic respiratory failure include recent onset of increased work of breathing, tachypnea, and anxiety. Cyanosis of the lips or fingers may be present when oxygenation of hemoglobin is severely compromised, often below 80%. Findings on auscultation such as crackles, wheezing, egophony, or rhonchi may suggest an underlying cause.

Management of hypoxemic respiratory failure centers on administration of supplemental oxygen and measures to open alveoli that are fluid-filled or collapsed, such as mechanical ventilation with administration of both positive inspiratory and positive end-expiratory pressure (PEEP). In extreme cases where the technology and expertise are available, extracorporeal membrane oxygenation (ECMO) can be used to provide external oxygenation of, and removal of carbon dioxide from, the blood. Disease-specific management is discussed below.

KEY POINTS

- The most common causes of hypoxemic respiratory failure in the ICU are ventilation-perfusion mismatch and shunt, which occurs when perfused areas of the lung are not ventilated, whether because of alveolar collapse (atelectasis) or filling of alveoli with blood, pus, protein, or water.
- Management of hypoxemic respiratory failure centers on administration of supplemental oxygen and measures to open alveoli that are fluid-filled or collapsed.

Acute Respiratory Distress Syndrome

Acute respiratory distress syndrome (ARDS) is characterized by a dysregulated inflammatory response within the lungs. The most common overall cause of ARDS is sepsis, but there are various other common causes of ARDS, including both direct and indirect pulmonary insults (**Table 45**).

In ARDS, disruption of surfactant production, vascular endothelial injury, and alveolar epithelial cell injury occur, leading to excess fluid and protein extravasation into interstitial and alveolar spaces. This results in interstitial and alveolar filling, microatelectasis, increased $\dot{V}/\dot{Q}$ mismatch, decreased lung compliance, and increases in both shunt and dead-space ventilation. Histology shows diffuse alveolar damage.

ARDS is a clinical diagnosis. The most recent guidelines defining ARDS were updated in the 2012 Berlin Definition of ARDS (**Table 46**). The Berlin definition emphasizes that ARDS occurs rapidly after an inciting event and is

TABLE 45. Common Causes of Acute Respiratory Distress Syndrome

Direct Pulmonary Injury	Indirect Pulmonary Injury
Aspiration of gastric contents	Disseminated intravascular coagulation
Fat embolism	Non-thoracic trauma
Near drowning	Pancreatitis
Pneumonia	Pulmonary reperfusion injury (following lung transplantation)
Smoke or chemical inhalation	Sepsis/septic shock
Thoracic trauma/thoracic contusion	Transfusion of blood products

TABLE 46. 2012 Berlin Definition of Acute Respiratory Distress Syndrome

The following criteria must be met:

Onset within 1 week of known ARDS insult (most cases occur within 72 hours)

Bilateral opacities on chest imaging consistent with pulmonary edema

Respiratory failure not related to cardiac failure or volume overload

Arterial PO_2/FIO_2 <300 on at least 5 cm H_2O PEEP from noninvasive or invasive mechanical ventilator

Once criteria for diagnosis are met, severity of ARDS is based on the following criteria:

Mild = Arterial PO_2/FIO_2 >200 to <300

Moderate = Arterial PO_2/FIO_2 100 to 200

Severe = Arterial PO_2/FIO_2 <100

ARDS = acute respiratory distress syndrome; PEEP = positive end-expiratory pressure.

Data from Ranieri VM, Rubenfeld GD, Thompson BT, Ferguson ND, Caldwell E, Fan E, et al; ARDS Definition Task Force. Acute respiratory distress syndrome: the Berlin definition. JAMA. 2012;307:2526-33. [PMID: 22797452] doi:10.1001/jama.2012.5669

CONT.

characterized by diffuse, bilateral, noncardiogenic pulmonary edema. Patients with ARDS are at high risk of mortality, which increases with ARDS severity. However, mortality is usually the result of the underlying disease that triggered ARDS, secondary infection, or multi-organ dysfunction rather than refractory hypoxemia.

Ventilatory Management

Most patients with ARDS are managed with invasive mechanical ventilation. PEEP and low tidal volume ventilation (LTVV) are the cornerstones of ARDS management, as they are associated with prevention of ventilator-associated lung injury. Because lungs affected by ARDS are frequently characterized by areas of noncompliant, diseased lung adjacent to lung with more normal compliance, high tidal volumes can lead to regional areas of lung overdistention and injury

(volutrauma). In 2000, the ARMA trial evaluated the benefits of LTVV (tidal volumes of 4 to 8 mL/kg) compared with higher tidal ventilation conventionally used at the time. The trial showed a significant, 11% absolute reduction in mortality with the use of LTVV. This trial also sought to prevent two other causes of ventilator-induced lung injury. Barotrauma, or lung injury due to high transpulmonary pressures, was prevented in the LTVV arm by avoiding plateau pressures greater than 30 cm H_2O. Current ARDS goals include both a tidal volume of ~6 mL/kg of predicted body weight and maintenance of the lowest possible plateau pressure. The ARMA trial also affirmed the utility of PEEP as having three benefits. First, it prevents lung injury associated with repeated opening and closing of distal airways and alveoli (atelectrauma). Second, it improves homogeneity of the lung parenchyma by reducing gross differences in regional lung compliance. Third, it improves $\dot{V}/\dot{Q}$ mismatch and shunt by maintaining alveolar recruitment. Although PEEP is now a standard part of lung protective ventilation, no definitive level of optimal PEEP has been designated for ventilation of patients with ARDS.

Despite the clear benefits of LTVV, adherence remains poor. Barriers to improved adherence include underrecognition of patients with ARDS, improper sedation of patients who do not initially tolerate LTVV, and a propensity for patients to develop respiratory acidosis from hypercapnia when using LTVV.

Ventilating patients in the prone position may reduce compression of portions of the lung behind the cardiac and mediastinal structures and improve $\dot{V}/\dot{Q}$ matching in ARDS patients. A recent large, randomized trial (PROSEVA) demonstrated improved mortality in patients with an arterial PO_2/FIO_2 ratio less than 150 who were treated with early prone positioning and LTVV. Early prone positioning for at least 12 hours a day should be considered in patients with severe ARDS.

The use of ECMO has been increasing, largely due to a single, prospective randomized controlled trial performed during the 2009 H1N1 influenza pandemic (CESAR trial). Although this trial suggested improved mortality in ARDS patients referred to a center capable of administering ECMO, many referred patients never received ECMO. This suggests that improved mortality may have simply been the result of referral to a center with improved expertise in ARDS management, not due to treatment with ECMO itself. In patients with severe, refractory hypoxemia, both prone positioning and ECMO may be considered; however, the effectiveness of prone positioning is better supported by data.

In patients with refractory hypoxemia, a recruitment maneuver—applying a high level of CPAP to open collapsed alveoli (for example, continuous pressure to 35 cm H_2O for 40 seconds)—may be considered. Although controversial, the 2017 ATS/ESICM/SCCM Guideline on Mechanical Ventilation in Adults with Acute Respiratory Distress Syndrome provides

H
CONT.

a conditional recommendation for recruitment maneuvers. The guideline cautions that recruitment maneuvers should not be used in patients with preexisting hypovolemia or shock due to a high propensity for hemodynamic deterioration during the maneuver.

Other methods to optimize ventilator management in ARDS have been suggested, including inverse ratio ventilation, esophageal pressure and driving pressure-guided titration of PEEP, and high-frequency oscillator ventilation (HFOV). None of these have demonstrated mortality benefit in ARDS. **H**

> **KEY POINT**
> • Treating patients with severe acute respiratory distress syndrome using early prone positioning and low tidal volume ventilation has demonstrated clinically important mortality benefit.

H **Nonventilatory Management**
Although mortality in ARDS has decreased, most of this is attributed to improved mechanical ventilation strategies. Mechanically ventilated patients often require sedation to improve patient-ventilator interactions and achieve LTVV goals. Data support minimizing sedation to intermittent, bolus administration when possible and daily awakening of patients who require continuous sedation. Use of nursing-led sedation protocols can decrease the overall sedation required and improve patient outcomes. Excessive sedation increases risk of delirium and nosocomial infection, increases length of ICU stays, and is a likely contributor to many long-term psychological and physical effects now associated with ARDS.

ICU patients receive volume resuscitation for a host of reasons. In ARDS, the FACCT trial suggested excessive fluid resuscitation is harmful to ARDS patients. This trial compared conservative to liberal fluid strategies based on central venous pressure and pulmonary artery occlusion pressure (a surrogate for left atrial pressure) in patients with ARDS. Although mortality did not differ between groups, patients who were treated with conservative fluid management showed improved oxygenation and decreased time on the ventilator and in the ICU. In patients who are hemodynamically stable and do not have end-organ hypoperfusion, minimizing fluid administration is warranted.

The use of paralytic agents in ARDS to improve oxygenation and decrease ventilator-induced lung injury is controversial, as there have been concerns about the potential association of paralytics with critical illness myopathy. However, a recent study in patients with ARDS who were paralyzed within 48 hours of starting mechanical ventilation found no difference in critical illness myopathy and a lower mortality. Although further study is warranted, this practice has been recommended as an early intervention strategy in patients with severe ARDS.

Other therapies, including nutritional modifications, glucocorticoid administration, macrolide antibiotics, inhaled nitric oxide, prostacyclin analogues, and stem cells or granulocyte-macrophage colony-stimulating factor have conflicting or limited evidence and are not recommended in the management of ARDS.

Heart Failure
Clinically, both acute cardiogenic pulmonary edema and ARDS present with pulmonary edema and hypoxemic respiratory failure. But unlike ARDS, cardiogenic pulmonary edema responds to aggressive diuresis and optimization of cardiac function. In patients who present with acute respiratory failure and features of ARDS, but no clear trigger, it is important to evaluate for cardiogenic causes, which include heart failure, mitral and aortic valve disease, myocardial ischemia, and arrhythmias (particularly atrial fibrillation with rapid ventricular rate). Evaluation for a cardiac cause of pulmonary edema should include an assessment for fluid overload (jugular venous distention, S_3, peripheral edema), an electrocardiogram, B-type natriuretic peptide, serial serum troponins, and an echocardiogram. **H**

> **KEY POINT**
> • Evaluation for a cardiac cause of pulmonary edema should include an assessment for fluid overload, an electrocardiogram, B-type natriuretic peptide, serial serum troponins, and an echocardiogram.

Atelectasis **H**
Atelectasis is a common postoperative complication. Inadequate postoperative analgesia or impaired respiratory mechanics following thoracic and abdominal surgeries can lead patients to adopt shallow breathing patterns or avoid airway clearance and cough. Presentation is often delayed following liberation from a ventilator and patients may be asymptomatic or present with diminished breath sounds at the lung bases, rhonchi, and labored breathing. Management of secretions with aggressive chest physiotherapy, suctioning, and incentive spirometry is recommended postoperatively. Bronchoscopy for airway mucous clearance offers no clear benefit compared to other methods of chest physiotherapy. If secretions are minimal, CPAP therapy to recruit collapsed alveoli may be considered. Use of mucolytics such as N-acetyl cysteine have not been adequately studied and are not indicated for treatment of atelectasis. **H**

> **KEY POINT**
> • Management of secretions with aggressive chest physiotherapy, suctioning, and incentive spirometry is recommended postoperatively to prevent atelectasis; bronchoscopy for airway mucous clearance offers no clear benefit compared to other methods of chest physiotherapy.

HVC

Pneumonia **H**
Pneumonia is a common cause of respiratory failure in the ICU and is the most common cause of ARDS that develops outside the hospital. In patients with an appropriate history, chest

CONT. radiograph is the standard for diagnosis. However, a negative clinical examination or chest radiograph does not necessarily rule out community-acquired pneumonia in symptomatic patients, especially in elderly individuals. Therefore, absence of typical features or focal infiltrates on chest radiograph should not preclude early antibiotic administration to individuals with an otherwise high probability of pneumonia. For further discussion of pneumonia see MKSAP 18 Infectious Disease. In patients who do not respond appropriately to antibiotics, repeat sputum cultures should be obtained, and both nonbacterial causes of infection and noninfectious causes should be considered. In addition, further evaluation with chest CT scan, bronchoscopy, or both should be considered to evaluate for complicating factors such as pleural effusion, abscess, or airway obstruction stemming from malignancy or foreign body aspiration. **H**

KEY POINT

- A negative clinical examination or chest radiograph does not necessarily rule out community-acquired pneumonia in symptomatic patients, especially in elderly individuals.

Diffuse Parenchymal Lung Disease

Acute exacerbations of diffuse parenchymal lung disease (DPLD), particularly idiopathic pulmonary fibrosis (IPF) can occur either as a complication of an inciting event, or in many cases, for unknown reason. See the Diffuse Parenchymal Lung Disease section earlier for a detailed discussion of diagnosis and management. The mortality in patients with hypoxemic respiratory failure due to an exacerbation of IPF exceeds 50%. Most patients with hypoxemic respiratory failure due to IPF are treated empirically with high dose glucocorticoids, but the data are insufficient to support dose, duration, or certainty of benefit. Outcomes following intubation and mechanical ventilation are very poor, as mortality can approach 100%. Therefore, many clinicians recommend that goals of care discussion and palliative care be involved early and other therapies, such as ECMO, only be offered as a bridge for patients eligible for lung transplantation.

Patients in the ICU with an exacerbation of IPF are frequently given broad spectrum antibiotics if infection has not been ruled out. Although the cause of most IPF exacerbations is unclear, new data suggest that aspiration and infection may play a significant role. **H**

KEY POINT

- Because outcomes following intubation and mechanical ventilation are very poor for patients with acute exacerbations of idiopathic pulmonary fibrosis, goals of care and palliative care should be discussed early, and other therapies, such as extracorporeal membrane oxygenation, should only be offered as a bridge for patients eligible for lung transplantation.

Pulmonary Embolism

Pulmonary embolism (PE) causes respiratory failure primarily through $\dot{V}/\dot{Q}$ mismatch, and to a less common extent through shunting or low mixed venous oxygen saturation. Following an acute PE, resistance to pulmonary blood flow increases, due to both thrombosis and to vasospasm of adjacent pulmonary blood vessels from activated inflammatory mediators. Subsequently, blood flow is directed to unembolized areas of normal lung, which become overperfused. If ventilation of the normal lung is insufficient to fully oxygenate blood in the overperfused vessels, hypoxemia ensues. In addition, regional atelectasis is common following PE and lung infarction. Chest radiograph or chest CT scan may demonstrate peripheral, ground-glass, wedge-shaped opacities (Hampton hump sign) signifying the presence of infarcted lung and surrounding atelectasis. Blood flow through atelectatic lung can result in shunt and hypoxemia.

Pulmonary emboli can also cause strain on the right ventricle (RV) if the PE is sufficiently large. In these cases, cardiac output may be impaired. Low cardiac output leads to reduced mixed venous oxygen saturations, especially when metabolic demands exceed cardiac capacity. If this occurs in conjunction with $\dot{V}/\dot{Q}$ mismatch and shunt, blood cannot fully saturate with oxygen before leaving the alveolar capillaries. This adds to hypoxemia and subsequent respiratory failure.

Although most patients with hypoxemia following PE can be managed with supplemental oxygen alone, some patients require intubation and positive pressure ventilation.

Mechanical ventilation produces several physiologic effects that need to be considered in the patient with PE and RV dysfunction. Increased pleural pressure from mechanical ventilation can cause decreased venous return and result in low RV preload. Additionally, overdistention of alveoli increases RV afterload. These effects can lead to further RV dysfunction and hemodynamic instability. Although there is no absolute contraindication to mechanical ventilation in patients with underlying PE, the risks and benefits should be weighed carefully. In patients with hemodynamic collapse, treatment with thrombolytics is associated with decreased mortality, and the vast majority of patients demonstrate improvement in clinical and echocardiographic parameters following thrombolytic administration.

Thrombolytics carry a significant side effect profile, including an up to 2% risk of intracranial hemorrhage, but this should be considered relative to the life-threatening risk of massive PE leading to hemodynamic collapse. In patients with contraindications to thrombolysis, and in those in whom thrombolysis has failed to improve the hemodynamic status, surgical embolectomy is recommended if resources are available. For further discussion of PE, see MKSAP 18 Hematology and Oncology.

Hypercapnic (Ventilatory) Respiratory Failure

Hypercapnic, or ventilatory, respiratory failure occurs when alveolar ventilation is inadequate to clear the CO_2 produced by cellular metabolism, and the level of CO_2 increases in the blood. Most commonly, hypercapnia reflects alveolar hypoventilation, but can also result from increased metabolic load (fever, increased work of breathing) that is not matched by an increase in alveolar ventilation. Alveolar hypoventilation occurs when the patient is unable to ventilate because of decreased respiratory drive, decreased tidal volume (V_T), or increased volume of dead space (V_D) relative to the overall tidal volume (V_D/V_T) (**Table 47**).

Clinical features of acute hypercapnic respiratory failure are variable and nonspecific. Symptoms may include somnolence and myoclonic jerks in the setting of CO_2 narcosis. In some cases, increased work of breathing may precede the development of acute hypercapnic respiratory failure. Underlying chest wall deformity, neurologic weakness, or polycythemia should also prompt evaluation for hypercapnia in the setting of respiratory failure.

Patients presenting with acute hypercapnic respiratory failure frequently have coexisting hypoxemia. Administration of supplemental oxygen may improve the hypoxemia, but will not necessarily improve hypercapnia. All patients who are suspected of acute hypercapnic respiratory failure should have

arterial blood gas analysis even if hypoxemia resolves with oxygen administration (**Table 48**). The pH helps to determine the acuity and severity of respiratory failure. In chronic hypercapnia, pH changes are less marked due to metabolic compensation resulting in increased serum bicarbonate levels. Management of an elevated arterial P_{CO_2} depends on the clinical situation and the resultant pH. For instance, a moderately elevated arterial P_{CO_2} may represent the baseline in patients with COPD; however, in an asthmatic, the development of elevated arterial P_{CO_2} may indicate imminent respiratory failure requiring emergent intubation.

KEY POINT

- All patients who are suspected of acute hypercapnic respiratory failure should have arterial blood gas analysis even if hypoxemia resolves with oxygen administration.

Management of Hypercapnic Respiratory Failure
Decreased Respiratory Drive

Decreased respiratory drive leads to diminished alveolar CO_2 clearance and hypercapnia. Patients often present with somnolence and difficulty protecting their airway. Noninvasive positive pressure ventilation (NIPPV) should be considered if the patient can protect his or her airway. This improves minute ventilation and gas exchange. If airway protection is compromised, or if there is either significant respiratory acidosis (generally pH less than 7.25) or hemodynamic instability, intubation and mechanical ventilation are indicated. See MKSAP 18 Nephrology for further discussion of respiratory acidosis.

Drug Overdose

Sedating drugs (illicit or prescribed), anesthetics, and severe alcohol intoxication can lead to depressed central respiratory drive. In cases of pharmacologic overdose, contact with a local poison control center is helpful to determine the most appropriate care of the patient. If opiate overdose is suspected, rapid reversal with naloxone is safe, effective, and may prevent the need for intubation. The benefits of flumazenil for patients with benzodiazepine overdose are less certain. Flumazenil carries the risk of precipitating withdrawal seizures in chronic users and is a short-acting agent, so several administrations

TABLE 47. Causes of Acute Hypercapnic Respiratory Failure

Decreased Respiratory Drive	Decreased V_T or Increased V_D/V_T
Anesthesia	Amyotrophic lateral sclerosis
Central apnea	Ankylosing spondylitis
Obesity hypoventilation syndrome	Asthma exacerbation
Drugs (such as opioids, benzodiazepines, ethanol)	Botulism
	Bronchiectasis flare (including cystic fibrosis)
Encephalitis	COPD exacerbation
Hypothermia	Critical illness myopathy
Hypothyroidism	Electrolyte disorder (low magnesium, low phosphate)
Meningitis	Guillain-Barré syndrome
Stroke	Multiple rib fractures (flail chest)
	Myasthenia gravis
	Myositis (such as polymyositis, dermatomyositis)
	Polio
	Spinal or phrenic nerve injury
	Thoracic cage deformity (kyphoscoliosis)

V_T = tidal volume; V_D = volume of dead space.

TABLE 48. Features of Acute and Chronic Hypercapnia

	Acute Hypercapnia	Chronic Hypercapnia
pH	<7.35	~7.35-7.40
Arterial P_{CO_2}	>45 mm Hg (6.0 kPa)	>45 mm Hg (6.0 kPa)
Bicarbonate concentration [HCO_3]	22-26 mEq/L (22-26 mmol/L)	>26 mEq/L (26 mmol/L)
Expected metabolic compensation	1.0 mEq/L ↑ [HCO_3] for each 10 mm Hg (1.3 kPa) ↑ in arterial P_{CO_2}	3.5 mEq/L ↑ [HCO_3] for each 10 mm Hg (1.3 kPa) ↑ arterial P_{CO_2}

may be required to keep respiratory failure from recurring, especially if long-acting benzodiazepines were ingested.

Obesity Hypoventilation Syndrome

Obesity hypoventilation syndrome (OHS) is characterized by the presence of obesity, sleep-disordered breathing, and persistent daytime hypercapnia (arterial P_{CO_2} greater than 45 mm Hg [5.9 kPa]). Hypercapnia stems from low tidal volumes and from inappropriate central respiratory response to hypoxemia and elevated P_{CO_2} levels. Acute hypercapnic respiratory failure due to OHS should be a diagnosis of exclusion. Positive pressure ventilation is the key to improving hypercapnia in patients with OHS.

NIPPV is reasonable in patients who can protect their airway, but high levels of positive pressure are often needed because of poor chest wall compliance from obesity, diminished lung compliance from atelectasis, and cephalad displacement of the diaphragm from central adiposity. If NIPPV is used, arterial blood gases should be monitored to ensure clinical improvement. If patients are not improving, early intubation is warranted. Respiratory stimulants, such as acetazolamide, a progestin, and theophylline offer a compelling theoretical benefit to patients with chronic hypercapnia or depressed respiratory drive, but have limited data supporting their use in this setting. **H**

KEY POINT

- Acute hypercapnic respiratory failure due to obesity hyperventilation syndrome is a diagnosis of exclusion; if airway protection is compromised, or there is significant respiratory acidosis or hemodynamic instability, intubation and mechanical ventilation are indicated.

Decreased Tidal Volume and Increased Dead Space
Neuromuscular Weakness

The diaphragm is the main muscle responsible for inspiration and accounts for more than two-thirds of the ventilatory work in humans. The C3-C5 cervical nerve roots form the phrenic nerves, which directly innervate the diaphragm. Patients with diaphragmatic weakness develop orthopnea, shallow breathing, and often paradoxical movement of the chest wall and abdomen. Although exhalation is generally a passive process, intercostal and abdominal wall muscles are required for coughing. Lower cervical and upper thoracic nerve roots supply the intercostal and abdominal wall muscles. Weak cough, difficulty managing secretions, or a change in voice, which can become softer or more "breathy," may point to weakness in these areas.

Assessment of cranial nerves and respiratory muscle function is important in a patient with suspected neurologic disease. Specific components of pulmonary function testing can be helpful (**Table 49**) but are effort-dependent, and facial or postural weakness can complicate accurate measurement.

Guillain-Barré syndrome and myasthenic crisis are the most common causes of acute neurologic respiratory failure in

TABLE 49. Pulmonary Function Value Suggestive of Neuromuscular Weakness

Function	Value
FVC	>20% decrement in supine position compared with upright position
Maximal inspiratory pressure (MIP)	Unable to achieve −30 cm H_2O
Maximal expiratory pressure (MEP)	Unable to achieve +40 cm H_2O

the ICU. Infection can precipitate myasthenic crisis or Guillain-Barré syndrome. Myasthenic crisis can occur following medication changes or significant stressors.

Patients with Guillain-Barré syndrome generally present with rapid onset of ascending, symmetric paralysis and areflexia occurring over the course of 2 to 4 weeks. Dysautonomia is common and can cause hemodynamic instability or cardiac arrhythmias. In myasthenic crisis, the hallmark feature is muscle fatigability. Diplopia, ptosis, dysarthria, limb weakness, and weak cough are common. See MKSAP 18 Neurology for further discussion of Guillain-Barré syndrome and myasthenic crisis.

In the 25% of patients with Guillain-Barré syndrome who develop respiratory failure, intubation is necessary because respiratory function can take days to weeks to recover. In myasthenic crisis, early NIPPV may prevent the need for intubation. Therapy for both diseases includes plasma exchange or intravenous immune globulin. Glucocorticoids have no benefit in Guillain-Barré syndrome, but are indicated in addition to cholinesterase inhibitors in myasthenic crisis.

Acute spinal cord injuries at or above the C5 level invariably require mechanical ventilation. In some cases (complete spinal cord injury below C3 or incomplete injury above C3), recovery of independent respiratory function can occur. However, atelectasis, aspiration pneumonia, and pulmonary emboli are common and can lead to recurrent acute hypercapnic respiratory failure. Aggressive chest physiotherapy and use of mechanical cough assist devices are helpful and may lower the risk of these events. **H**

KEY POINTS

- Guillain-Barré syndrome and myasthenic crisis are the most common causes of acute neurologic respiratory failure in the ICU.

- Evaluation of maximum inspiratory and expiratory pressures and positional changes in vital capacity are helpful in assessing neuromuscular weakness as a cause of hypercapnic respiratory failure.

Restrictive Chest Wall Disease

Restrictive disease from disorders affecting the pulmonary parenchyma (such as the various causes of diffuse parenchymal lung disease primarily leads to hypoxemia without hypercapnia. Acute hypercapnic respiratory failure is more common in patients with extrapulmonary chest wall restriction (pectus deformity, scoliosis, kyphosis), which causes compromised respiratory mechanics. Ascites and severe bowel distention can also compromise respiratory mechanics by exerting a significant cephalad force on the diaphragm. Commonly, extrapulmonary chest wall restriction causes poor ventilatory reserve without overt respiratory failure. However, acute insults such as infection or sedating medications can upset this delicate balance and precipitate hypercapnic respiratory failure. NIPPV and invasive positive pressure mechanical ventilation are both appropriate while the precipitating condition is managed. In patients with thoracic cage deformity, NIPPV in the outpatient setting is frequently beneficial. Improved V_T, especially during sleep when respiratory drive and minute ventilation decrease, can reduce the incidence of acute hypercapnic respiratory failure and improve patient function and quality of life.

Obstructive Lung Diseases (Asthma and COPD)

Abnormal mechanical properties of the airways and the lung parenchyma cause both static and dynamic hyperinflation. A decrease in the lung's elastic recoil (as seen in emphysema) results in increased total lung capacity and is one of the factors leading to an increase in functional residual capacity (lung volume after a normal, not forced, exhalation). In addition, the ability to exhale is dependent on the elastic recoil of the lung, the degree of airflow obstruction (associated with structural changes, inflammation, increases in cholinergic tone, and mucous plugging), and the rate of breathing.

The degree of airflow obstruction and the respiration rate can each vary and cause greater air trapping during periods of exertion and exacerbation of disease, leading to increased lung volumes at the end of exhalation. This complication of airflow obstruction and insufficient time for exhalation is called dynamic hyperinflation and can result in intrathoracic pressure remaining positive at the end of exhalation, a phenomenon called auto-PEEP. Dynamic hyperinflation, auto-PEEP, and decreased elastic recoil of the lung all contribute to disordered lung mechanics, increased work of breathing, and respiratory muscle fatigue. Auto-PEEP may also decrease venous return and contribute to hemodynamic instability in patients receiving mechanical ventilation who are not given sufficient time for exhalation.

At the time of a COPD exacerbation, patients may present with signs of increased respiratory work. They may also have findings related to the presence of hypercapnia, such as altered sensorium or somnolence. See Airways Disease for more detailed information about management of COPD exacerbations.

In patients with COPD, excessive oxygen can increase $\dot{V}/\dot{Q}$ mismatch by disrupting compensatory vasoconstriction in poorly ventilated regions of lung, potentially leading to further elevation in P_{CO_2}. Therefore, in patients with COPD

exacerbation, oxygen therapy should be titrated to 88% to 92% oxyhemoglobin saturation. In patients with hypercapnic respiratory failure due to COPD exacerbation, NIPPV is preferred as the initial means to reduce P_{CO_2}. If patients cannot protect their airway, are hemodynamically unstable, or do not improve on NIPPV, intubation and mechanical ventilation are necessary. Strategies for mechanical ventilation in COPD include assuring sufficient expiratory time during the respiratory cycle to minimize auto-PEEP.

In patients with asthma, upright posture, inability to speak in full sentences, flaring of the nares, and contraction of the sternocleidomastoid muscles during inspiration, are signs of increased respiratory work and may herald respiratory failure. Blood gases usually demonstrate respiratory alkalosis due to rapid, shallow breathing patterns. Therefore, the presence of a normal or elevated arterial P_{CO_2} may signal impending respiratory failure. Oxygen should be given to maintain a hemoglobin saturation of 90% to 95%. Hypoxemia can result from $\dot{V}/\dot{Q}$ mismatch, but should correct with oxygen. If oxygen saturation does not readily correct, other factors should be considered, including pneumonia, pneumothorax, or pulmonary embolism.

In cases of severe asthma exacerbation, magnesium sulfate may be used in addition to standard therapies to promote further bronchodilation. Adjunctive therapies, including anesthetics with bronchodilator properties (ketamine, isoflurane, sevoflurane), inhalation of a helium-oxygen mixture, mucolytics, and leukotriene receptor antagonists are not recommended because of lack of clear efficacy.

There is little objective evidence to support use of NIPPV in management of asthma exacerbations. Therefore, in asthmatic patients with respiratory failure, intubation is recommended. In these patients, efforts should be directed at maximizing expiratory time, as this improves dynamic hyperinflation and reduces auto-PEEP. The most effective way to do this is to minimize the patient's respiration rate. Doing so often requires sedation or paralytics and can lower a patient's overall minute ventilation. Because this may increase arterial P_{CO_2}, arterial blood gas analysis should be performed frequently in these patients.

KEY POINTS

- Patients with hypercapnic respiratory failure and COPD exacerbation benefit from NIPPV provided they can protect their airway and are hemodynamically stable.

- In asthmatic patients with respiratory failure, intubation and mechanical evaluation are recommended rather than NIPPV.

- Adjunctive therapies for severe asthma exacerbation, including anesthetics with bronchodilator properties (ketamine, isoflurane, sevoflurane), inhalation of a helium-oxygen mixture, mucolytics, and leukotriene receptor antagonists are not recommended because of lack of clear efficacy.

HVC

Shock

Shock occurs when systemic tissue perfusion is inadequate. In early states of tissue hypoperfusion, aerobic metabolism is supplanted by anaerobic metabolism and tissue injury is reversible. As compensatory mechanisms fail, sustained organ hypoperfusion can lead to cellular dysfunction and death. There are three primary mechanisms of shock: decreased circulating volume (hypovolemic), decreased cardiac output (cardiogenic), and inappropriate vasodilation (distributive).

Low blood pressure alone should not be considered diagnostic of end-organ hypoperfusion. Instead, blood pressure should be considered in the context of other physical examination findings that may suggest end-organ hypoperfusion (**Table 50**), as well as other general considerations for early shock assessment (**Figure 20**).

Treatment of a patient in shock is predicated on distinguishing the type of shock present and directing treatment toward correcting the root cause of the shock state (**Table 51**). Although many tools are available to aid in shock assessment and management, the use of bedside echocardiography has increased significantly during the last 10 years. Echocardiography can provide useful data regarding cardiac function and cardiac response to treatment. Other tools such as pulmonary artery catheters or those that predict response to volume replacement such as pulse pressure or stroke volume variation can also be considered; however, these technologies often carry higher risk due to their invasive nature, and the assessment of pulse pressure and stroke volume have procedural limitations (mechanical ventilation, receiving 8 mL/kg or greater of tidal volume, need for sinus rhythm, not triggering the ventilator) that may make them impractical. Pulmonary artery catheters have lost favorability in recent years because several large studies and meta-analyses that suggest no benefit, and in some cases increased risk to patients when used to guide therapy. Technologies that employ pulse contour, pulse pressure, or stroke volume variation assessment should be used with caution as well, given a broad array of clinical scenarios that can skew results and limited data to support their benefit in guiding therapy. **H**

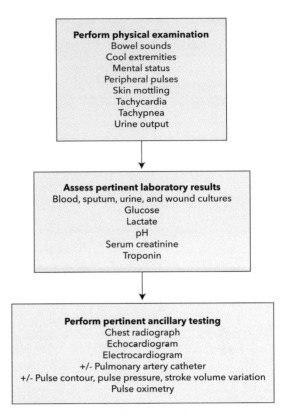

FIGURE 20. Early assessment of suspected shock.

KEY POINTS

- Treatment of a patient in shock is predicated on distinguishing the type of shock present and directed toward the root cause of the shock state.

- Pulmonary artery catheters have lost favorability in recent years because several large studies and meta-analyses that suggest no benefit, and in some cases increased risk to patients when used to guide therapy.

HVC

Distributive Shock

In distributive shock, the blood volume is generally normal, but a state of "relative" hypovolemia occurs from excessive vasodilation and microvascular dysfunction. This causes blood to bypass vital capillary beds, leading to tissue hypoxia. Cardiac output is often increased, but still cannot maintain a pressure sufficient for normal tissue perfusion. Initial treatment of distributive shock should focus on fluid resuscitation. Several studies have compared the effectiveness of crystalloid versus colloid administration, with no clear evidence that one is better than the other. Given the relative expense of colloids, crystalloid administration is generally preferred and recommended by guidelines. Vasopressor support is warranted if fluid administration alone is insufficient to support tissue perfusion. The selection of a vasopressor should be based on the patient's comorbidities and underlying cause of shock (see Table 39). **H**

TABLE 50. Common Clinical Findings in Patients with Shock
Altered mentation
Hypotension (SBP < 90 mm Hg) or 30 mm Hg drop in SBP from baseline
Mottled skin
Tachycardia (heart rate >100/min)
Tachypnea (respiration rate >25/min)
Urine output <0.5 mL/kg/h
Weak or absent peripheral pulses
Elevated serum lactate (>3 mEq/L [3 mmol/L])
SBP = systolic blood pressure.

TABLE 51. Selected Causes of Shock

Distributive
Anaphylaxis
Sepsis
Spinal injury (usually above T4 level)
Drugs (peripheral vasodilators, nitrates)
Hypovolemic
Acute blood loss (trauma, GI bleeding, surgery, uterine bleeding, obstetrical, retroperitoneal bleeding, aortic rupture)
Crush injury, metabolic rhabdomyolysis
Cutaneous losses (burns, toxic epidermal necrolysis, erythroderma, excessive sweating)
Drugs (diuretics, laxatives)
GI losses (vomiting/diarrhea)
Kidney losses (diabetic ketoacidosis, hyperglycemic hyperosmolar syndrome, adrenal insufficiency, post-ATN osmotic diuresis)
Cardiogenic (Including Noncardiac Causes of Decreased Cardiac Output)
Abdominal compartment syndrome
Arrhythmia (tachycardia, bradycardia)
Atrial myxoma
Heart failure
Left ventricular infarction, right ventricular infarction
Pericardial tamponade, constrictive pericarditis
Pulmonary embolism
Tension pneumothorax, severe dynamic hyperinflation (for example, excessive PEEP)
Valvular heart disease (severe insufficiency, valve or chordae rupture, critical stenosis)
Ventricular septal rupture, free ventricular wall rupture

ATN = acute tubular necrosis; GI = gastrointestinal; PEEP = positive end-expiratory pressure; T4 = fourth thoracic vertebra.

KEY POINT

HVC

- Several studies have compared the effectiveness of crystalloid versus colloid administration for treatment of distributive shock, with no clear evidence that one is better than the other; given the relative expense of colloids, crystalloid administration is generally preferred and recommended by guidelines.

Hypovolemic Shock

Hypovolemic shock occurs when decreased intravascular blood volume causes decreased preload, decreased ventricular filling, and diminished stroke volume. Initially, tachycardia and peripheral vasoconstriction help to preserve perfusion of vital organs but cannot compensate in the setting of severe hypovolemia. Treatment of hypovolemic shock includes aggressive volume or blood product replacement and, if

possible, control of bleeding. Patients with hemorrhage may initially receive intravenous fluids to maintain hemodynamic stability, but ultimately need erythrocyte transfusion to prevent tissue ischemia. In stable ICU patients, hemoglobin levels should be maintained at about 7 g/dL (70 g/L); however, different thresholds and hemoglobin levels may trigger transfusion in actively bleeding patients who are in shock. Higher values may be necessary in patients with underlying cardiovascular disease. In patients with severe trauma, massive blood replacement requirements, and coagulopathy, evidence supports early resuscitation with a 1:1:1 ratio of erythrocytes, platelets, and fresh frozen plasma.

Cardiogenic Shock

Cardiogenic shock occurs when a primary cardiac insult causes decreased cardiac output. This can result from any combination of obstructed filling or emptying of the ventricles, high or low heart rates, and decreased ejection fraction. It is essential to promptly identify the cause of cardiogenic shock to ensure appropriate medical therapy, surgical therapy, or both. In addition to a physical examination, evaluation should include laboratory testing for myocardial ischemia and heart failure, chest radiograph, electrocardiogram, and echocardiogram. In patients presenting with severe cardiogenic shock, additional supportive measures may include short-term mechanical support to allow a bridge toward definitive therapy. These include ECMO, intraaortic balloon pump, temporary pacemaker, and left or right ventricular assist device. However, recent technological advances have allowed many of these devices to be used for longer durations and even as destination therapy.

Sepsis
Definition, Pathophysiology, and Clinical Presentation of Sepsis

The Third International Definitions for Sepsis and Septic Shock (Sepsis-3) were published in 2016 and reflect evolving understanding of sepsis. Sepsis-3 defines sepsis as life-threatening organ dysfunction caused by a dysregulated host response to infection. Septic shock is defined as a subset of sepsis in which profound circulatory, cellular, and metabolic abnormalities are associated with a greater risk of mortality than with sepsis alone. The previous definition, combining known or suspected infection and systemic inflammatory response syndrome criteria, which can be appropriate (not necessarily dysregulated) responses to infection, is neither sensitive nor specific enough to diagnose sepsis. The terms *severe sepsis* and *septicemia* should no longer be used.

Infections giving rise to sepsis can include any agent and involve any organ, and need not be disseminated. The pathophysiology of sepsis is complex and involves dysfunction at many levels, from subcellular mitochondrial dysfunction to failure of entire organ systems. Loss of regulation of the body's finely balanced proinflammatory and antiinflammatory mediators and unregulated coagulation in the microvasculature are characteristic of the syndrome, although these features are difficult to assess clinically.

Operationally, sepsis can be identified whenever infection is known or suspected and clinical criteria defining organ dysfunction are met. The recommended criteria to assess organ dysfunction are included in the Sequential Organ Failure Assessment (SOFA) score, which assigns a value of 0-4 for each of six organ systems assessed: respiratory, coagulation, hepatic, cardiovascular, central nervous, and kidney, with increasing scores for more severe dysfunction (online SOFA score calculators are available: http://clincalc.com/IcuMortality/SOFA.aspx; https://www.mdcalc.com/sequential-organ-failure-assessment-sofa-score). An initial SOFA score of 2 or greater or an increase in SOFA score of 2 or more correlates with acute organ dysfunction and predicts hospital mortality of greater than 10%. The SOFA score should be used to assess patients in the ICU.

In the pre-ICU arena, Sepsis-3 guidelines recommend the use of the quick SOFA (qSOFA) score, a simplified clinical scoring system that includes only three criteria: respiration rate of 22/min or greater, altered mentation, and systolic blood pressure 100 mm Hg or less (**Table 52**). A qSOFA score of 2 or greater in the setting of known or suspected infection predicts increased mortality and should prompt evaluation for resuscitation and consideration of ICU admission. Failure to meet two or more qSOFA criteria should not be construed as ruling out sepsis, and investigation or treatment of infection should be pursued as deemed necessary by the responsible physicians. Although there is no definitive test for sepsis, the qSOFA score (specific but not sensitive) and the systemic inflammatory response syndrome (SIRS) criteria (sensitive but not specific) are complementary and can be used together to inform clinical judgment when diagnosing sepsis.

The criteria for diagnosing septic shock include hypotension requiring pressors to maintain a mean arterial pressure of greater than 65 mm Hg and serum lactate level of greater than 2 mEq/L (2 mmol/L) after adequate volume resuscitation. Patients who meet these criteria have a 40% or greater risk of in-hospital mortality. **H**

TABLE 52.	qSOFA Score	
Criterion	**Value**	**qSOFA Points**
Respiration rate	>22/min	1
Systolic blood pressure	<100 mm Hg	1
Mental status	Altered from baseline	1
qSOFA score	**Predicted mortality**	
0	<1%	
1	2-3%	
≥2	≥10%	
qSOFA = quick sequential organ failure assessment.		

KEY POINTS

- Sepsis is defined as life-threatening organ dysfunction caused by a dysregulated host response to infection.

- Septic shock is defined as a subset of sepsis in which profound circulatory, cellular, and metabolic abnormalities are associated with a greater risk of mortality than with sepsis alone.

Epidemiology of Sepsis

The epidemiology of sepsis is difficult to judge accurately because of its evolving definition, challenges with clinical recognition of the syndrome, and lack of standardized reporting. However, it is possible to estimate its incidence and clinical and economic effects. There are disparities in sepsis rates among different demographic groups. For example, sepsis is more common among black men than other racial groups or women. Sepsis is also more common among elderly patients, with incidence increasing with each year after the age of 65. Mortality from sepsis is high. A patient who is septic has a mortality rate 4 or more times greater for the same underlying condition and comorbidities without sepsis. Mortality increases by roughly 15% for each sepsis-related organ system failure.

Management of Sepsis

Early diagnosis and timely treatment of sepsis are important to improve survival. In settings where sepsis is suspected, cultures and other investigations to identify infection, as well as the use of diagnostic instruments like the SOFA and qSOFA scoring tools to identify organ dysfunction, are helpful. Once sepsis is diagnosed, the two main pillars of management are: 1) supporting organ perfusion and function; and 2) controlling the infection. Various other adjunctive therapies may also affect survival. **H**

KEY POINT

- The two main pillars of sepsis management are: 1) supporting organ perfusion and function; and 2) controlling the infection.

Initial Resuscitation

Sepsis can have serious hemodynamics effects, with decreased preload (due to capillary leak), impaired cardiac contractility, and decreased vascular tone. Patients may present in shock, sometimes with profound hypotension requiring large volume resuscitation with intravenous fluids and often vasopressor therapy.

The fourth iteration of the Surviving Sepsis Guidelines, published in 2016, recommends early and aggressive fluid resuscitation for patients with hypoperfusion due to sepsis, with an initial bolus of 30 mL/kg of body weight. Additional fluids may be needed, and physiologic markers such as mean arterial pressure, pulse pressure variation, change in serum lactate level, bedside echocardiographic assessment of inferior vena cava filling, or other techniques are used as indicators of adequate fluid resuscitation. Although experts agree that aggressive fluid resuscitation is essential, the adequacy of fluid resuscitation requires clinical judgment in conjunction with the available data.

Fluid resuscitation should be with crystalloid, using normal saline or a balanced crystalloid solution. A balanced crystalloid solution has an electrolyte composition similar to plasma with the addition of a buffer, such as lactate (for example, Ringer's lactate solution). Data are emerging that suggest a balanced crystalloid solution may be associated with improved outcomes compared to normal saline, particularly in patients receiving a large volume of fluid, but current guidelines recommend either. There is weak evidence suggesting benefit from the use of albumin in patients requiring large volume resuscitation; however, sepsis guidelines offer this as a consideration rather than a recommendation. **H**

KEY POINT

- Early and aggressive fluid resuscitation for patients with hypoperfusion due to sepsis begins with an initial bolus of 30 mL/kg body weight of normal saline or a balanced crystalloid solution.

Antibiotic Therapy

Early administration of antibiotic therapy is crucial in treating sepsis. Broad spectrum antibiotics should be given within the first hour of suspected sepsis, and the regimen adjusted based on culture results. A delay in the first dose of antibiotic therapy increases sepsis mortality. The Surviving Sepsis Guidelines recommend empiric combination therapy for the initial management of septic shock, or when broad empiric coverage is needed for initial management of sepsis, bacteremia, or both. However, they recommend against combination therapy for the routine or ongoing treatment of sepsis and bacteremia without shock, even in the setting of neutropenia. The guidelines define combination therapy as the use of two different classes of antibiotics for a single putative pathogen expected to be sensitive to both, for purposes of accelerating pathogen clearance. The term is not used when the purpose of a multidrug strategy is to strictly broaden the range of antimicrobial activity. Antibiotic therapy should usually be continued for 7 to 10 days, depending on the clinical situation, and continually reassessed for efficacy and possible deescalation.

Procalcitonin, a serum marker for bacterial infection, should be measured when the probability of infection is estimated to be low. If the procalcitonin level is low, bacterial infection is unlikely and antibiotic therapy may not be warranted. There is no role for procalcitonin measurement in sepsis likely due to infection.

Prompt identification and control of any potential source of infection is essential in the management of sepsis. Examples include drainage of abscesses and removal of possibly infected intravenous catheters (once alternative intravenous access has

been established). One exception is necrotizing pancreatitis, for which definitive resection should be delayed until the extent of necrosis is clear. **H**

KEY POINTS

- Antibiotic therapy for patients with sepsis should usually be continued for 7 to 10 days, depending on the clinical situation, and continually reassessed for efficacy and for possible deescalation.

- Procalcitonin, a serum marker for infection, should be measured when the probability of infection is estimated to be low.

- There is no role for procalcitonin measurement in sepsis **HVC** likely due to infection.

- Prompt identification and control of any potential source of infection is essential in the management of sepsis.

Adjunctive Therapies

Norepinephrine is the vasopressor of choice for shock due to **H** sepsis. Vasopressin at a fixed dose of 0.03 or 0.04 units per minute can be added to norepinephrine to further raise blood pressure or reduce the dose of norepinephrine. Vasopressin should generally not be used in cardiogenic or hypovolemic shock and is not recommended as a first pressor agent in septic shock (see Table 39). If possible, all patients receiving vasopressor therapy should have an arterial catheter for continuous blood pressure monitoring.

The use of glucocorticoids in the setting of sepsis is suggested to achieve hemodynamic stability when not achieved using intravenous fluids and vasopressor therapies. They have no role in sepsis without shock. If used, glucocorticoids can be added at a dose of not more than 200 mg daily of hydrocortisone (usually 50 mg intravenously every 6 hours). An adrenocorticotropic hormone stimulation test is not recommended. **H**

KEY POINTS

- Norepinephrine is the vasopressor of choice in treatment of shock due to sepsis; vasopressin can be added to further raise the blood pressure or reduce the dose of norepinephrine.

- The use of glucocorticoids in the setting of sepsis is sug- **HVC** gested if adequate fluid resuscitation and vasopressor therapy are unable to restore hemodynamic stability; there is no role for glucocorticoids in sepsis without shock.

Specific Critical Care Topics **H**
Anaphylaxis

Anaphylaxis is a severe reaction caused by acute mediator release into the circulation, usually triggered by IgE-linked

CONT. immunological responses to specific foods, medications, insect venom, latex, or other antigens, but sometimes occurring without an allergic trigger. The mediator release results in various clinical manifestations including pruritus, hypotension, and tissue swelling (known as angioedema) caused by capillary leak from widespread inflammatory mediator release (**Table 53**). Onset of symptoms may be immediate after antigen exposure or delayed, sometimes for hours or even days, although more rapid onset usually signals a more severe reaction. This capillary leak can result in distributive shock with many of the same features as septic shock. Angioedema can be life-threatening when it compromises the airway.

Initial treatment is with epinephrine, which may be administered intramuscularly or intravenously. Adjunctive therapy with antihistamine medications may be used to relieve symptoms of pruritus and rash. Although commonly administered, evidence that glucocorticoids are useful in the treatment of anaphylaxis is sparse. Sometimes epinephrine must be given many times or continuously to achieve clinical stability. Patients should be given supplemental oxygen and watched closely for signs of airway compromise, which may require intubation to maintain airway patency. Patients often require fluid resuscitation, with or without vasopressor therapy. Removal of the precipitating antigen is also important if exposure is ongoing. Fortunately, anaphylaxis is rarely fatal but successful management requires early recognition and prompt attention to supportive and disease-reversing therapies, especially when shock or airway compromise is present.

Angioedema can occur without allergic stimulus (bradykinin-mediated), sometimes in response to medications (notably ACE inhibitors, even after long-term use), and sometimes for no identifiable reason. Nonallergic angioedema usually has slower onset and is not associated with urticaria, pruritus, or hypotension, but the tissue swelling can be clinically significant, especially in the airway, and may require intubation. Recurrent angioedema can be hereditary or acquired, as in C1 inhibitor deficiency. As in other forms of angioedema, treatment is supportive, sometimes with additional measures to control abnormal bradykinin, complement activation, or both. For more detail on angioedema see MKSAP 18 Dermatology.

KEY POINT

- Initial treatment of anaphylaxis is with epinephrine, which may be administered intramuscularly or intravenously.

Hypertensive Emergencies

Hypertensive emergency refers to elevated blood pressure significantly above the normal range causing acute organ damage or dysfunction. The end-organ damage is the defining characteristic, particularly clinical dysfunction of the central nervous system (ischemic or hemorrhagic stroke, encephalopathy), the renal system (acute kidney injury), or the cardiovascular system (acute myocardial infarction, aortic dissection, acute heart failure). These effects often occur at blood pressures above 180/120 mm Hg, but there is no specific pressure threshold above which the syndrome is defined. When blood pressure is significantly elevated without evidence of end-organ damage, this is often labeled hypertensive urgency.

Hypertensive emergency should be treated by rapidly lowering the blood pressure, usually using intravenous short-acting agents in the ICU setting (**Table 54** and **Table 55**). The 2017 blood pressure guidelines from the American College of Cardiology/American Heart Association and nine other organizations recommend that for adults with a compelling condition (such as aortic dissection, severe preeclampsia or eclampsia, or pheochromocytoma crisis), systolic blood pressure (SBP) should be reduced to less than 140 mm Hg during the first hour and to less than 120 mm Hg in aortic dissection. For adults without a compelling condition, SBP should be reduced by no more than 25% within the first hour; then, if stable, to 160/100 mm Hg within the next 2 to 6 hours; and then cautiously to normal during the following 24 to 48 hours. See MKSAP 18 Neurology for further discussion of the treatment of hypertension associated with ischemic stroke and intracerebral hemorrhage.

TABLE 53.	Organ System Involvement in Anaphylaxis		
Organ System	**Symptoms**	**Signs**	**Patients with Organ Involved**
Skin and mucosa	Pruritus of skin, oropharynx, genitals, palms, soles	Flushing, urticaria, morbilliform rash, angioedema	85%
Respiratory	Dyspnea, chest and throat tightness, stridor, cough, hoarseness, sneezing, rhinorrhea	Wheeze, stridor, respiratory distress	70%
Cardiovascular	Lightheadedness, chest pain, palpitations	Hypotension, tachycardia > bradycardia	45%
Gastrointestinal	Pain, nausea, vomiting, diarrhea		45%
Neurologic	Anxiety, headache	Encephalopathy	15%

TABLE 54. Intravenous Antihypertensive Drugs for Treatment of Hypertensive Emergencies without a Compelling Comorbidity

Class	Examples	Comments
Dihydropyridine calcium channel blockers	Nicardipine	Nicardipine: Contraindicated in patients with severe aortic stenosis
	Clevidipine	Clevidipine: Contraindicated in patients with soy allergy, egg allergy, hyperlipidemia, lipoid nephrosis, and acute pancreatitis
Vasodilator-nitric oxide dependent	Sodium nitroprusside	Sodium nitroprusside: Intraarterial blood pressure monitoring recommended. Tachyphylaxis common with prolonged use. Irreversible cyanide toxicity possible with prolonged use
	Nitroglycerin	Nitroglycerin: Use only for patients with acute coronary syndrome or acute pulmonary edema; avoid in patients with right ventricular infarction and those taking PDE-5 inhibitors
Vasodilator-direct	Hydralazine	Not first-line drug due to unpredictable response and long duration of action
Adrenergic blocker-β_1 selective	Esmolol	Contraindicated with concurrent β-blocker therapy, bradycardia, pulmonary edema, severe HF
Adrenergic blocker-combined α_1 and nonselective β blocker	Labetalol	Useful in hyperadrenergic syndromes. Contraindicated in patients with asthma, COPD, heart block. May worsen heart failure
Adrenergic blocker-nonselective α-blocker	Phentolamine	Useful in patients with pheochromocytoma, cocaine toxicity, amphetamine overdose, clonidine withdrawal
Dopamine$_1$-agonist	Fenoldopam	Contraindicated in patients with glaucoma or increased intracerebral pressure
ACE inhibitor	Enalaprilat	Useful in situations associated with high plasma renin activity (scleroderma renal crisis). Contraindicated in pregnancy, acute MI, bilateral renal artery stenosis

HF = heart failure; MI = myocardial infarction; PDE = phosphodiesterase.

Data from Whelton PK, Carey RM, Aronow WS, Casey DE Jr, Collins KJ, Dennison Himmelfarb C, et al. 2017 ACC/AHA/AAPA/ABC/ACPM/AGS/APhA/ASH/ASPC/NMA/PCNA guideline for the prevention, detection, evaluation, and management of high blood pressure in adults: executive summary: A report of the American College of Cardiology/American Heart Association task force on clinical practice guidelines. Hypertension. 2018;71:1269-1324. [PMID: 29133354] doi:10.1161/HYP.0000000000000066

TABLE 55. Intravenous Antihypertensive Drugs for Treatment of Hypertensive Emergencies in Patients with a Compelling Comorbidity

Comorbidity	Preferred Drugs[a]	Comments
Acute aortic dissection	Esmolol, labetalol	Rapid SBP lowering to ≤120 mm Hg. β-Blockade should precede vasodilator (such as with nicardipine or nitroprusside) administration.
Acute pulmonary edema	Nitroglycerin, nitroprusside, clevidipine	β-Blockers contraindicated
Acute coronary syndromes	Esmolol, labetalol, nicardipine, nitroglycerin	Esmolol and nitroglycerin are first-line drugs.
Acute kidney injury	Clevidipine, fenoldopam, nicardipine	
Eclampsia or preeclampsia	Hydralazine, labetalol, nicardipine	ACE inhibitors, ARBs, renin inhibitors, nitroprusside contraindicated

[a]See Table 54 for specific drug contraindications.

ARB = angiotensin receptor blocker; SBP = systolic blood pressure.

Data from Whelton PK, Carey RM, Aronow WS, Casey DE Jr, Collins KJ, Dennison Himmelfarb C, et al. 2017 ACC/AHA/AAPA/ABC/ACPM/AGS/APhA/ASH/ASPC/NMA/PCNA guideline for the prevention, detection, evaluation, and management of high blood pressure in adults: executive summary: A report of the American College of Cardiology/American Heart Association task force on clinical practice guidelines. Hypertension. 2018;71:1269-1324. [PMID: 29133354] doi:10.1161/HYP.0000000000000066

KEY POINTS

- For adults with a hypertensive emergency and a compelling condition (such as aortic dissection, severe preeclampsia or eclampsia, or pheochromocytoma crisis), systolic blood pressure should be reduced to less than 140 mm Hg during the first hour and to less than 120 mm Hg in aortic dissection.

- For adults with a hypertensive emergency but without a compelling condition, systolic blood pressure should be reduced by no more than 25% within the first hour; then, if stable, to 160/100 mm Hg within the next 2 to 6 hours; and then cautiously to normal during the following 24 to 48 hours.

Hyperthermic Emergencies

Hyperthermic emergency is defined as elevation of core body temperature, usually above 40°C (104°F), causing end-organ dysfunction or damage, which may include alteration in mental status, seizures, kidney injury, muscle rigidity, rhabdomyolysis, acute respiratory distress syndrome, and disseminated intravascular coagulation. Common causes of hyperthermia include heat stroke, malignant hyperthermia, and neuroleptic malignant syndrome, all of which can be fatal if not recognized and treated appropriately (**Table 56**).

Heat Stroke

Heat stroke is a failure of the body's thermal regulatory system caused by dysfunction, as in elderly patients taking

TABLE 56. Causes of Severe Hyperthermia

Diagnosis	Suggestive History	Key Examination Findings	Treatment	Notes
Heat stroke	Environmental exposure	Encephalopathy and fever	Evaporative cooling Ice water immersion	Avoid ice water immersion if nonexertional
Malignant hyperthermia	Exposure to volatile anesthetic or succinylcholine	Masseter muscle rigidity; ↑ arterial P_{CO_2}	Stop inciting drug Dantrolene	Monitor and treat ↑ K^+ and ↑ arterial P_{CO_2}
Neuroleptic malignant syndrome	Typical > atypical antipsychotic agent; onset over days to weeks	Altered mentation, severe rigidity, ↑ HR, ↑ BP, hyporeflexia, no clonus	Stop the inciting drug Dantrolene Bromocriptine	Resolves over days to weeks Mentation change first
Severe serotonin syndrome[a]	Onset within 24 hours of initiation or increasing dose, gastrointestinal prodrome	Agitation, clonus, ↑ reflexes, rigidity	Stop inciting drug Benzodiazepines Cyproheptadine	Resolves in 24 hours

[a]Not routinely considered a cause of severe hyperthermia but commonly confused with neuroleptic malignant syndrome.

BP = blood pressure; HR = heart rate; K^+ = potassium.

anticholinergic medications; volume depletion (diuretics, insensible water loss); or because the system is overwhelmed, as in athletes or military recruits who train strenuously in hot, humid weather. When the core temperature rises above 40°C patients develop encephalopathy. They may also experience hypotension, nausea, and muscle weakness.

If untreated, mortality in heat stroke can be up to 60%. Centrally acting antipyretics such as NSAIDs or acetaminophen are not effective. For patients with nonexertional heat stroke, evaporative cooling with or without ice packs can be used to lower the core temperature to a safe target level, usually 38.5°C (101°F). For exertional heat stroke, evaporative cooling may be effective, but patients who remain severely symptomatic despite evaporative cooling efforts sometimes require immersion in ice water to bring the core temperature down rapidly. Because immersion therapy may be complicated by hypothermia, it is not recommended as first-line treatment. **H**

KEY POINT

- For patients with nonexertional heat stroke, evaporative cooling with or without ice packs can be used to lower the core temperature to a safe target level; for exertional heat stroke, immersion in ice water is sometimes required for severe cases.

Malignant Hyperthermia

Malignant hyperthermia is a rare cause of severe hyperthermia in response to inhaled anesthetic agents (such as halothane and isoflurane) or depolarizing paralytic agents (such as succinylcholine). When a patient with inherited susceptibility is exposed to one of these agents, he or she may develop muscle rigidity, rhabdomyolysis, cardiac arrhythmias, and core body temperature elevation to 45°C

(113°F) or more. Mortality can reach 10%. Treatment consists of discontinuing the triggering agent, active cooling, and administration of the muscle relaxant dantrolene every 5 to 10 minutes until muscle rigidity and hyperthermia resolve.

Neuroleptic Malignant Syndrome and Serotonin Syndrome

Neuroleptic malignant syndrome is an idiosyncratic response to neuroleptic agents such as haloperidol. It can occur with any neuroleptic medication, even after prolonged use, although it is more common at times of initiation or dose escalation. It can also occur with rapid withdrawal of dopaminergic medications for Parkinson disease. Dehydration may increase the risk of the syndrome, which includes fever, mental status changes, and rigidity. Mortality may exceed 10%. Treatment includes stopping the triggering agent (or reinstating the withdrawn dopaminergic agent), active cooling, and rehydration. Evidence for using dantrolene is weak. Neuroleptic medications can be reintroduced after a waiting period of at least 2 weeks, usually at lower dose, with care to avoid dehydration and concomitant administration with lithium.

Serotonin syndrome is a less severe hyperthermic reaction triggered by simultaneous use of two or more medications that affect release or reuptake of serotonin. Unlike neuroleptic malignant syndrome, serotonin syndrome usually includes hyperreflexia and myoclonus, and generally resolves after 24 hours. **H**

KEY POINT

- Treatment of neuroleptic malignant syndrome includes stopping the triggering agent, active cooling, and rehydration.

Accidental Hypothermia

Accidental hypothermia results from heat loss significant enough to overwhelm the body's ability to maintain its core temperature. Shivering is the body's usual mechanism for raising a low core temperature and is quite effective. In the mild stage of hypothermia, shivering occurs, and patients may develop tachycardia, hyperventilation, poor judgment, loss of coordination, and diuresis. Clinical findings may progress to include hypotension, bradycardia, and further depression of mental status. As hypothermia worsens, victims stop shivering, lose consciousness, and can develop life-threatening complications, including pulmonary edema and ventricular arrhythmias (**Table 57**). In moderate to severe hypothermia Osborne waves may be present on electrocardiogram tracings (**Figure 21**).

If a severely hypothermic patient becomes pulseless and requires resuscitation, it is reasonable to continue cardiopulmonary resuscitation for a prolonged period of time until the patient can be rewarmed. There are reports of cardiopulmonary resuscitation lasting hours and resulting in full recovery when a severely hypothermic patient has a cardiac arrest.

Hypothermic patients who are shivering will passively rewarm themselves if they are removed from the cold environment and given adequate insulation to prevent heat loss, but as hypothermia progresses, shivering stops, usually when the core temperature drops below 32°C (89.6°F). At this point, a patient must be actively rewarmed to prevent complications. Active rewarming techniques include surface methods, such as heating pads and forced-air warming systems, as well as invasive methods such as rewarming by peritoneal or pleural space irrigation using peritoneal catheters or thoracostomy tubes. Extracorporeal support, including cardiopulmonary bypass, is recommended for patients in cardiac arrest because it maximizes the rewarming rate and can provide hemodynamic support. During active rewarming, core temperature should be monitored with an esophageal temperature probe, as rectal and bladder temperatures will lag behind the rising core temperature during the rewarming process.

Toxicology

Alcohol Poisoning

Ethanol and other ingested alcohols activate the γ-aminobutyric acid receptor, which is the primary central nervous system (CNS) inhibitor, thus leading to CNS depression, including loss of consciousness and suppression of respiratory drive at high doses. In addition to this acute toxicity, which can lead to life-threatening apnea or aspiration events, alcohol withdrawal can also be fatal, and patients should be monitored for signs of withdrawal, including seizures. Ethanol is the most commonly ingested alcohol and the most often encountered toxicity (**Table 58**). For further discussion of alcohol withdrawal see MKSAP 18 General Internal Medicine.

Other alcohols ingested include ethylene glycol (antifreeze), methanol (wood alcohol), and isopropyl alcohol (rubbing alcohol). These all have similar CNS depressant effects to those of ethanol. However, after ingestion, ethylene glycol is metabolized by alcohol dehydrogenase to oxalic acid, which crystalizes in the renal tubules and can lead to permanent kidney damage. Methanol is metabolized to formic acid, which is toxic to the retina and leads to blindness. When either of these alcohols has been ingested, there is an elevated anion gap metabolic acidosis as well as an osmolal gap (see MKSAP 18 Nephrology: Increased Anion Gap Metabolic Acidosis). Therapy includes elimination but also prevention of metabolism by alcohol dehydrogenase to toxic metabolites. The enzymatic process can be competitively inhibited by administering fomepizole.

Isopropyl alcohol has no toxic metabolites and does not elevate the anion gap, although it does increase the osmolal gap. Treatment is supportive. Dialysis removes all alcohols effectively, but is not necessary for patients who are inebriated but otherwise stable.

Carbon Monoxide Poisoning

Carbon monoxide (CO) is a colorless, odorless product of hydrocarbon combustion that is readily absorbed into the circulation when inhaled, and binds avidly to hemoglobin to form carboxyhemoglobin, displacing oxygen and causing clinical tissue hypoxia and ischemia. CO toxicity occurs almost exclusively in enclosed areas where combustion is occurring and is often accidental, but may be intentional in suicide attempts. Exposed patients present with headache, nausea,

TABLE 57.	Symptoms and Signs of Hypothermia	
Severity	**Temperature**	**Findings**
Mild	32.0-35.0 °C (89.6-95.0 °F)	↑ HR, ↑ BP, ↑ RR, shivering, alert, poor judgment
Moderate	28.0-32.0 °C (82.4-89.6 °F)	↓ HR, ↓ BP, ↓ RR, ↓ CO, ↓ O_2 consumption, ↓ kidney function, somnolence, no shivering, supraventricular arrhythmia
Severe	<28.0 °C (82.4 °F)	Coma, absent reflexes, ventricular arrhythmia, asystole, apnea

BP = blood pressure; CO = cardiac output; HR = heart rate; RR = respiration rate.

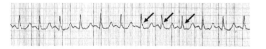

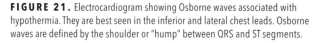

FIGURE 21. Electrocardiogram showing Osborne waves associated with hypothermia. They are best seen in the inferior and lateral chest leads. Osborne waves are defined by the shoulder or "hump" between QRS and ST segments.

TABLE 58. Presentation and Treatment of Alcohol Poisoning

Alcohol	Common Sources	Major Findings	Anion Gap	Osmolar Gap	Antidote
Ethanol	Alcoholic beverages	CNS depression Nausea, emesis	Possible	Yes	Supportive care
Isopropyl alcohol	Rubbing alcohol Disinfectants Antifreeze	CNS depression Ketone elevation	No	Yes	Supportive care
Methanol	Windshield wiper fluid De-icing solutions Solvents "Moonshine"	CNS depression Vision loss Hypotension	Yes	Yes	Fomepizole HD for severe acidemia, very large ingestions, severe CNS depression, and any visual impairment
Ethylene glycol	Antifreeze De-icing solutions Solvents	CNS depression AKI Hypocalcemia Hypotension	Yes	Yes	Fomepizole HD for severe acidemia, very large ingestions, severe CNS depression, AKI, and systemic collapse

AKI = acute kidney injury; CNS = central nervous system; HD = hemodialysis.

malaise, confusion, syncope, seizures, or coma. Patients with coronary artery disease may develop signs and symptoms of cardiac ischemia.

Pulse oximetry is not helpful, as current transcutaneous oximetry technology does not differentiate between oxyhemoglobin and carboxyhemoglobin. Blood gas analysis, including cooximetry, will provide the carboxyhemoglobin level, which is less than 3% in normal individuals. Smokers may have up to 10% to 15% carboxyhemoglobin, and anything higher is consistent with CO poisoning.

The primary treatment is displacement of CO on the hemoglobin molecule with oxygen, which depends on the alveolar concentration of oxygen and the minute ventilation. Once the CO exposure has been stopped, the half-life of carboxyhemoglobin is 300 minutes if patients are breathing ambient air, 90 minutes if breathing 100% oxygen, and 30 minutes if given hyperbaric oxygen in a chamber where the pressure is gradually increased to 2 to 3 times the normal atmospheric pressure. Patients with high levels of carboxyhemoglobin (25% and greater) and evidence of organ ischemia should be treated with hyperbaric oxygen if possible.

Besides the immediate complications resulting from tissue hypoxia in the setting of CO toxicity, there are also delayed neurologic sequelae in approximately 40% of severe cases of CO poisoning. The mechanism is poorly understood, but probably relates to ischemic damage sustained in specific, oxygen-sensitive areas of the brain. These delayed neurocognitive and personality defects usually appear within 20 days of the exposure, but can appear later. They can last for a year or longer. There is weak evidence that hyperbaric oxygen therapy reduces the risk and severity of these delayed neurologic sequelae.

KEY POINTS

- Pulse oximetry is not helpful in diagnosing carbon monoxide poisoning, as it does not differentiate between oxyhemoglobin and carboxyhemoglobin.

- Patients with high levels of carboxyhemoglobin (25% or higher) and evidence of organ dysfunction should be treated with hyperbaric oxygen if possible.

Cyanide Poisoning

Cyanide is one of the most lethal poisons known. It inhibits cellular respiration by binding to cytochrome oxidase a_3 in the mitochondria, blocking the cells' ability to use oxygen for aerobic metabolism. This results in clinical signs of hypoxia, despite normal oxyhemoglobin saturation. Symptoms often include headache, anxiety, nausea, and either a metallic or bitter almond odor and taste. More severe or prolonged exposure can lead to coma, seizures, liver or kidney injury, vomiting, ischemic pain, rhabdomyolysis, and death. Serum lactate elevation is a sensitive but nonspecific marker for cyanide toxicity. A normal lactate concentration effectively rules out significant cyanide exposure.

Cyanide can be ingested or inhaled and is absorbed readily and acts quickly to inhibit cellular metabolism. Inhalation exposure is common in house fires where cyanide is produced and aerosolized when vinyl burns. Cyanide is a common co-exposure with carbon monoxide.

Successful treatment depends on early recognition of cyanide toxicity, elimination of ongoing exposure (for example, removal of contaminated clothing), and either neutralization or competitive binding of the cyanide to remove it from the mitochondrial respiration system. Hydroxocobalamin avidly binds to cyanide to produce

CONT.

cyanocobalamin, which is soluble, nontoxic, and readily excreted. The usual dose is 5 g for an adult. Other antidotes include nitrites (amyl nitrite and sodium nitrite) to induce methemoglobin, which in turn binds cyanide, as well as sodium thiosulfate, which donates sulfur to combine with cyanide, producing harmless thiocyanate. Inducing methemoglobinemia in inhalation-injury victims who may also have high levels of carboxyhemoglobin is not safe, so nitrite therapy should be avoided. Of these potential treatment strategies, hydroxocobalamin is the most commonly recommended due to ease and safety of administration. **H**

KEY POINT

- Successful treatment of cyanide poisoning depends on early recognition of cyanide toxicity, elimination of ongoing exposure, and administration of hydroxocobalamin to remove the cyanide from the mitochondrial respiration system.

Toxicity of Drugs of Abuse

Drugs of abuse may be taken singly or in combination, and an accurate history may be impossible to obtain due to alteration of mental status, reluctance on the part of the patient or others to admit what was taken, and insufficient or incorrect knowledge about the composition of illicit drugs. Clinical toxic syndromes, or constellations of symptoms and signs indicative of certain classes of drugs, can be recognized and provide clues as to what should be done for effective medical management of overdose (**Table 59** and **Table 60**).

In addition to seeking to identify the specific agent(s) or class(es) of drugs taken, care of overdose patients is primarily supportive; critically important is maintenance of airway patency and ventilation in patients with decreased mental status. Patients are often intubated to prevent aspiration and allow for mechanical ventilation in cases where respiratory drive is impaired by drugs.

An early empiric trial of the opioid antagonist naloxone is warranted when opioid overdose is suspected to reverse respiratory depression and depressed mental status. It is important to remember that naloxone has a very short half-life, and its antidote effects will usually wear off before the opioid effects are gone; patients should be observed for signs of opioid withdrawal (which is not fatal and requires only supportive care) and for continued or recurrent signs of respiratory distress, which may require repeated dosing of naloxone.

Administration of flumazenil for suspected benzodiazepine overdose is more problematic, as reversing the effect of benzodiazepines can lead to life-threatening CNS activation, including seizures, which are most likely in patients taking benzodiazepines chronically. It is usually best to manage patients with ventilator support and allow elimination of the agent over time.

In patients who have taken sympathomimetic agents, such as cocaine or amphetamines, benzodiazepines are the

TABLE 59. Toxic Syndromes and Their Manifestations

Syndrome	Manifestations	Representative Drugs
Sympathomimetic	Tachycardia Hypertension Diaphoresis Agitation Seizures Mydriasis	Cocaine Amphetamines Ephedrine Caffeine
Cholinergic	"SLUDGE" (Salivation, Lacrimation, increased Urination and Defecation, Gastrointestinal upset, and Emesis) Confusion Bronchorrhea Bradycardia Miosis	Organophosphates (insecticides, sarin) Carbamates Physostigmine Edrophonium Nicotine
Anticholinergic	Hyperthermia Dry skin and mucous membranes Agitation, delirium Tachycardia, tachypnea Hypertension Mydriasis	Antihistamines Tricyclic antidepressants Anti-Parkinson agents Atropine Scopolamine
Opioids	Miosis Respiratory depression Lethargy, confusion Hypothermia Bradycardia Hypotension	Morphine, fentanyl, oxycodone and related drugs Heroin

cornerstone of therapy for agitation. Beta-blocker medications should be avoided, as they will block the beta-adrenergic receptors and theoretically leave the activated alpha receptors unopposed, thus leading to severe hypertension.

Hallucinogenic agents have no antidote, so care is supportive, including maintaining the airway, ventilation, and hemodynamic support. These patients may be extremely agitated and combative, requiring physical restraints or sedation to prevent them from harming themselves and others.

Overdose of Therapeutic Drugs

Patients may overdose on prescribed medications either inadvertently or intentionally, and often many medications

TABLE 60. Presentation and Toxicity of Some Drugs of Abuse

Drug Class	Examples	Examination Findings	Antidote
Opioids	Heroin, oxycodone, fentanyl analogs	↓ HR, ↓ temp, ↓ BP, ↓ RR, miosis	Naloxone
Benzodiazepines	Lorazepam	CNS depression, usually normal vital signs and eye examination	Flumazenil (may be complicated by seizure)
Sympathomimetics		Shared findings: ↑ HR, ↑ BP, ↑ temp, diaphoresis, mydriasis, agitation, seizure, ↑ CK, ↑ liver chemistry studies, ↑ Cr	Benzodiazepines are first line for agitation Avoid β-blockers for hypertension Haloperidol may worsen hyperthermia
	Cocaine	30-minute duration, myocardial infarction prominent	
	Methamphetamine	Violent agitation prominent, ↓ Na, duration 20 hours	
	MDMA ("ecstasy")	↓ Na, serotonin syndrome	
	Bath salts ("plant food")	Hallucinations, violent agitation common, duration up to 48 hours, negative urine drug screen	
Hallucinogens	Dextromethorphan	↑ HR, ↑ BP, agitation, coma	Benzodiazepines are first line for agitation Haloperidol is second line
	Lysergic acid diethylamide (LSD)	Mild ↑ HR, ↑ BP; rare ↑ temp and hemodynamic instability	
	Phencyclidine (PCP)	Variable mental status: ↑ agitation, CNS depression, nystagmus	
	Synthetic cannabinoids ("Spice," "K-2")	↑ HR, agitation > marijuana, ↑Cr, negative urine drug screen	

BP = blood pressure; CK = creatine kinase; CNS = central nervous system; Cr = creatinine; ECG = electrocardiogram; HR = heart rate; MDMA = 3-4 methylenedioxymethamphetamine; Na = sodium; RR = respiration rate; temp = temperature.

are taken together, sometimes with alcohol. Information about suicidal ideation or intent, what medications a patient and family members have been prescribed, what prescriptions were filled, events reported by the patient or bystanders, and clinical signs and symptoms are all important in determining the nature of an overdose. If patients are alert and cooperative enough to protect their airway, administration of activated charcoal may be beneficial if it can be given within 1 to 2 hours of ingestion (**Table 61**). Acetaminophen overdose is discussed in MKSAP 18 Gastroenterology and Hepatology, and salicylate overdose in MKSAP 18 Nephrology.

Acute Abdominal Surgical Emergencies

A large number of conditions can cause abdominal pain, distention, and rigidity. Although many of them can and should be managed medically, some require surgery, and timely diagnosis followed by surgical intervention is needed to improve survival. Imaging decisions should be based on history and examination findings, and should not delay intervention

(**Table 62**). For further discussion of abdominal compartment syndrome see MKSAP 18 Nephrology.

Encephalopathy

Alterations in mental status are common in the ICU because of both critical illness and the ICU environment, which can provide sick patients few contextual clues to reorient themselves to time, place, and events. There are many situations that involve mental status change, but three are most important in the context of critical care medicine: delirium (addressed earlier in Principles of Critical Care), coma, and anoxic brain injury.

Coma

Coma describes a condition of absent cortical function of the CNS, with intact brainstem function, whether due to illness, trauma, or medication. Patients in a coma do not respond to external stimuli. The Glasgow Coma Scale (GCS) is an instrument for assessing the severity of deficit based on three categories of stimulus response: eye response, verbal response, and motor response (**Table 63**). A GCS score of 15 means a normal,

TABLE 61.	Presentation and Treatment of Therapeutic Drug Toxicities		
Medication	**Key Clinical Findings**	**Treatment**	**Notes**
Nonopioid analgesics			
Acetaminophen	↑ liver chemistry studies, ↑Cr, ↑INR, encephalopathy, cerebral edema, vomiting	N-acetylcysteine	Transfer to liver transplant center if severe
Salicylates	Mixed respiratory alkalosis/anion gap metabolic acidosis, tinnitus, agitation, confusion, hyperthermia	Bicarbonate infusion, dextrose	Target urine pH 7.5 to 8.0; hemodialysis if acute kidney injury or severe toxicity
Cardiovascular			
β-Blocker, calcium channel blocker	↓ HR, ↓ BP, heart block, altered mental status if β-blocker	Atropine 1 mg IV up to 3 doses, glucagon, calcium chloride, vasopressors, cardiac pacemaker (if indicated), high-dose insulin and glucose, IV lipid emulsion	Treatments may be added sequentially or initiated simultaneously depending on severity of case and response to treatment
Digoxin	↓ HR, arrhythmia, nausea, emesis, abdominal pain, confusion, weakness	Digoxin-specific antibody	Use of antibody lowers K^+; hemodialysis not effective
Anticholinergics			
Tricyclic antidepressants	↓ BP, sedation, seizure, anticholinergic signs, arrhythmia	Bicarbonate infusion titrated to QRS duration; benzodiazepines for seizure	Physostigmine contraindicated
Antihistamines	Anticholinergic signs including agitation and seizures	Benzodiazepines; physostigmine if isolated anticholinergic overdose	Physostigmine use requires continuous cardiac monitor and bedside atropine
Hypoglycemic			
Sulfonylurea	↓ glucose, confusion, seizure, anxiety, diaphoresis, tremor	Dextrose + octreotide, glucagon IM = temporizing	Monitor for ↓ glucose for 48 hours if large ingestion
Metformin	↑ lactate, abdominal pain	Hemodialysis for severe ↓ pH or acute kidney injury	Glucose usually normal if isolated metformin ingestion
Others			
Lithium	GI distress, confusion, ataxia, tremor, myoclonic jerks, diabetes insipidus	Hemodialysis if lithium level >4 mEq/L or severe symptoms	Serum level can guide need for hemodialysis, confirm diagnosis
SSRI/SNRI	Agitation, clonus, ↑ reflexes, rigidity, fever, ↑ HR	Benzodiazepines, cyproheptadine if severe	Venlafaxine has ↑ cardiac toxicity

BP = blood pressure; Cr = creatinine; GI = gastrointestinal; HR = heart rate; IM = intramuscular; IV = intravenous; K^+ = potassium; SNRI = serotonin norepinephrine reuptake inhibitor; SSRI = selective serotonin reuptake inhibitor.

alert (or fully arousable) patient, and a score of 3 means no response at all. Comatose patients are often hyperreflexic. In addition to a clinical examination, lumbar puncture and CNS imaging with MRI or CT scan are useful in diagnosing the cause of coma. Treatment is supportive with efforts to reverse the specific cause of the coma if possible.

Anoxic Brain Injury

Anoxic brain injury refers to damage to the CNS caused by prolonged, profound tissue hypoxia. There are many possible causes of such hypoxia, including near drowning, seizures, obstructed airway, lung disease, cardiac arrest, asphyxiation, and other inhalational injury. Brain imaging shows edema and loss of grey-white matter demarcation. Electroencephalographic monitoring shows various patterns,

from diffuse slowing (typical of many types of encephalopathy) to burst suppression or seizure activity (indicative of more severe injury) to absence of brain electrical activity (which can indicate brain death). Prognosis is often not immediately apparent, and patients with anoxic brain injury require supportive care for 3 to 5 days or longer before the extent of injury can be understood well enough to be declared irreversible. **H**

KEY POINT

- Prognosis for patients with anoxic brain injury is often not immediately apparent, and patients require supportive care for 3 to 5 days or longer before the extent of injury can be understood well enough to be declared irreversible.

TABLE 62. Acute Abdominal Emergencies

Diagnosis	Presentation	Diagnostic Imaging	Notes
Acute cholecystitis and cholangitis	Persistent peritoneal RUQ or epigastric pain, fever, emesis, positive Murphy sign	Ultrasound EUS and ERCP for diagnosis and treatment of cholangitis	↑ alkaline phosphatase, ↑ bilirubin suggests cholangitis but typically not cholecystitis
Bowel obstruction	Cramping pain, emesis, distention, obstipation, dehydration	Radiograph: dilated loops of bowel with air-fluid levels CT scan: identifies cause, complications	Top causes: incarcerated hernia, adhesions, volvulus, intussusception
Acute appendicitis	Classic: periumbilical then RLQ pain, emesis, ↑ leukocyte count	Often unnecessary CT or ultrasound if unclear	Pain quality and location vary with appendix location
Peptic ulcer perforation	Abrupt peritoneal pain, later distention and hypovolemia	Radiograph: free air CT scan if unclear	Surgery necessary in majority of cases
Acute mesenteric ischemia	Pain > examination findings, vomiting, hypotension, risk factors for clotting, embolism	CT angiography or conventional arteriography	↑ amylase, ↑ phosphate common Regular CT and lactate can be normal early in course
Toxic megacolon	Pain, diarrhea, fever, ↑ HR, ↓ BP, confusion	Radiograph: dilated colon, air-fluid levels in colon CT scan if unclear	Causes: inflammatory bowel disease, *Clostridium difficile* infection
Ruptured abdominal aortic aneurysm	↓ BP, abdominal and/or flank pain, pulsatile mass	Unnecessary if high suspicion and unstable CT or ultrasound if unclear	Risk factors: older age, male, smoking, hypertension, family history of aneurysm
Ectopic pregnancy with tubal rupture	↓ BP, ↓ Hb, ↑ hCG, abdominal pain, vaginal bleeding	Transvaginal ultrasound	High mortality without early surgery

BP = blood pressure; ERCP = endoscopic retrograde cholangiopancreatography; EUS = endoscopic ultrasound; Hb = hemoglobin; hCG = human chorionic gonadotropin; HR = heart rate; RLQ = right lower quadrant; RUQ = right upper quadrant; temp = temperature.

TABLE 63. Glasgow Coma Scale

Eyes	Score
Does not open eyes	1
Opens eyes in response to painful stimuli (when given pain)	2
Opens eyes in response to voice	3
Opens eyes spontaneously	4
Verbal	
Makes no sound	1
Incomprehensible sounds (mumbles)	2
Utters inappropriate words	3
Confused, disorientated	4
Oriented, chats normally	5
Motor (physical reflexes)	
Makes no movements	1
Extension (straightens limb when given painful stimulus)	2
Abnormal flexion (flexes limbs indiscriminately when given painful stimulus)	3
Flexion/withdrawal to painful stimuli (moves away when given painful stimulus)	4
Localizes painful stimuli (can pinpoint where pain is)	5
Obeys commands	6
Brain Injury as Classified in the Glasgow Coma Scale (Eyes + Verbal + Motor)	
Coma	3 to 8
Moderate brain injury	9 to 12
Mild brain injury	13 to 15

Bibliography

Pulmonary Diagnostic Tests

Berrizbeitia LD. The lower limit of normal in the evaluation of pulmonary function [Editorial]. Heart Lung. 2014;43:267-8. [PMID: 24856225] doi:10.1016/j.hrtlng.2014.04.011

Johnson JD, Theurer WM. A stepwise approach to the interpretation of pulmonary function tests. Am Fam Physician. 2014;89:359-66. [PMID: 24695507]

Little BP. Approach to chest computed tomography. Clin Chest Med. 2015;36:127-45, vii. [PMID: 26024596] doi:10.1016/j.ccm.2015.02.001

Murgu SD. Diagnosing and staging lung cancer involving the mediastinum. Chest. 2015;147:1401-12. [PMID: 25940251] doi:10.1378/chest.14-1355

Parreira VF, Janaudis-Ferreira T, Evans RA, Mathur S, Goldstein RS, Brooks D. Measurement properties of the incremental shuttle walk test. a systematic review. Chest. 2014;145:1357-69. [PMID: 24384555]

Pellegrino R, Viegi G, Brusasco V, Crapo RO, Burgos F, Casaburi R, et al. Interpretative strategies for lung function tests. Eur Respir J. 2005;26:948-68. [PMID: 16264058]

Singh SJ, Puhan MA, Andrianopoulos V, Hernandes NA, Mitchell KE, Hill CJ, et al. An official systematic review of the European Respiratory Society/American Thoracic Society: measurement properties of field walking tests in chronic respiratory disease [Editorial]. Eur Respir J. 2014;44:1447-78. [PMID: 25359356] doi:10.1183/09031936.00150414

Airways Disease

Altenburg J, de Graaff CS, Stienstra Y, Sloos JH, van Haren EH, Koppers RJ, et al. Effect of azithromycin maintenance treatment on infectious exacerbations among patients with non-cystic fibrosis bronchiectasis: the BAT randomized controlled trial. JAMA. 2013;309:1251-9. [PMID: 23532241] doi:10.1001/jama.2013.1937

Bel EH, Wenzel SE, Thompson PJ, Prazma CM, Keene ON, Yancey SW, et al; SIRIUS Investigators. Oral glucocorticoid-sparing effect of mepolizumab in eosinophilic asthma. N Engl J Med. 2014;371:1189-97. [PMID: 25199060] doi:10.1056/NEJMoa1403291

Boulet LP, O'Byrne PM. Asthma and exercise-induced bronchoconstriction in athletes. N Engl J Med. 2015;372:641-8. [PMID: 25671256] doi:10.1056/NEJMra1407552

Daniels JM, Snijders D, de Graaff CS, Vlaspolder F, Jansen HM, Boersma WG. Antibiotics in addition to systemic corticosteroids for acute exacerbations of chronic obstructive pulmonary disease. Am J Respir Crit Care Med. 2010;181:150-7. [PMID: 19875685] doi:10.1164/rccm.200906-0837OC

Evensen AE. Management of COPD exacerbations. Am Fam Physician. 2010;81:607-13. [PMID: 20187597]

Fishman A, Fessler H, Martinez F, McKenna RJ Jr, Naunheim K, Piantadosi S, et al; National Emphysema Treatment Trial Research Group. Patients at high risk of death after lung-volume-reduction surgery. N Engl J Med. 2001;345:1075-83. [PMID: 11596586]

Gilljam M, Ellis L, Corey M, Zielenski J, Durie P, Tullis DE. Clinical manifestations of CF among patients with diagnosis in adulthood. Chest. 2004;126:1215-24. [PMID: 15486385]

Global Strategy for Asthma. Global Strategy for Asthma Web site. www.ginasthma.org. Accessed May 9, 2018.

Herth FJ, Gompelmann D, Ernst A, Eberhardt R. Endoscopic lung volume reduction. Respiration. 2010;79:5-13. [PMID: 19923881] doi:10.1159/000256510

Leuppi JD, Schuetz P, Bingisser R, Bodmer M, Briel M, Drescher T, et al. Short-term vs conventional glucocorticoid therapy in acute exacerbations of chronic obstructive pulmonary disease: the REDUCE randomized clinical trial. JAMA. 2013;309:2223-31. [PMID: 23695200] doi:10.1001/jama.2013.5023

Maguire G. Bronchiectasis—a guide for primary care. Aust Fam Physician. 2012;41:842-50. [PMID: 23145413]

McShane PJ, Naureckas ET, Tino G, Strek ME. Non-cystic fibrosis bronchiectasis. Am J Respir Crit Care Med. 2013;188:647-56. [PMID: 23898922] doi:10.1164/rccm.201303-0411CI

Most Recent Asthma Data. Centers for Disease Control and Prevention Web site. https://www.cdc.gov/asthma/most_recent_data.htm. Updated February 13, 2018. Accessed May 9, 2018.

Mulhall P, Criner G. Non-pharmacological treatments for COPD. Respirology. 2016;21:791-809. [PMID: 27099216] doi:10.1111/resp.12782

Ong T, Ramsey BW. Update in cystic fibrosis 2014. Am J Respir Crit Care Med. 2015;192:669-75. [PMID: 26371812] doi:10.1164/rccm.201504-0656UP

Pakhale S, Baron J, Dent R, Vandemheen K, Aaron SD. Effects of weight loss on airway responsiveness in obese adults with asthma: does weight loss lead to reversibility of asthma? Chest. 2015;147:1582-90. [PMID: 25763936] doi:10.1378/chest.14-3105

Prasad Kerlin M. In the clinic. Asthma. Ann Intern Med. 2014;160:ITC3 2-15; quiz ITC3 16-9. [PMID: 24737276] doi:10.7326/0003-4819-160-5-201403040-01003

Qaseem A, Wilt TJ, Weinberger SE, Hanania NA, Criner G, van der Molen T, et al; American College of Physicians. Diagnosis and management of stable chronic obstructive pulmonary disease: a clinical practice guideline update from the American College of Physicians, American College of Chest Physicians, American Thoracic Society, and European Respiratory Society. Ann Intern Med. 2011;155:179-91. [PMID: 21810710] doi:10.7326/0003-4819-155-3-201108020-00008

Scheinberg P, Shore E. A pilot study of the safety and efficacy of tobramycin solution for inhalation in patients with severe bronchiectasis. Chest. 2005;127:1420-6. [PMID: 15821224]

Skloot GS, Busse PJ, Braman SS, Kovacs EJ, Dixon AE, Vaz Fragoso CA, et al; ATS ad hoc Committee on Asthma in the Elderly. An official American Thoracic Society Workshop report: evaluation and management of asthma in the elderly. Ann Am Thorac Soc. 2016;13:2064-2077. [PMID: 27831798]

Tarlo SM, Lemiere C. Occupational asthma. N Engl J Med. 2014;370:640-9. [PMID: 24521110] doi:10.1056/NEJMra1301758

Teodorescu M, Broytman O, Curran-Everett D, Sorkness RL, Crisafi G, Bleecker ER, et al; National Institutes of Health, National Heart, Lung and Blood Institute Severe Asthma Research Program (SARP) investigators. Obstructive sleep apnea risk, asthma burden, and lower airway inflammation in adults in the severe asthma research program (SARP) II. J Allergy Clin Immunol Pract. 2015;3:566-75.e1. [PMID: 26004304] doi:10.1016/j.jaip.2015.04.002

The Global Strategy for the Diagnosis, Management and Prevention of COPD, Global Initiative for Chronic Obstructive Lung Disease (GOLD) 2017. Available from: goldcopd.org. Accessed May 25, 2018.

Vogelmeier CF, Criner GJ, Martinez FJ, Anzueto A, Barnes PJ, Bourbeau J, et al. Global Strategy for the Diagnosis, Management, and Prevention of Chronic Obstructive Lung Disease 2017 Report. GOLD Executive Summary. Am J Respir Crit Care Med. 2017;195:557-582. [PMID: 28128970] doi:10.1164/rccm.201701-0218PP

Wechsler ME. Getting control of uncontrolled asthma. Am J Med. 2014;127:1049-59. [PMID: 24844737] doi:10.1016/j.amjmed.2014.05.006

Diffuse Parenchymal Lung Disease

Collard HR, Ryerson CJ, Corte TJ, Jenkins G, Kondoh Y, Lederer DJ, et al. Acute exacerbation of idiopathic pulmonary fibrosis. An international working group report. Am J Respir Crit Care Med. 2016;194:265-75. [PMID: 27299520] doi:10.1164/rccm.201604-0801CI

Fischer A, Antoniou KM, Brown KK, Cadranel J, Corte TJ, du Bois RM, et al; ERS/ATS Task Force on Undifferentiated Forms of CTD-ILD. An official European Respiratory Society/American Thoracic Society research statement: interstitial pneumonia with autoimmune features. Eur Respir J. 2015;46:976-87. [PMID: 26160873] doi:10.1183/13993003.00150-2015

Hansell DM, Bankier AA, MacMahon H, McLoud TC, Müller NL, Remy J. Fleischner Society: glossary of terms for thoracic imaging. Radiology. 2008;246:697-722. [PMID: 18195376] doi:10.1148/radiol.2462070712

Hutchinson JP, Fogarty AW, McKeever TM, Hubbard RB. In-hospital mortality after surgical lung biopsy for interstitial lung disease in the United States. 2000 to 2011. Am J Respir Crit Care Med. 2016;193:1161-7. [PMID: 26646481] doi:10.1164/rccm.201508-1632OC

Raghu G, Chen SY, Hou Q, Yeh WS, Collard HR. Incidence and prevalence of idiopathic pulmonary fibrosis in US adults 18-64 years old. Eur Respir J. 2016;48:179-86. [PMID: 27126689] doi:10.1183/13993003.01653-2015

Raghu G, Rochwerg B, Zhang Y, Garcia CA, Azuma A, Behr J, et al; American Thoracic Society. An official ATS/ERS/JRS/ALAT Clinical Practice Guideline: treatment of idiopathic pulmonary fibrosis. An update of the 2011 Clinical Practice Guideline. Am J Respir Crit Care Med. 2015;192:e3-19. [PMID: 26177183] doi:10.1164/rccm.201506-1063ST

Schwaiblmair M, Behr W, Haeckel T, Märkl B, Foerg W, Berghaus T. Drug-induced interstitial lung disease. Open Respir Med J. 2012;6:63-74. [PMID: 22896776] doi:10.2174/1874306401206010063

Tashkin DP, Elashoff R, Clements PJ, Goldin J, Roth MD, Furst DE, et al; Scleroderma Lung Study Research Group. Cyclophosphamide versus placebo in scleroderma lung disease. N Engl J Med. 2006;354:2655-66. [PMID: 16790698]

Tashkin DP, Roth MD, Clements PJ, Furst DE, Khanna D, Kleerup EC, et al; Scleroderma Lung Study II Investigators. Mycophenolate mofetil versus oral cyclophosphamide in scleroderma-related interstitial lung disease (SLS II): a randomised controlled, double-blind, parallel group trial. Lancet Respir Med. 2016;4:708-19. [PMID: 27469583] doi:10.1016/S2213-2600(16)30152-7

Travis WD, Costabel U, Hansell DM, King TE Jr, Lynch DA, Nicholson AG, et al; ATS/ERS Committee on Idiopathic Interstitial Pneumonias. An official

American Thoracic Society/European Respiratory Society statement: update of the international multidisciplinary classification of the idiopathic interstitial pneumonias. Am J Respir Crit Care Med. 2013;188:733-48. [PMID: 24032382] doi:10.1164/rccm.201308-1483ST

Weill D, Benden C, Corris PA, Dark JH, Davis RD, Keshavjee S, et al. A consensus document for the selection of lung transplant candidates: 2014–an update from the Pulmonary Transplantation Council of the International Society for Heart and Lung Transplantation. J Heart Lung Transplant. 2015;34:1-15. [PMID: 25085497] doi:10.1016/j.healun.2014.06.014

Occupational Lung Disease

Bacchus L, Shah RD, Chung JH, Crabtree TP, Heitkamp DE, Iannettoni MD, et al; Expert Panel on Thoracic Imaging. ACR appropriateness criteria review ACR appropriateness criteria® occupational lung diseases. J Thorac Imaging. 2016;31:W1-3. [PMID: 26656194] doi:10.1097/RTI.0000000000000194

Curti S, Sauni R, Spreeuwers D, De Schryver A, Valenty M, Rivière S, et al. Interventions to increase the reporting of occupational diseases by physicians. Cochrane Database Syst Rev. 2015:CD010305. [PMID: 25805310] doi:10.1002/14651858.CD010305.pub2

Laney AS, Weissman DN. The classic pneumoconioses: new epidemiological and laboratory observations. Clin Chest Med. 2012;33:745-58. [PMID: 23153613] doi:10.1016/j.ccm.2012.08.005

Sauler M, Gulati M. Newly recognized occupational and environmental causes of chronic terminal airways and parenchymal lung disease. Clin Chest Med. 2012;33:667-80. [PMID: 23153608] doi:10.1016/j.ccm.2012.09.002

Seaman DM, Meyer CA, Kanne JP. Occupational and environmental lung disease. Clin Chest Med. 2015;36:249-68, viii-ix. [PMID: 26024603] doi:10.1016/j.ccm.2015.02.008

Pleural Disease

Baumann MH, Strange C, Heffner JE, Light R, Kirby TJ, Klein J, et al; AACP Pneumothorax Consensus Group. Management of spontaneous pneumothorax: an American College of Chest Physicians Delphi consensus statement. Chest. 2001;119:590-602. [PMID: 11171742]

Bhatnagar R, Corcoran JP, Maldonado F, Feller-Kopman D, Janssen J, Astoul P, et al. Advanced medical interventions in pleural disease. Eur Respir Rev. 2016;25:199-213. [PMID: 27246597] doi:10.1183/16000617.0020-2016

Davies HE, Davies RJ, Davies CW; BTS Pleural Disease Guideline Group. Management of pleural infection in adults: British Thoracic Society Pleural Disease Guideline 2010. Thorax. 2010;65 Suppl 2:ii41-53. [PMID: 20696693] doi:10.1136/thx.2010.137000

Davies HE, Mishra EK, Kahan BC, Wrightson JM, Stanton AE, Guhan A, et al. Effect of an indwelling pleural catheter vs chest tube and talc pleurodesis for relieving dyspnea in patients with malignant pleural effusion: the TIME2 randomized controlled trial. JAMA. 2012;307:2383-9. [PMID: 22610520] doi:10.1001/jama.2012.5535

Feller-Kopman D, Light R. Pleural disease. N Engl J Med. 2018;378:740-751.

MacDuff A, Arnold A, Harvey J; BTS Pleural Disease Guideline Group. Management of spontaneous pneumothorax: British Thoracic Society Pleural Disease Guideline 2010. Thorax. 2010;65 Suppl 2:ii18-31. [PMID: 20696690] doi:10.1136/thx.2010.136986

Rahman NM, Maskell NA, West A, Teoh R, Arnold A, Mackinlay C, et al. Intrapleural use of tissue plasminogen activator and DNase in pleural infection. N Engl J Med. 2011;365:518-26. [PMID: 21830966] doi:10.1056/NEJMoa1012740

Rahman NM, Mishra EK, Davies HE, Davies RJ, Lee YC. Clinically important factors influencing the diagnostic measurement of pleural fluid pH and glucose. Am J Respir Crit Care Med. 2008;178:483-90. [PMID: 18556632] doi:10.1164/rccm.200801-062OC

Roberts ME, Neville E, Berrisford RG, Antunes G, Ali NJ; BTS Pleural Disease Guideline Group. Management of a malignant pleural effusion: British Thoracic Society Pleural Disease Guideline 2010. Thorax. 2010;65 Suppl 2:ii32-40. [PMID: 20696691] doi:10.1136/thx.2010.136994

Wilcox ME, Chong CA, Stanbrook MB, Tricco AC, Wong C, Straus SE. Does this patient have an exudative pleural effusion? The Rational Clinical Examination systematic review. JAMA. 2014;311:2422-31. [PMID: 24938565] doi:10.1001/jama.2014.5552

Pulmonary Vascular Disease

Galiè N, Humbert M, Vachiery JL, Gibbs S, Lang I, Torbicki A, et al; ESC Scientific Document Group. 2015 ESC/ERS Guidelines for the diagnosis and treatment of pulmonary hypertension: The Joint Task Force for the Diagnosis and Treatment of Pulmonary Hypertension of the European Society of Cardiology (ESC) and the European Respiratory Society (ERS): Endorsed by: Association for European Paediatric and Congenital Cardiology (AEPC), International Society for Heart and Lung

Transplantation (ISHLT). Eur Heart J. 2016;37:67-119. [PMID: 26320113] doi:10.1093/eurheartj/ehv317

Lung Tumors

Aberle DR, Adams AM, Berg CD, Black WC, Clapp JD, Fagerstrom RM, et al; National Lung Screening Trial Research Team. Reduced lung-cancer mortality with low-dose computed tomographic screening. N Engl J Med. 2011;365:395-409. [PMID: 21714641] doi:10.1056/NEJMoa1102873

Gould MK, Donington J, Lynch WR, Mazzone PJ, Midthun DE, Naidich DP, et al. Evaluation of individuals with pulmonary nodules: when is it lung cancer? Diagnosis and management of lung cancer, 3rd ed: American College of Chest Physicians evidence-based clinical practice guidelines. Chest. 2013;143:e93S-e120S. [PMID: 23649456] doi:10.1378/chest.12-2351

Husain AN, Colby T, Ordonez N, Krausz T, Attanoos R, Beasley MB, et al; International Mesothelioma Interest Group. Guidelines for pathologic diagnosis of malignant mesothelioma: 2012 update of the consensus statement from the International Mesothelioma Interest Group. Arch Pathol Lab Med. 2013;137:647-67. [PMID: 22929121] doi:10.5858/arpa.2012-0214-OA

MacMahon H, Naidich DP, Goo JM, Lee KS, Leung ANC, Mayo JR, et al. Guidelines for management of incidental pulmonary nodules detected on CT images: from the Fleischner Society 2017. Radiology. 2017;284:228-243. [PMID: 28240562] doi:10.1148/radiol.2017161659

McWilliams A, Tammemagi MC, Mayo JR, Roberts H, Liu G, Soghrati K, et al. Probability of cancer in pulmonary nodules detected on first screening CT. N Engl J Med. 2013;369:910-9. [PMID: 24004118] doi:10.1056/NEJMoa1214726

Naidich DP, Bankier AA, MacMahon H, Schaefer-Prokop CM, Pistolesi M, Goo JM, et al. Recommendations for the management of subsolid pulmonary nodules detected at CT: a statement from the Fleischner Society. Radiology. 2013;266:304-17. [PMID: 23070270] doi:10.1148/radiol.12120628

Sholl LM. Biomarkers in lung adenocarcinoma: a decade of progress. Arch Pathol Lab Med. 2015;139:469-80. [PMID: 25255293] doi:10.5858/arpa.2014-0128-RA

Silvestri GA, Gonzalez AV, Jantz MA, Margolis ML, Gould MK, Tanoue LT, et al. Methods for staging non-small cell lung cancer: Diagnosis and management of lung cancer, 3rd ed: American College of Chest Physicians evidence-based clinical practice guidelines. Chest. 2013;143:e211S-e250S. [PMID: 23649440] doi:10.1378/chest.12-2355

Strollo DC, Rosado de Christenson ML, Jett JR. Primary mediastinal tumors. Part 1: tumors of the anterior mediastinum. Chest. 1997;112:511-22. [PMID: 9266892]

Strollo DC, Rosado-de-Christenson ML, Jett JR. Primary mediastinal tumors: part II. Tumors of the middle and posterior mediastinum. Chest. 1997;112:1344-57. [PMID: 9367479]

Sleep Medicine

Aurora RN, Chowdhuri S, Ramar K, Bista SR, Casey KR, Lamm CI, et al. The treatment of central sleep apnea syndromes in adults: practice parameters with an evidence-based literature review and meta-analyses. Sleep. 2012;35:17-40. [PMID: 22215916] doi:10.5665/sleep.1580

Caples SM, Rowley JA, Prinsell JR, Pallanch JF, Elamin MB, Katz SG, et al. Surgical modifications of the upper airway for obstructive sleep apnea in adults: a systematic review and meta-analysis. Sleep. 2010;33:1396-407. [PMID: 21061863]

Cowie MR, Woehrle H, Wegscheider K, Angermann C, d'Ortho MP, Erdmann E, et al. Adaptive servo-ventilation for central sleep apnea in systolic heart failure. N Engl J Med. 2015;373:1095-105. [PMID: 26323938] doi:10.1056/NEJMoa1506459

Kapur VK, Auckley DH, Chowdhuri S, Kuhlmann DC, Mehra R, Ramar K, et al. Clinical practice guideline for diagnostic testing for adult obstructive sleep apnea: an American Academy of Sleep Medicine clinical practice guideline. J Clin Sleep Med. 2017;13:479-504. [PMID: 28162150] doi:10.5664/jcsm.6506

Ramar K, Dort LC, Katz SG, Lettieri CJ, Harrod CG, Thomas SM, et al. Clinical practice guideline for the treatment of obstructive sleep apnea and snoring with oral appliance therapy: an update for 2015. J Clin Sleep Med. 2015;11:773-827. [PMID: 26094920] doi:10.5664/jcsm.4858

Sack RL. Clinical practice. jet lag. N Engl J Med. 2010;362:440-7. [PMID: 20130253] doi:10.1056/NEJMcp0909838

Xie W, Zheng F, Song X. Obstructive sleep apnea and serious adverse outcomes in patients with cardiovascular or cerebrovascular disease: a PRISMA-compliant systematic review and meta-analysis. Medicine (Baltimore). 2014;93:e336. [PMID: 25546682] doi:10.1097/MD.0000000000000336

High-Altitude–Related Illnesses

Ahmedzai S, Balfour-Lynn IM, Bewick T, Buchdahl R, Coker RK, Cummin AR, et al; British Thoracic Society Standards of Care Committee. Managing passengers with stable respiratory disease planning air travel: British Thoracic

Society recommendations. Thorax. 2011;66 Suppl 1:i1–30. [PMID: 21856702] doi:10.1136/thoraxjnl-2011-200295

Bärtsch P, Swenson ER. Clinical practice: acute high-altitude illnesses. N Engl J Med. 2013;368:2294-302. [PMID: 23758234] doi:10.1056/NEJMcp1214870

Hu X, Cowl CT, Baqir M, Ryu JH. Air travel and pneumothorax. Chest. 2014;145:688-694. [PMID: 24687705] doi:10.1378/chest.13-2363

Silverman D, Gendreau M. Medical issues associated with commercial flights. Lancet. 2009;373:2067-77. [PMID: 19232708] doi:10.1016/S0140-6736(09)60209-9

West JB; American College of Physicians. The physiologic basis of high-altitude diseases. Ann Intern Med. 2004;141:789-800. [PMID: 15545679]

Principles of Critical Care

Barr J, Fraser GL, Puntillo K, Ely EW, Gélinas C, Dasta JF, et al; American College of Critical Care Medicine. Clinical practice guidelines for the management of pain, agitation, and delirium in adult patients in the intensive care unit. Crit Care Med. 2013;41:263-306. [PMID: 23269131] doi:10.1097/CCM.0b013e3182783b72

Connolly B, O'Neill B, Salisbury L, Blackwood B; Enhanced Recovery After Critical Illness Programme Group. Physical rehabilitation interventions for adult patients during critical illness: an overview of systematic reviews. Thorax. 2016;71:881-90. [PMID: 27220357] doi:10.1136/thoraxjnl-2015-208273

Girard TD, Alhazzani W, Kress JP, Ouellette DR, Schmidt GA, Truwit JD, et al; ATS/CHEST Ad Hoc Committee on Liberation from Mechanical Ventilation in Adults. An Official American Thoracic Society/American College of Chest Physicians Clinical Practice Guideline: Liberation from Mechanical Ventilation in Critically Ill Adults. Rehabilitation Protocols, Ventilator Liberation Protocols, and Cuff Leak Tests. Am J Respir Crit Care Med. 2017;195:120-133. [PMID: 27762595] doi:10.1164/rccm.201610-2075ST

Hermans G, Van den Berghe G. Clinical review: intensive care unit acquired weakness. Crit Care. 2015;19:274. [PMID: 26242743] doi:10.1186/s13054-015-0993-7

Schweickert WD, Pohlman MC, Pohlman AS, et al: Early physical and occupational therapy in mechanically ventilated, critically ill patients: A randomised controlled trial. Lancet 2009; 373:1874–1882. PMID 19446324

Taylor BE, McClave SA, Martindale RG, Warren MM, Johnson DR, Braunschweig C, et al; Society of Critical Care Medicine. Guidelines for the Provision and Assessment of Nutrition Support Therapy in the Adult Critically Ill Patient: Society of Critical Care Medicine (SCCM) and American Society for Parenteral and Enteral Nutrition (A.S.P.E.N.). Crit Care Med. 2016;44:390-438. [PMID: 26771786] doi:10.1097/CCM.0000000000001525

Common ICU Conditions

Briel M, Meade M, Mercat A, Brower RG, Talmor D, Walter SD, et al. Higher vs lower positive end-expiratory pressure in patients with acute lung injury and acute respiratory distress syndrome: systematic review and meta-analysis. JAMA. 2010;303:865-73. [PMID: 20197533] doi:10.1001/jama.2010.218

Brower RG, Matthay MA, Morris A, Schoenfeld D, Thompson BT, Wheeler A; Acute Respiratory Distress Syndrome Network. Ventilation with lower tidal volumes as compared with traditional tidal volumes for acute lung injury and the acute respiratory distress syndrome. N Engl J Med. 2000;342:1301-8. [PMID: 10793162]

Fan E, Del Sorbo L, Goligher EC, Hodgson CL, Munshi L, Walkey AJ, et al; American Thoracic Society, European Society of Intensive Care Medicine, and Society of Critical Care Medicine. An official American Thoracic Society/European Society of Intensive Care Medicine/Society of Critical Care Medicine clinical practice guideline: mechanical ventilation in adult patients with acute respiratory distress syndrome. Am J Respir Crit Care Med. 2017;195:1253-1263. [PMID: 28459336] doi:10.1164/rccm.201703-0548ST

Global Strategy for the Diagnosis, Management and Prevention of COPD, Global Initiative for Chronic Obstructive Lung Disease (GOLD) 2017. http://goldcopd.org. Accessed May 25, 2018.

Guérin C, Reignier J, Richard JC, Beuret P, Gacouin A, Boulain T, et al; PROSEVA Study Group. Prone positioning in severe acute respiratory distress syndrome. N Engl J Med. 2013;368:2159-68. [PMID: 23688302] doi:10.1056/NEJMoa1214103

National Heart, Lung and Blood Institute. National Asthma Education and Prevention Program. Expert Panel Report 3: Guidelines for the Diagnosis and Management of Asthma. August 28, 2007: www.nhlbi.nih.gov/guidelines/asthma/asthgdln.pdf. Accessed May 25, 2018.

Papazian L, Forel JM, Gacouin A, Penot-Ragon C, Perrin G, Loundou A, et al; ACURASYS Study Investigators. Neuromuscular blockers in early acute respiratory distress syndrome. N Engl J Med. 2010;363:1107-16. [PMID: 20843245] doi:10.1056/NEJMoa1005372

Ranieri VM, Rubenfeld GD, Thompson BT, Ferguson ND, Caldwell E, Fan E, et al; ARDS Definition Task Force. Acute respiratory distress syndrome: the berlin definition. JAMA. 2012;307:2526-33. [PMID: 22797452] doi:10.1001/jama.2012.5669

Rhodes A, Evans LE, Alhazzani W, Levy MM, Antonelli M, Ferrer R, et al. Surviving sepsis campaign: international guidelines for management of sepsis and septic shock: 2016. Crit Care Med. 2017;45:486-552. [PMID: 28098591] doi:10.1097/CCM.0000000000002255

Singer M, Deutschman CS, Seymour CW, Shankar-Hari M, Annane D, Bauer M, et al. The third international consensus definitions for sepsis and septic shock (Sepsis-3). JAMA. 2016;315:801-10. [PMID: 26903338] doi:10.1001/jama.2016.0287

Wiedemann HP, Wheeler AP, Bernard GR, Thompson BT, Hayden D, deBoisblanc B, et al; National Heart, Lung, and Blood Institute Acute Respiratory Distress Syndrome (ARDS) Clinical Trials Network. Comparison of two fluid-management strategies in acute lung injury. N Engl J Med. 2006; 354:2564-75. [PMID: 16714767]

Specific Critical Care Topics

Brooks DE, Levine M, O'Connor AD, French RNE, Curry SC. Toxicology in the ICU: part 2: specific toxins. Chest. 2011;140:1072-1085. [PMID: 21972388] doi:10.1378/chest.10-2726

Elmer J, Callaway CW. The brain after cardiac arrest. Semin Neurol. 2017;37:19-24. [PMID: 28147414] doi:10.1055/s-0036-1597833

Leon LR, Bouchama A. Heat stroke. Compr Physiol. 2015;5:611-47. [PMID: 25880507] doi:10.1002/cphy.c140017

Levine M, Brooks DE, Truitt CA, Wolk BJ, Boyer EW, Ruha AM. Toxicology in the ICU: Part 1: general overview and approach to treatment. Chest. 2011;140:795-806. [PMID: 21896525] doi:10.1378/chest.10-2548

Lieberman PL. Recognition and first-line treatment of anaphylaxis. Am J Med. 2014;127:S6-11. [PMID: 24384138] doi:10.1016/j.amjmed.2013.09.008

Rainer C, Scheinost NA, Lefeber EJ. Neuroleptic malignant syndrome. When levodopa withdrawal is the cause. Postgrad Med. 1991;89:175-8, 180. [PMID: 2008397]

Whelton PK, Carey RM, Aronow WS, Casey DE Jr, Collins KJ, Dennison Himmelfarb C, et al. 2017 ACC/AHA/AAPA/ABC/ACPM/AGS/APhA/ASH/ASPC/NMA/PCNA guideline for the prevention, detection, evaluation, and management of high blood pressure in adults: executive summary: A report of the American College of Cardiology/American Heart Association task force on clinical practice guidelines. Hypertension. 2018;71:1269-1324. [PMID: 29133354] doi:10.1161/HYP.0000000000000066

Pulmonary and Critical Care Medicine Self-Assessment Test

This self-assessment test contains one-best-answer multiple-choice questions. Please read these directions carefully before answering the questions. Answers, critiques, and bibliographies immediately follow these multiple-choice questions. The American College of Physicians (ACP) is accredited by the Accreditation Council for Continuing Medical Education (ACCME) to provide continuing medical education for physicians.

The American College of Physicians designates MKSAP 18 Pulmonary and Critical Care Medicine for a maximum of 25 *AMA PRA Category 1 Credits*™. Physicians should claim only the credit commensurate with the extent of their participation in the activity.

Successful completion of the CME activity, which includes participation in the evaluation component, enables the participant to earn up to 25 medical knowledge MOC points in the American Board of Internal Medicine's Maintenance of Certification (MOC) program. It is the CME activity provider's responsibility to submit participant completion information to ACCME for the purpose of granting MOC credit.

Earn Instantaneous CME Credits or MOC Points Online

Print subscribers can enter their answers online to earn instantaneous CME credits or MOC points. You can submit your answers using online answer sheets that are provided at mksap.acponline.org, where a record of your MKSAP 18 credits will be available. To earn CME credits or to apply for MOC points, you need to answer all of the questions in a test and earn a score of at least 50% correct (number of correct answers divided by the total number of questions). Please note that if you are applying for MOC points, you must also enter your birth date and ABIM candidate number. Take either of the following approaches:

- Use the printed answer sheet at the back of this book to record your answers. Go to mksap.acponline.org, access the appropriate online answer sheet, transcribe your answers, and submit your test for instantaneous CME credits or MOC points. There is no additional fee for this service.

- Go to mksap.acponline.org, access the appropriate online answer sheet, directly enter your answers, and submit your test for instantaneous CME credits or MOC points. There is no additional fee for this service.

Earn CME Credits or MOC Points by Mail or Fax

Pay a $20 processing fee per answer sheet and submit the printed answer sheet at the back of this book by mail or fax, as instructed on the answer sheet. Make sure you calculate your score and enter your birth date and ABIM candidate number, and fax the answer sheet to 215-351-2799 or mail the answer sheet to Member and Customer Service, American College of Physicians, 190 N. Independence Mall West, Philadelphia, PA 19106-1572, using the courtesy envelope provided in your MKSAP 18 slipcase. You will need your 10-digit order number and 8-digit ACP ID number, which are printed on your packing slip. Please allow 4 to 6 weeks for your score report to be emailed back to you. Be sure to include your email address for a response.

If you do not have a 10-digit order number and 8-digit ACP ID number, or if you need help creating a username and password to access the MKSAP 18 online answer sheets, go to mksap.acponline.org or email custserv@acponline.org.

CME credits and MOC points are available from the publication date of December 31, 2018, until December 31, 2021. You may submit your answer sheet or enter your answers online at any time during this period.

Item 1

A 52-year-old woman is evaluated in the emergency department for wheezing, dyspnea, and cough productive of clear sputum, which have worsened during the past 3 days despite use of her albuterol inhaler up to four times daily. She has no environmental triggers or recent respiratory infection. She smokes two packs of cigarettes per day and is unable to quit. History is notable for anxiety and a 20-year history of asthma. She has had two exacerbations in the past year and was hospitalized and briefly intubated for one of them. Her prescription for budesonide/formoterol controller inhaler ran out 2 weeks ago, and she has been unable to refill it. Other medications are albuterol, montelukast, and alprazolam.

On physical examination, temperature is 37.0 °C (98.6 °F), blood pressure is 140/82 mm Hg, pulse rate is 140/min, and respiration rate is 32/min with increased work of breathing. Oxygen saturation is 89% breathing ambient air. Chest examination demonstrates poor air movement with faint expiratory wheezing. The remainder of the examination is normal.

Chest radiograph demonstrates hyperinflation without infiltrates.

Albuterol improves her symptoms.

Which of the following is the most appropriate management?

(A) Admit patient to the hospital for inpatient management

(B) Begin prednisone and schedule outpatient follow-up

(C) Refill patient's prescription for budesonide/formoterol and schedule outpatient follow-up

(D) Refill patient's prescription for budesonide/formoterol, begin prednisone, and schedule outpatient follow-up

Item 2

A 37-year-old man is evaluated for a 1-month history of worsening cough and wheezing requiring use of rescue therapy several times per week, as well as increasing nasal congestion and rhinorrhea. He has a history of moderate persistent asthma and rhinitis since his early twenties. One month ago the patient underwent repair of a traumatic anterior cruciate ligament tear and has some residual daily knee pain. His medical history is notable for sinusitis. He has no symptoms of gastroesophageal reflux disease. Medications are albuterol, budesonide/formoterol, and ibuprofen.

On physical examination, vital signs are normal. Oxygen saturation is 97% breathing ambient air. Examination demonstrates conjunctival injection and nasal polyps in both nostrils. Chest examination reveals wheezing on expiration. The remainder of the examination is noncontributory.

Laboratory studies reveal IgE is 265 U/mL (265 kU/L). Complete blood count reveals a leukocyte count of 4000/μL (4×10^9/L) with 10% eosinophils.

Office spirometry demonstrates moderate airflow obstruction.

Which of the following is the most appropriate initial management?

(A) 24-Hour esophageal pH monitoring

(B) Add montelukast

(C) Discontinue ibuprofen, begin prednisone

(D) Nasal polypectomy

Item 3

A 69-year-old man is evaluated for a 3-year history of dyspnea and chronic productive cough. He was diagnosed with COPD 2 years ago after spirometry confirmed severe airflow obstruction. He discontinued smoking at that time but in the past year he was treated for three COPD exacerbations, one requiring hospitalization. Medications are tiotropium, fluticasone/salmeterol, and albuterol inhalers.

On physical examination, vital signs are normal; oxygen saturation is 92% on ambient air. He intermittently coughs during the examination. He has a prolonged expiratory phase. The remainder of the examination is unremarkable.

Chest radiograph shows the lungs to be clear.

Spirometry demonstrates a postbronchodilator FEV_1 of 45% of predicted.

Which of the following long-term treatments is most likely to reduce this patient's exacerbations of COPD?

(A) Prednisone

(B) Roflumilast

(C) Theophylline

(D) Trimethoprim-sulfamethoxazole

Item 4

A 57-year-old man is evaluated for a 6-month history of daytime sleepiness. His wife complains of his loud snoring and has observed breathing pauses; he sometimes awakens with a gasp. He has nocturia twice per night. He takes no medications.

On physical examination, vital signs are normal. Oxygen saturation is 96% breathing ambient air. BMI is 33. He has a crowded oropharynx with a low-lying soft palate; his neck is 46 cm (18 in) in circumference; he has trace edema at the ankles. Cardiovascular and neurologic examinations are normal.

Which of the following is the most appropriate management?

(A) Auto-adjusting positive airway pressure

(B) Home sleep testing

(C) Multiple sleep latency testing

(D) Overnight pulse oximetry

Item 5

A 72-year-old man is evaluated during a follow-up visit. He was evaluated in the emergency department 2 weeks ago for the sudden onset of chest pain. A CT scan was negative for pulmonary embolism but demonstrated an 8-mm ground-glass nodule in the right upper lobe. He has had no recurrence of chest pain. His history is significant for hypertension treated with lisinopril.

Upon physical examination, vital signs are normal. The remainder of the physical examination is normal. The patient undergoes follow-up CT scans of his lung at 12 months and also at 2 years. The nodule is unchanged.

Which of the following is the most appropriate management of the lung nodule?

(A) Chest CT scans every 2 years for 5 years
(B) PET/CT scan
(C) Tissue sampling
(D) No further follow-up is needed

Item 6

A 72-year-old man is hospitalized for progressive dyspnea and cough following a sore throat 3 weeks ago. Medical history is significant for idiopathic pulmonary fibrosis diagnosed 4 years ago that required 2 L/min of oxygen at rest. He is disabled because of his lung disease and is homebound. His only medication is pirfenidone.

On physical examination, blood pressure is 150/95 mm Hg, pulse rate is 105/min, and respiration rate is 28/min. Oxygen saturation is 89% on 6 L/min of oxygen. Lung examination demonstrates diffuse inspiratory crackles in all zones that are worse at the bases. He has clubbing and trace edema but no jugular venous distention.

Bronchoalveolar lavage is positive only for rhinovirus.
B-type natriuretic peptide is 20 pg/mL.

High-resolution CT scan with contrast demonstrates new bilateral ground-glass opacities on a background of basal-predominant septal line thickening with traction bronchiectasis and honeycomb changes. CT angiography demonstrates no evidence of pulmonary embolism.

Which of the following is the most likely diagnosis?

(A) Acute exacerbation of idiopathic pulmonary fibrosis
(B) Acute heart failure
(C) Acute hypersensitivity pneumonitis
(D) Nonspecific interstitial pneumonia

Item 7

A 32-year-old man is evaluated in the hospital for symptoms of persistent asthma. He was evaluated in the emergency department 2 days ago for dyspnea accompanied by wheezing, dysphonia, and upper chest and throat tightness. Symptoms persisted despite use of albuterol inhaler every 3 to 4 hours and intravenous methylprednisolone, and he was hospitalized. He was diagnosed with asthma in high school and generally requires several courses of prednisone per year. Current medications are albuterol and fluticasone/salmeterol inhalers, prednisone, and montelukast.

On physical examination, blood pressure is 130/85 mm Hg, pulse rate is 110/min, and respiration rate is 18/min. Oxygen saturation is 100% on 2 L/min of oxygen through nasal cannula. BMI is 25. Chest examination demonstrates monophonic wheezing on inspiration.

Laboratory studies, including complete blood count, metabolic panel, and IgE, are normal.

Chest radiograph is clear and bedside spirometry is normal.

Which of the following is the most appropriate management?

(A) CT scan of the sinuses
(B) Increase prednisone dosage
(C) Laryngoscopy
(D) Polysomnography

Item 8

A 56-year-old man hospitalized for respiratory failure is evaluated for new-onset confusion. He has acute respiratory distress syndrome secondary to community-acquired pneumonia. He has been in the critical care unit for 3 days. He is orally intubated and placed on mechanical ventilation. Current medications are ceftriaxone, azithromycin, and propofol for light sedation according to protocol.

On physical examination, temperature is 38.3 °C (100.9 °F), blood pressure is 100/45 mm Hg, pulse rate is 112/min, and respiration rate is 24/min. He cannot focus his attention, does not follow simple commands, and has demonstrated fluctuating mental status during the past 8 hours. The neurological examination is otherwise normal. He appears to be comfortable and shows no signs of pain.

Arterial blood gas studies show a pH of 7.41, a P_{CO_2} of 38 mm Hg (5.1 kPa), and a P_{O_2} of 62 mm Hg (8.2 kPa). Serum sodium, serum creatinine, and blood urea nitrogen are normal.

Chest radiograph shows multifocal opacities consistent with pneumonia and acute respiratory distress syndrome.

In addition to orientation strategies and promoting a normal sleep-wake cycle, which of the following is the most appropriate management?

(A) Add haloperidol
(B) Add lorazepam
(C) Early mobilization
(D) Increase propofol

Item 9

A 62-year-old man is evaluated during a general medical exam. He is a current smoker with a 42-pack-year history. He has a chronic cough but no shortness of breath or chronic health conditions.

On physical examination, vital signs and the remainder of the physical examination are normal.

Which of the following interventions is most likely to improve this patient's long-term survival?

(A) Annual chest radiograph
(B) Annual low-dose CT scan
(C) Annual sputum cytology
(D) Smoking cessation

Item 10

A 56-year-old man is hospitalized for hematemesis. He vomited 300 mL of bright red blood 15 minutes ago. He has a history of heavy alcohol use and cirrhosis. He takes no medications.

On physical examination, blood pressure is 99/50 mm Hg, pulse rate is 110/min, and respiration rate is 25/min. Oxygen saturation is 93% breathing ambient air. He is only responsive to painful stimuli. He is jaundiced. His breathing is shallow but without accessory muscle use. Lung examination reveals rhonchi. There are telangiectasias on his chest. Ascites is present. The remainder of the examination is unremarkable.

Laboratory studies reveal a hemoglobin level of 8 g/dL (80 g/L), total bilirubin of 6.8 mg/dL (116.3 μmol/L), aspartate aminotransferase of 154 U/L, and alanine aminotransferase of 54 U/L.

Two large-bore intravenous lines have been placed and crystalloid resuscitation has been initiated.

Which of the following should be done next?

(A) Administer a nonselective β-blocker
(B) Administer oxygen by nasal cannula
(C) Emergency upper endoscopy
(D) Initiate noninvasive bilevel positive airway pressure
(E) Insert an endotracheal tube

Item 11

A 30-year-old man presents for a refill on his albuterol inhaler. In the past he only needed albuterol once or twice a month, generally related to exercise. Over the last 4 to 5 months, he has noted that he needs his albuterol inhaler at least 3 or 4 times weekly for symptoms not associated with exercise. There are no apparent environmental triggers, symptoms of reflux, sinus symptoms, or recent respiratory infections. His medical and family history is otherwise unremarkable.

On physical examination, vital signs are normal. Oxygen saturation is 97% breathing ambient air. He has expiratory wheezing. Cardiac examination is normal.

Laboratory studies, including complete blood count and IgE level, are normal.

On spirometry FEV_1 is 82% of predicted and improves significantly following inhaled albuterol. His inhaler technique is excellent.

Which of the following is the most appropriate treatment?

(A) Beclomethasone
(B) Fluticasone/salmeterol
(C) Ipratropium
(D) Montelukast

Item 12

A 72-year-old man is evaluated for nonproductive cough and progressively worsening dyspnea on exertion during the past year. He has no history of dry eyes, dry mouth, Raynaud phenomenon, arthralgia, myalgia, or arthritis. He has a 30-pack-year smoking history and quit 15 years ago.

Currently retired, he worked as a car insurance adjustor and reports no environmental exposures.

On physical examination, vital signs are normal. Oxygen saturation is 95% breathing ambient air. Findings on lung examination include late velcro inspiratory crackles at the bases. Bilateral clubbing is present. The remainder of the physical examination is normal.

Spirometry shows an FVC of 82% of predicted, an FEV_1 of 90% of predicted, an FEV_1/FVC ratio of 0.85, and a D_{LCO} of 65% of predicted.

Chest radiograph shows an increase in reticular markings at the lung bases. High-resolution CT scan shows bilateral peripheral and basal predominant septal line thickening with honeycombing at the bases.

Which of the following is the most likely diagnosis?

(A) Desquamative interstitial pneumonia
(B) Hypersensitivity pneumonitis
(C) Idiopathic pulmonary fibrosis
(D) Pulmonary Langerhans cell histiocytosis
(E) Respiratory bronchiolitis–associated interstitial lung disease

Item 13

A 38-year-old woman is evaluated for 24 hours of fever, myalgia, and confusion. She returned from a camping trip in the woods 5 days ago.

On physical examination, temperature is 39.0 °C (102.2 °F), blood pressure is 80/34 mm Hg, pulse rate is 125/min, and respiration rate is 24/min. Oxygen saturation is 95% breathing ambient air. She has right axillary lymphadenopathy. She is confused. The skin is warm and dry. Her right hand is erythematous and has a wound with purulent drainage. Lung examination reveals scattered basilar crackles. Cardiac examination shows no gallops, murmurs, or jugular venous distention. The remainder of the physical examination is noncontributory.

Which of the following is required to assess this patient's intravascular volume status before fluid administration?

(A) Central venous catheter measure of venous pressure
(B) Inferior vena cava collapsibility on echocardiography
(C) Pulmonary artery catheter measurements
(D) Pulse pressure variation
(E) No additional testing

Item 14

A 67-year-old man is evaluated in the emergency department with a 3-day history of weakness and nausea and a 2-week history of difficulty swallowing. He has lost 22.7 kg (50 lb) during the past year. He has no other symptoms. History is significant for a 30-pack-year history of smoking. He quit smoking 4 years ago. He takes no medications.

On physical examination, vital signs are normal. Lung examination reveals decreased tactile fremitus above the lower portion of the right lung as well as dullness to percussion and decreased breath sounds. His neurologic examination is normal.

Laboratory studies reveal a serum sodium concentration of 127 mEq/L (127 mmol/L).

A chest CT scan is shown.

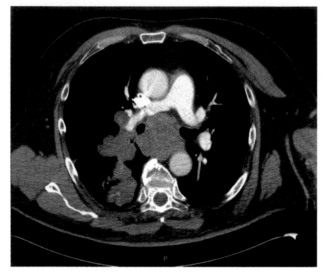

Which of the following is the most likely diagnosis?

(A) Adenocarcinoma of the lung
(B) Malignant pleural mesothelioma
(C) Small cell lung cancer
(D) Squamous cell carcinoma of the lung

Item 15

A 62-year-old woman is evaluated in the emergency department for worsening dyspnea on exertion during the last 2 weeks. She has a history of severe COPD and an FEV_1 of 45% of predicted. She has a cough productive of yellow sputum and wheezing during the same time period. She has a 20-pack-year history of smoking but quit 10 years ago. Her albuterol inhaler and nebulizer have provided temporary relief at home. Current medications are umeclidinium/vilanterol, mometasone, and albuterol.

On physical examination, temperature is normal, blood pressure is 132/64 mm Hg, pulse rate is 110/min, and respiration rate is 30/min. Oxygen saturation is 90% on 6 L/min of oxygen by nasal cannula. Cardiopulmonary examination reveals tachycardia, tachypnea with accessory muscle use, and decreased breath sounds throughout with a prolonged expiratory phase and end expiratory wheezes. She has no jugular venous distention or edema.

Laboratory studies reveal an arterial P_{CO_2} of 46 mm Hg (6.11 kPa). Complete blood count, serum electrolytes, and blood glucose are normal.

A chest radiograph shows hyperinflated lungs with flattening of the diaphragms but no infiltrate.

Which of the following is the most appropriate next additional test?

(A) CT pulmonary angiogram
(B) Electrocardiogram
(C) Sputum culture
(D) Sputum Gram stain

Item 16

A 62-year-old man is evaluated for sleep apnea. He was recently hospitalized for atrial fibrillation with rapid ventricular rate. He sleeps 8 hours most nights but awakens feeling unrested. He is likely to doze off during the day while watching TV and reading the newspaper. He has hypertension and type 2 diabetes mellitus. Current medications are apixaban, lisinopril, metoprolol, and metformin.

On physical examination, blood pressure is 154/90 mm Hg and pulse rate is 82/min. Oxygen saturation is 98% breathing ambient air. BMI is 29. He has a low-lying soft palate, prominent tongue base, and an irregular heart rhythm. Cardiac examination reveals an irregular rhythm and variable intensity of S_1. There are no findings of heart failure.

Polysomnography demonstrates moderate obstructive sleep apnea (apnea–hypopnea index 18/hour).

Hemoglobin A_{1c} measurement is 7.5%.

Which of the patient's conditions is the strongest indication for positive airway pressure therapy?

(A) Atrial fibrillation
(B) Diabetes
(C) Excessive daytime sleepiness
(D) Hypertension

Item 17

A 39-year-old man with obesity hypoventilation syndrome is hospitalized for hypoxemia and altered mental status. Three hours ago he was placed on bilevel positive airway pressure (BPAP) with 50% oxygen. History is significant for obesity, diabetes, and obesity hypoventilation syndrome for which he is receiving home nocturnal BPAP ventilation and metformin. He has been unsuccessful in losing weight with diet and medications; he is being evaluated for bariatric surgery.

On physical examination, blood pressure is 150/78 mm Hg, pulse rate is 90/min, and respiration rate is 16/min. BMI is 42. Oxygen saturation is 96% on 50% oxygen. His respirations are shallow without wheezing. He is somnolent but awakens to light touch. He has an intact cough and gag reflex.

Chest radiograph shows small lung volumes, normal heart, and normal vascularization of the lung parenchyma.

Arterial blood gas studies on BPAP and 50% oxygen:

	3 Hours Ago	Now
Bicarbonate	29 mEq/L (29 mmol/L)	28 mEq/L (28 mmol/L)
pH	7.21	7.17
P_{O_2}	114 mm Hg (15.1 kPa)	108 mm Hg (14.4 kPa)
P_{CO_2}	74 mm Hg (9.8 kPa)	80 mm Hg (10.6 kPa)

Which of the following is the most appropriate treatment?

(A) Acetazolamide
(B) Endotracheal intubation
(C) Prednisone
(D) Theophylline

Item 18

A 42-year-old man is evaluated in the office for follow-up of progressive dyspnea of 2 years' duration. He first noted dyspnea with exercise but now has symptoms when walking up a flight of stairs. He has intermittent wheezing but no coughing or nocturnal respiratory symptoms. At the time of his initial evaluation 2 years ago, pulmonary function tests demonstrated moderate airflow obstruction. He has a 1-pack-year smoking history but has not smoked in 20 years. He has no environmental exposures. His father and uncle both have emphysema without a history of smoking. He takes no medications.

On physical examination, vital signs are normal. Oxygen saturation is 94% breathing ambient air. Examination reveals no clubbing or jugular venous distention, extra cardiac sounds, edema, pulmonary crackles, or wheezing.

A chest radiograph shows hyperinflation and diaphragmatic flattening.

Which of the following is the most appropriate test to perform next?

(A) α_1-Antitrypsin level
(B) Exhaled nitric oxide test
(C) High-resolution CT scan of the chest
(D) Vascular endothelial growth factor-D

Item 19

A 46-year-old man is evaluated for problems with auto-adjusting positive airway pressure therapy that was prescribed 3 weeks ago for severe obstructive sleep apnea. He awakens with a sore throat, nasal congestion, and an occasional headache. Download from the device shows a residual apnea-hypopnea index of 3, which correlates with a decrease in his daytime sleepiness.

On physical examination, vital signs are normal. BMI is 33. He has a crowded oropharynx; low-hanging soft palate; 1+ tonsils; and boggy, erythematous nasal mucosa.

Which of the following is the most appropriate treatment?

(A) Bilevel positive airway pressure
(B) Eszopiclone
(C) Heated humidification
(D) Nasal fluticasone spray

Item 20

A 49-year-old woman is evaluated in the office following a recent hospitalization for an asthma exacerbation. Her symptoms have improved but she continues to have dyspnea and intermittent wheezing. She has had two other hospitalizations within the past year for asthma exacerbations despite the chronic use of oral glucocorticoids. Other than a 3-year history of asthma, her medical history is unremarkable. Medications are mometasone/formoterol, montelukast, albuterol, tiotropium, and prednisone.

On physical examination, vital signs are normal. Oxygen saturation is 95% on ambient air. Pulmonary examination reveals expiratory wheezes with good air movement. The remainder of the physical examination is unremarkable.

Laboratory studies reveal leukocyte count of 10,000/μL (10×10^9/L) with 650 eosinophils/μL (0.65×10^9/L). Serum IgE level is 12 U/mL (12 kU/L) (normal range, 0-90 U/mL [0-90 kU/L]).

FEV_1 is 56% of predicted.

Chest radiograph is normal.

Which of the following is the most appropriate treatment?

(A) Begin doxycycline
(B) Change mometasone/formoterol to fluticasone/salmeterol
(C) Initiate a trial of mepolizumab therapy
(D) Initiate a trial of omalizumab therapy

Item 21

A 79-year-old woman is brought into the emergency department after she was found unconscious in her apartment by a neighbor. She had been using a propane-fueled heater to heat her small apartment. No other medical history is available.

On physical examination, blood pressure is 100/64 mm Hg, pulse rate is 70/min, and respiration rate is 16/min. Pulse oximetry shows 100% oxygen saturation on mechanical ventilation using 50% oxygen. She is unresponsive to pain or voice but has intact normal deep tendon and brainstem reflexes.

Co-oximetry shows a carboxyhemoglobin level of 50%. CT scan of the head shows no acute changes.

Which of the following is the most appropriate treatment?

(A) Continue current management
(B) Decrease oxygen to 30%
(C) Hydroxocobalamin administration
(D) Hyperbaric oxygen therapy

Item 22

A 55-year-old man with COPD is evaluated in the emergency department for worsening dyspnea. He was doing well until 3 days ago when he developed fever, myalgia, increased cough productive of yellow sputum, and progressive dyspnea. He has no headaches, hypersomnolence, tremors, or extremity edema. Pulmonary function tests obtained 4 months ago demonstrated severe obstruction with air trapping. Current medications are albuterol and umeclidinium/vilanterol.

On physical examination, temperature is 38.2 °C (100.9 °F), blood pressure is 142/82 mm Hg, pulse rate is 94/min, and respiration rate is 18/min. Oxygen saturation is 90% breathing ambient air. He has end-expiratory wheezing throughout. There is no jugular venous distention or extra cardiac sounds.

A complete blood count and comprehensive metabolic profile are normal.

Other than tachycardia, an electrocardiogram is normal. Chest radiograph shows the lungs to be clear.

Therapy for a COPD exacerbation is initiated.

Which of the following is the most appropriate next diagnostic test?

(A) Arterial blood gas analysis
(B) B-type natriuretic peptide measurement
(C) CT pulmonary angiography
(D) Echocardiogram

Item 23

A 35-year-old woman is evaluated for a 4-month history of exertional dyspnea and a 1-week history of chest pressure. She has no sputum production, cough, or wheezes. She has never smoked.

On physical examination, vital signs are normal. Oxygen saturation is 91% breathing ambient air. Cardiopulmonary examination reveals a widened split S_2 with a prominent pulmonic component and neck vein distention. Lungs are clear to auscultation.

Laboratory studies, including complete blood count and comprehensive metabolic profile, are normal.

Electrocardiogram is normal.

Chest radiograph shows clear lung fields and prominent hilae.

Which of the following is the most appropriate initial test?

(A) High resolution CT of the chest
(B) Pulmonary function testing
(C) Transthoracic echocardiogram
(D) Ventilation-perfusion ($\dot{V}/\dot{Q}$) scan

Item 24

A 58-year-old man is evaluated for follow-up of an asthma exacerbation with no clear trigger, which improved with oral glucocorticoids and a short-acting β_2-agonist in addition to his outpatient medications. The patient has a 30-year history of asthma and has had two previous exacerbations during the preceding 12 months. He has no environmental triggers, allergies, atopy, symptoms of reflux, sinus symptoms, snoring, or recent respiratory infections. A recent sleep study was negative for obstructive sleep apnea. Medications are albuterol, budesonide/formoterol, montelukast, tiotropium, and prednisone.

On physical examination, vital signs are normal. Oxygen saturation is 97% breathing ambient air. BMI is 36. Pulmonary examination reveals scattered expiratory wheezing. Cardiac examination is normal.

Bedside spirometry demonstrates moderate airflow obstruction; FEV_1 improves by 15% following inhaled albuterol.

Laboratory studies, including IgE level and complete blood count, are normal.

CT scan of the sinuses is normal.

Which of the following is the most appropriate management?

(A) Add beclomethasone
(B) Perform methacholine challenge testing
(C) Start mepolizumab
(D) Start omalizumab
(E) Supervised weight loss program

Item 25

A 71-year-old man is evaluated during a follow-up visit for sleep-related breathing pauses observed by the hospital staff when he was admitted for implantation of a cardioverter-defibrillator for ischemic cardiomyopathy (left ventricular ejection fraction of 30%). He has recently experienced dyspnea, a few episodes of which have awakened him from sleep. He has no insomnia or daytime sleepiness. He has dyslipidemia, stable coronary artery disease, and hypertension. Current medications are aspirin, atorvastatin, valsartan, metoprolol, and nitroglycerin as needed.

On physical examination, vital signs are normal. Oxygen saturation is 93% breathing ambient air. BMI is 23. Lung examination reveals bibasilar crackles, faint end-expiratory wheezing, neck vein distention, and 1+ ankle edema.

Polysomnography demonstrates central sleep apnea with a Cheyne-Stokes breathing pattern.

Which of the following is the most appropriate treatment of the patient's central sleep apnea?

(A) Adaptive servo-ventilation
(B) Auto-adjusting positive airway pressure
(C) Furosemide
(D) Supplemental oxygen

Item 26

A 60-year-old woman is evaluated during a follow-up visit. She has a lifelong history of intermittent asthma previously provoked by exertion and exposure to cold air. During the past 2 years her symptoms have progressed, and she now has dyspnea after walking one block or going up any incline. COPD was diagnosed 4 days ago after spirometry revealed an FEV_1 of 65% of predicted that was only partially reversible with bronchodilator therapy. She has no history of acute exacerbations. She has recently discontinued cigarette smoking. She currently takes albuterol as needed.

On physical examination, vital signs are normal; oxygen saturation is 95% breathing ambient air. Lungs are clear to auscultation.

Laboratory studies reveal normal hemoglobin concentration and leukocyte count with 8% eosinophils.

Chest radiograph shows clear lungs.

Which of the following is the most appropriate initial treatment?

(A) Chronic macrolide therapy
(B) Inhaled glucocorticoid and long-acting β_2-agonist
(C) Long-acting β_2-agonists
(D) Long-acting muscarinic agent and long-acting β_2-agonists

Item 27

A 68-year-old man develops abrupt, pleuritic, right-sided chest pain, and dyspnea 90 minutes into a flight from Nashville to Phoenix. He is on the second week of a prednisone taper for a recent COPD exacerbation in the setting of bullous emphysema. He is on supplemental oxygen at home at 2 L/min, which was augmented to 4 L/min for the flight. Current medications are a long-acting β_2-agonist, a long-acting muscarinic agent, and prednisone.

On physical examination, blood pressure is 138/78 mm Hg, pulse rate is 114/min, and respiration rate is 24/min. He appears moderately distressed. Lung examination reveals diminished breath sounds bilaterally, tympany to percussion bilaterally, and end-expiratory wheezing. He has strong symmetric peripheral pulses but no neck vein distention. Cardiac examination is unremarkable.

Which of the following is the most likely diagnosis?

(A) Descending aortic dissection
(B) *Pneumocystis jirovecii* pneumonia
(C) Pneumothorax
(D) Pulmonary embolism

Item 28

A 58-year-old man with a history of severe COPD is evaluated for his chronic exertional dyspnea. He is taking his inhalers and medications as prescribed with excellent technique and has completed a pulmonary rehabilitation program within the last 6 months and is continuing his exercise program. He is using supplemental oxygen but despite adequate oxygenation still has significant exertional dyspnea. Current medications are umeclidinium/vilanterol, mometasone, and albuterol. He feels that his current quality of life is poor and would like other treatment options.

On physical examination, vital signs are normal. Oxygen saturation is 90% on 2 L/min of oxygen. BMI is normal. Pulmonary examination reveals decreased breath sounds throughout with a prolonged expiratory phase but no wheezing.

Spirometry demonstrates severe airflow obstruction. A recent chest CT shows heterogeneous emphysema without any nodules. A recent echocardiogram shows diastolic dysfunction but no evidence of pulmonary hypertension.

Which of the following is the most appropriate management?

(A) Add daily roflumilast
(B) Evaluation for lung volume reduction surgery
(C) Obtain a right heart catheterization
(D) Repeat pulmonary rehabilitation program

Item 29

A 58-year-old man is evaluated for a 2-year history of slowly progressive exertional dyspnea with intermittent wheezing and a cough that is occasionally productive of clear sputum. He has no chest pain, palpitations, or lower extremity edema. He has a 40-pack-year history of smoking but quit 3 years ago. He has a history of coronary artery disease. He currently takes aspirin, metoprolol, rosuvastatin, and lisinopril.

On physical examination, vital signs are normal; oxygen saturation is 94% on ambient air. Pulmonary examination reveals a prolonged expiratory phase. The remainder of the physical examination is normal.

Chest radiograph shows the lungs to be clear. Electrocardiogram is normal.

Which of the following is the most appropriate test to perform next?

(A) Echocardiogram
(B) Exercise stress test
(C) High-resolution chest CT
(D) Spirometry

Item 30

A 78-year-old woman is evaluated in the hospital for progressive dyspnea requiring increased oxygen. She was diagnosed with idiopathic pulmonary fibrosis 5 years ago. She was evaluated in the clinic 2 months ago; at that time she required 5 L/min of supplemental oxygen at rest and daily activities were limited to dressing and eating, both of which caused severe dyspnea. Currently, despite broad spectrum antibiotics and intravenous methylprednisolone, 1 g daily for 5 days, she is in severe respiratory distress requiring high-flow oxygen at 80%. She is alert and breathless, and understands her condition and treatment options.

On physical examination, blood pressure is 150/85 mm Hg, pulse rate is 110/min, and respiration rate is 36/min. Oxygen saturation is 88% on 80% high-flow oxygen. BMI is 24. Pulmonary examination reveals diffuse inspiratory crackles. She has clinical findings of pulmonary hypertension on cardiac examination, unchanged from 2 months ago. She has no edema or jugular venous distention.

Chest radiograph is unchanged.

Which of the following is the most appropriate management?

(A) Increase methylprednisolone
(B) Initiate albuterol
(C) Mechanical ventilation
(D) Palliative care

Item 31

A 41-year-old woman is evaluated for nonproductive cough with dyspnea on exertion for the past 6 months. Her medical history is significant for diffuse cutaneous systemic sclerosis, gastroesophageal reflux disease, and Raynaud phenomenon. Her medications are omeprazole, nifedipine, and lisinopril.

On physical examination, vital signs are normal. Oxygen saturation is 98% breathing ambient air at rest but drops to 93% with exertion. She has sclerodactyly. The lung examination is normal.

Pulmonary function tests demonstrate restriction with a total lung capacity of 70% of predicted and D_{LCO} of 65% of predicted.

Chest radiograph is normal.

Which of the following is the most appropriate diagnostic test to perform next?

(A) 6-Minute walk test
(B) Cardiopulmonary exercise testing
(C) High-resolution chest CT scan
(D) PET/CT scan

Item 32

A 62-year-old woman is evaluated for a 1-year history of cough. She works in an office and has no environmental exposures, and cannot recall any specific initiating event. Her cough seems to be triggered by temperature changes, exercise, laughter, and strong scents and perfumes. She has no sputum production, rhinitis, postnasal drip, wheezing, or gastroesophageal reflux disease. She has recently been treated with intranasal fluticasone and oral antihistamines without significant improvement. She is not taking any medications currently.

On physical examination, oxygen saturation is 97% on ambient air. All vital signs and pulmonary and cardiac examinations are normal.

Laboratory studies, including complete blood count, are normal.

Chest radiograph is normal. Pulmonary function testing shows a normal FEV_1 and FEV_1/FVC ratio.

Which of the following is the most appropriate management?

(A) Begin daily inhaled budesonide and albuterol

(B) Obtain esophageal manometry and 24-hour pH monitoring study

(C) Obtain high-resolution CT scan of the chest

(D) Obtain methacholine challenge testing

Item 33

A 45-year-old woman with hypovolemic shock is evaluated for rapid resuscitation in the ICU. She has sickle cell disease with recurrent pain and hemolytic crises, and osteoporosis.

On physical examination, temperature is 39 °C (102.3 °F), blood pressure is 70/40 mm Hg, pulse rate is 142/min and weak, and respiration rate is 22/min. Oxygen saturation is 99% breathing ambient air. There is a subcutaneous port in the right anterior chest wall.

Which of the following is the most appropriate type of venous access for this patient?

(A) Intraosseous port

(B) Peripheral wide-bore catheter

(C) Subcutaneous intravenous port

(D) Triple-lumen central catheter

Item 34

A 66-year-old man is hospitalized in December for a 1-week history of increasing dyspnea on exertion, wheezing, and a nonproductive cough despite outpatient treatment with antibiotics and steroids. He now has awakenings with nocturnal dyspnea, which are only partially relieved by the use of his albuterol inhaler. He has started using his albuterol nebulizer four times a day, which provides only temporary relief. He does not have fever, headache, myalgia, runny nose, sputum production, chest pain, lower extremity edema, or palpitations. He has a history of COPD with an FEV_1 of 42% of predicted on spirometry obtained 3 months ago. In addition to albuterol, he takes umeclidinium and vilanterol and was started on azithromycin and prednisone 3 days ago.

On physical examination, temperature is 37.1 °C (98.8 °F), blood pressure is 135/80 mm Hg, pulse rate is 110/min, and respiration rate is 22/min. Oxygen saturation is 90% on ambient air. The patient is not using his accessory muscles. He has decreased breath sounds throughout, with diffuse end-expiratory wheezes. Other than tachycardia, the cardiovascular examination is normal without jugular venous distention or edema.

Laboratory studies, including complete blood count with differential, basic metabolic panel, B-type natriuretic peptide, and arterial blood gases, are unremarkable.

Electrocardiogram demonstrates sinus tachycardia, and a chest radiograph shows hyperinflation but no infiltrates.

Which of the following is the most appropriate diagnostic test to perform next?

(A) Bedside spirometry

(B) CT pulmonary angiography

(C) Polymerase chain reaction testing for influenza A and B

(D) Sputum culture

Item 35

A 72-year-old woman is evaluated during a routine visit. She has a 30-pack-year smoking history and quit 5 years ago. She has a history of mild COPD and breast cancer diagnosed 15 years ago, currently in remission. A chest radiograph from 5 years ago showed no signs of disease recurrence. Medications are albuterol and tiotropium inhalers.

On physical examination, vital signs are normal. Lung examination reveals prolonged expiration and diminished breath sounds throughout. The breast examination is unremarkable.

A screening low-dose chest CT scan shows a peripheral 9-mm solid pulmonary nodule in the left upper lobe and emphysema but no mediastinal or hilar lymphadenopathy and no pleural effusion. A PET/CT scan using fluorodeoxyglucose (FDG) is performed and the nodule is intensely hypermetabolic. There is no evidence of distant uptake.

Which of the following is the most appropriate management?

(A) Bronchoscopy with biopsy

(B) Serial chest CT scans

(C) Surgical wedge resection

(D) Transthoracic needle aspiration

Item 36

A 75-year-old man is evaluated for a 6-month history of dyspnea on exertion. He was a construction worker between 1972 and 1986. He notes that he was often in buildings with high levels of dust without respiratory protection. He finished his working career providing janitorial services for the public school system. He is an avid wood worker and has a shop in his garage. He has never smoked. He has no other medical problems and takes no medications.

On physical examination, vital signs are normal. Lung examination reveals inspiratory crackles at the lung bases bilaterally.

Spirometry shows an FVC of 80% of predicted, an FEV_1 of 85% of predicted, and a DL_{CO} of 75% of predicted. CT scan shows pleural plaques, peripheral and basal predominant septal line thickening without ground-glass opacities, micronodules, or honeycombing.

Which of the following is the most likely diagnosis?

(A) Asbestosis

(B) Chronic hypersensitivity pneumonitis

(C) Idiopathic pulmonary fibrosis

(D) Respiratory bronchiolitis-associated interstitial lung disease

Item 37

A 24-year-old woman is treated in the emergency department for an acute asthma exacerbation. She has received continuous albuterol and ipratropium nebulization and intravenous methylprednisolone. She has persistent wheezing and dyspnea. Her outpatient medications are inhaled albuterol and fluticasone/salmeterol.

On physical examination, blood pressure is 164/84 mm Hg, pulse rate is 121/min, and respiration rate is 28/min. Oxygen saturation is 95% on 4 L/min of oxygen through nasal cannula. Peak flow is less than 40% of her baseline. She is sitting upright and is using accessory muscles of respiration and can speak four words of a sentence. Lung examination demonstrates diffuse wheezing throughout both lungs.

Which of the following is the most appropriate treatment?

(A) Ketamine infusion

(B) Magnesium sulfate, intravenously

(C) Montelukast sodium

(D) Theophylline

Item 38

A 65-year-old woman is admitted to the ICU with sepsis. She has become increasingly hypotensive despite intravenous fluid resuscitation of 30 mL/kg and the administration of increasing doses of norepinephrine and a standard dose of vasopressin. She has an arterial catheter in place. Appropriate antibiotics have been administered.

On physical examination, temperature is 37.7 °C (100 °F), blood pressure is 88/45 mm Hg, pulse rate is 116/min. Oxygen saturation is 98% on 2 L/min of oxygen through nasal cannula. She is alert and oriented. Her skin is cool. The remainder of the examination is normal.

Telemetry shows premature ventricular complexes.

Which of the following is the most appropriate treatment?

(A) Change norepinephrine to dopamine

(B) Hydrocortisone

(C) Increase the vasopressin infusion rate

(D) Intravenous immune globulin

Item 39

A 73-year-old man is evaluated for a 6-month history of right-sided chest discomfort, fatigue, nonproductive cough, and progressive dyspnea. He has lost 9 kg (20 lb) during the last 6 months. His history is significant for COPD. He was a brake mechanic for 30 years. Medications are an albuterol inhaler as needed and tiotropium inhaler.

On physical examination, vital signs are normal. Lung examination reveals dullness to percussion and diminished breath sounds above the lower half of the right hemithorax. The physical examination is otherwise normal.

Laboratory studies, including complete blood count, are normal.

Chest radiograph shows a moderate right-sided loculated pleural effusion with pleural thickening.

A thoracentesis is performed that removes 600 mL of serosanguineous fluid.

Pleural fluid analysis:

Cytology	Atypical mesothelial cells, negative for malignancy
Gram stain	Negative
Lactate dehydrogenase	425 U/L
pH	7.35
Total protein	4.6 g/dL (46 g/L)

Which of the following is the most likely diagnosis?

(A) Empyema

(B) Heart failure

(C) Malignant pleural mesothelioma

(D) Rheumatoid pleuritis

Item 40

A 60-year-old woman is evaluated for a 2-year history of dyspnea on exertion. She has dyspnea and wheezing when walking up an incline, especially if she is carrying something, but no other symptoms. She quit smoking 5 years ago and has a history of hypertension. Current medications are hydrochlorothiazide and ramipril.

On physical examination, vital signs are normal; oxygen saturation is 95% on ambient air. Lungs are clear on auscultation. Cardiovascular examination is unremarkable.

Laboratory studies reveal normal hemoglobin.

Spirometry shows a postbronchodilator FEV_1 of 75% of predicted and an FEV_1/FVC ratio of 0.65. Electrocardiogram and chest radiograph are normal.

Which of the following is the most appropriate initial treatment?

(A) Roflumilast

(B) Short-acting and long-acting bronchodilator

(C) Short-acting bronchodilator

(D) Short-acting bronchodilator and inhaled glucocorticoid

(E) Short course of prednisone

Item 41

A 54-year-old man is evaluated during a follow-up visit 1 month after an emergency appendectomy. He was diagnosed with amyotrophic lateral sclerosis 9 months ago. He was placed on supplemental oxygen for 2 nights after surgery because of nocturnal oxyhemoglobin desaturations.

Arterial blood gas studies revealed a pH of 7.42, P_{CO_2} of 53 mm Hg (7.0 kPa), P_{O_2} of 53 mm Hg (7.0 kPa), and bicarbonate of 33 mEq/L (33 mmol/L).

On physical examination, vital signs are normal. Oxygen saturation is 92% breathing ambient air. He has no difficulty managing his secretions. Examination reveals upper limb weakness, muscle fasciculations, hyperactive deep tendon reflexes, and dysarthria. Lung examination is unremarkable.

In-office measurement of FVC is 49% of predicted.

Which of the following is the most appropriate management?

(A) Bilevel positive airway pressure
(B) Continuous positive airway pressure
(C) Hypoglossal nerve stimulation
(D) Supplemental oxygen
(E) Tracheostomy

Item 42

A 21-year-old man is hospitalized for sudden onset of dyspnea with chest pain that worsens with inspiration. He has a 3-pack-year history of smoking, but his medical history is otherwise unremarkable.

On physical examination, vital signs are normal. Oxygen saturation is 95% breathing ambient air. BMI is 18. Lung examination reveals reduced lung expansion, hyperresonance to percussion, and diminished breath sounds on the left side.

Chest radiograph demonstrates a large left-sided pneumothorax.

A thoracostomy tube is inserted that provides good lung reexpansion. Repeat chest radiograph is normal.

Avoidance of which of the following is the most appropriate measure to prevent long-term recurrence of pneumothorax?

(A) Air travel
(B) Mountain climbing
(C) Smoking
(D) Strenuous exercise

Item 43

A 32-year-old woman is evaluated for a 10-day history of severe cough with increased sputum production, fever, wheezing, and dyspnea. She has a 12-year history of recurrent abdominal pain with watery stools and poor weight gain, recurrent sinusitis, and chronic cough that is productive of foul sputum. She takes no medications chronically.

On physical examination, temperature is 38.2 °C (100.8 °F), blood pressure is 92/64 mm Hg, pulse rate is 101/min, and respiration rate is 24/min. Oxygen saturation is 91% on ambient air. BMI is 18.2. Pulmonary examination reveals wheezes. Additional findings include a scaphoid abdomen and clubbing.

Laboratory studies reveal a leukocyte count of 16,000/μL (16×10^9/L), hemoglobin of 10 g/dL (100 g/L), and serum creatinine of 0.7 mg/dL (61.9 μmol/L). Serum immunoglobulin levels are normal.

Pulmonary function testing reveals an FVC of 80% of predicted, an FEV_1 of 50% of predicted, and an FEV_1/FVC ratio of 0.55.

Chest radiograph is shown.

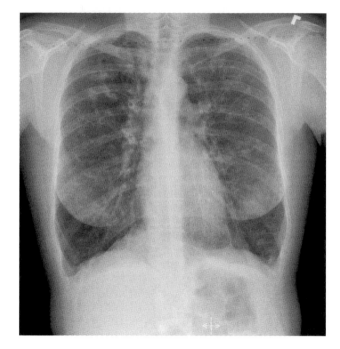

Which of the following is the most likely underlying diagnosis?

(A) Common variable immunodeficiency
(B) Complement component deficiency
(C) COPD
(D) Cystic fibrosis

Item 44

A 62-year-old woman with a history of moderate COPD is evaluated in the emergency department for increasing dyspnea, cough, and sputum production. She had been doing well until 4 days ago when she developed rhinorrhea and a cough productive of purulent sputum. During the past two days she has noted increasing dyspnea on exertion that responds transiently to her albuterol inhaler. This is the patient's first episode of this nature. She stopped smoking 18 months ago. Current medications are albuterol and tiotropium inhalers.

On physical examination, temperature is 38.1 °C (100.6 °F), blood pressure is 130/80 mm Hg, pulse rate is 102/min, and respiration rate is 22/min. Oxygen saturation is 90% on ambient air. The patient is tachypneic and catches her breath between sentences but improves after a treatment of albuterol. She has diffuse end-expiratory wheezing.

A chest radiograph shows the lungs to be clear but hyperinflated.

Arterial blood gases on 2L/min of oxygen through nasal cannula show a pH 7.38, a P_{CO_2} of 42 mm Hg (5.58 kPa), and a P_{O_2} of 70 mm Hg (9.31 kPa).

Which of the following is the most appropriate treatment?

(A) Azithromycin and prednisone
(B) Mometasone inhaler
(C) Noninvasive positive pressure ventilation
(D) Roflumilast

Item 45

A 62-year-old woman is evaluated for increasing exertional dyspnea during the past 6 months. She is a former smoker who was diagnosed with severe COPD 3 years ago (FEV_1 is 35% of predicted). For the past 18 months, she has used tiotropium and salmeterol; inhaled fluticasone was added 4 months ago, but without any perceived benefit. She takes no other medications.

On physical examination, blood pressure is 130/79 mm Hg, pulse rate is 88/min, and respiration rate is 18/min. Oxygen saturation is 89% breathing ambient air. Lung examination demonstrates diminished breath sounds. A prominent pulmonic sound is heard on cardiac examination.

Arterial blood gas studies breathing ambient air show a pH of 7.41, a P_{CO_2} of 43 mm Hg (5.7 kPa), and a P_{O_2} of 55 mm Hg (7.3 kPa).

Chest radiograph reveals hyperinflation. Echocardiography shows an estimated right ventricular systolic pressure of 58 mm Hg. Polysomnography showed an apnea–hypopnea index of 2 and a mean oxygen saturation of 87%.

Which of the following is the most appropriate treatment?

(A) Bilevel positive airway pressure
(B) Prednisone
(C) Sildenafil
(D) Supplemental oxygen

Item 46

A 46-year-old man is evaluated for 6 months of exertional dyspnea, fatigue, and ankle edema. Recently he experienced near-syncope walking up two flights of stairs. He has no other medical problems and takes no medications.

On physical examination, blood pressure is 106/70 mm Hg, pulse rate is 94/min, and respiration rate is 18/min. Oxygen saturation is 90% breathing ambient air. On cardiac examination, a prominent jugular venous *a* wave is present along with widened splitting of S_2. Lung examination is unremarkable.

A transthoracic echocardiogram demonstrates a normal size left ventricle with ejection fraction of 65% and right ventricular enlargement. The estimated pulmonary artery systolic pressure is 58 mm Hg. Spirometry, lung volumes, and ventilation–perfusion scan are unremarkable; D_{LCO} is 42% of predicted. CT angiogram of the chest is negative for pulmonary embolism and interstitial lung disease. Right heart catheterization demonstrates a mean pulmonary arterial pressure of 36 mm Hg, with no change with inhaled nitric oxide. Pulmonary capillary wedge pressure is normal.

Which of the following is the most appropriate treatment?

(A) Bosentan
(B) Diltiazem
(C) Metoprolol
(D) Pirfenidone

Item 47

A 27-year-old woman is evaluated for concern about a 3-week history of a new chemical odor in her workplace.

She has a history of mild asthma since childhood that is well-controlled with infrequent use of an albuterol inhaler. The plant safety manager at her job said there is no need for protective equipment, but she is experiencing increased cough and now uses her albuterol inhaler once daily.

On physical examination, vital signs are normal. Lungs are clear on auscultation with no wheeze.

Office spirometry shows an FVC of 98% of predicted, an FEV_1 of 93% of predicted, and an FEV_1/FVC ratio of 0.78 of predicted.

Which of the following is the most appropriate management?

(A) Chest CT scan
(B) Obtain hair sample for toxic analysis
(C) Review employer Material Safety Data Sheet
(D) Transfer patient to other area of plant

Item 48

A 49-year-old man is evaluated for a 4-month history of cough, chest pressure, and double vision. He has no fever, night sweats, or weight loss. He has never smoked.

On physical examination, vital signs are normal. There is ptosis bilaterally. The remainder of the physical examination is normal.

A CT scan of the chest is shown.

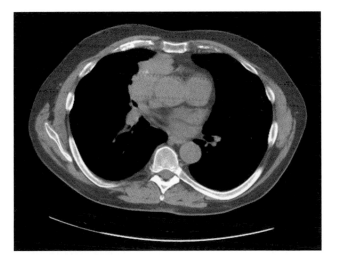

Which of the following is the most appropriate test to perform next?

(A) Acetylcholine receptor antibody
(B) α-Fetoprotein
(C) β-Human chorionic gonadotropin
(D) Lactate dehydrogenase

Item 49

A 60-year-old woman is evaluated in the hospital for respiratory failure. She was hospitalized 3 weeks ago after a house fire. She suffered significant third-degree burns covering 40% of her body and mucosal burns to her nose. She was intubated, but was successfully liberated from the ventilator last week. A surveillance bronchoscopy performed before extubation was unremarkable. Last night she became progressively dyspneic and hypoxic, eventually requiring reintubation. Current medications are topical antibiotics and subcutaneous heparin.

On physical examination, temperature is 37.9 °C (100.2 °F), blood pressure is 104/60 mm Hg, pulse rate is 95/min, and respiration rate is 26/min. Oxygen saturation is 91% breathing from a ventilator (F_{IO_2} of 0.6). Copious yellow sputum is present in the endotracheal tube when suctioned.

Laboratory studies reveal a leukocyte count of 16,000/μL (16×10^9/L), increased from 12,000/μL (12×10^9/L) yesterday.

A chest radiograph shows a focal consolidation in the lower left lobe.

Which of the following is the most appropriate treatment?

(A) Administer hydroxocobalamin
(B) Administer intravenous antibiotics
(C) Bronchoscopic airway stenting
(D) Insert a thoracostomy tube

Item 50

A 30-year-old man with a history of alcohol and drug abuse is brought to the emergency department. He was found unresponsive and on arrival he was intubated and placed on mechanical ventilation for poor respiratory effort. Witnesses confirmed that he had been drinking alcohol and had also taken drugs at a party.

On physical examination, vital signs are normal. Respiration rate is 14/min on mechanical ventilation. He is not triggering the ventilator. Oxygen saturation is 100% on 35% oxygen. He responds to pain only. His pupils are dilated and reactive to light. He shows no signs of trauma.

Blood toxicology screening is positive for alcohol; urine toxicology screening is positive for benzodiazepines. Arterial pH and electrolyte anion gap are normal.

Which of the following is the most appropriate management?

(A) Administer flumazenil
(B) Administer fomepizole
(C) Administer hemodialysis
(D) Monitor for signs of agitation

Item 51

A 22-year-old man is evaluated for acute onset of fever, chills, dyspnea, and nonproductive cough. He is a college student and spends summers using a combine to harvest wheat. He does not wear respiratory protective equipment. His symptoms start at the beginning of a work week, progress to the point that he must miss several days of work, and then the cycle begins again.

On physical examination, temperature is 37.8 °C (100.1 °F), blood pressure is 120/80 mm Hg, pulse rate is 98/min, and respiration rate is 22/min. Oxygen saturation is 94% breathing ambient air. Lung examination reveals diffuse crackles.

Chest radiograph demonstrates diffuse upper-lobe micronodular opacities.

Which of the following is the most appropriate treatment?

(A) Counsel the patient not to return to work
(B) Inhaled glucocorticoids
(C) Pirfenidone
(D) Sirolimus

Item 52

A 64-year-old woman is evaluated during a posthospital visit for severe COPD with an FEV_1 of 30% of predicted. She has been admitted three times during the last year with acute exacerbations characterized by cough, increased purulent sputum production, and dyspnea. She is now at baseline of her exertional dyspnea and has no cough. She has already participated in a pulmonary rehabilitation program. She currently takes tiotropium, budesonide/formoterol, and albuterol.

On physical examination, vital signs are normal. Oxygen saturation is 90% on 3 L/min of supplemental oxygen at rest and with exertion. Pulmonary examination reveals decreased breath sounds throughout. The remainder of the examination is noncontributory.

Which of the following is the most appropriate treatment to reduce this patient's COPD exacerbations?

(A) Chronic low-dose oral glucocorticoid
(B) Chronic macrolide therapy
(C) Increase supplemental oxygen
(D) Nebulized hypertonic saline

Item 53

A 52-year-old man is evaluated in the ICU for dyspnea that developed after aspiration of gastric contents during an upper endoscopy. The endoscopy was performed for evaluation of upper gastric bleeding due to peptic ulcer disease. His only medication is pantoprazole.

On physical examination, temperature is 37.3 °C (99.1 °F), blood pressure is 150/99 mm Hg, pulse rate is 110/min, and respiration rate is 28/min. Oxygen saturation is 90% on a 100% oxygen nonrebreather mask. He is awake, diaphoretic, and anxious. Lung examination reveals scant bilateral crackles and rhonchi as well as use of accessory muscles. The remainder of the physical examination is normal.

Arterial blood gas studies on a 100% oxygen nonrebreather mask show a pH of 7.35, a P_{CO_2} of 46 mm Hg (6.1 kPa), and a P_{O_2} of 55 mm Hg (7.3 kPa).

Chest radiograph reveals new bilateral opacities.

Which of the following is the most appropriate treatment?

(A) Continue current therapy
(B) High-flow humidified nasal cannula
(C) Intubation and mechanical ventilation
(D) Noninvasive mechanical ventilation

Item 54

A 38-year-old man is evaluated for a 6-month history of dyspnea on exertion. He has gastroesophageal reflux disease and Raynaud phenomenon. He does not smoke and has no cough or wheezing. Current medications are lansoprazole and amlodipine.

On physical examination, vital signs are normal. Oxygen saturation is 91% breathing ambient air. He has scattered telangiectasias on the face and trunk and sclerodactyly. Lung fields are clear on auscultation.

The only abnormality on pulmonary function testing is a D$_{LCO}$ of 43% of predicted.

High-resolution CT of the chest shows no evidence of parenchymal lung disease.

Which of the following is the most likely diagnosis?

(A) Cryptogenic organizing pneumonia
(B) Lymphangioleiomyomatosis
(C) Lymphoid interstitial pneumonia
(D) Pulmonary arterial hypertension

Item 55

A 58-year-old man is evaluated in the hospital for fever, hypotension, and altered mental status. He was hospitalized 2 days ago for an infected arm wound and was treated with intravenous piperacillin/tazobactam and vancomycin. This morning he developed new pain in the middle of his back and difficulty urinating. His medical history is significant for type 2 diabetes mellitus treated with metformin.

On physical examination, temperature is 39.1 °C (102.4 °F), blood pressure is 83/48 mm Hg, pulse rate is 109/min, and respiration rate is 21/min. Oxygen saturation is 98% breathing 2 L/min of oxygen through nasal cannula. He is somnolent but arousable and oriented when awake. There is erythema surrounding the wound on his right upper arm with no drainage or tenderness. There is tenderness to percussion in the middle of his back and a palpable bladder.

Laboratory studies reveal a blood serum leukocyte count of 22,000/µL (22 × 10⁹/L), and plasma glucose of 160 mg/dL (8.88 mmol/L).

Chest radiograph is unremarkable.

Which of the following is the most appropriate next step in management?

(A) Intravenous fluid bolus
(B) Intravenous insulin
(C) MRI of the spine
(D) Surgical exploration of the arm wound

Item 56

A 72-year-old woman is evaluated in the hospital for a pneumothorax. The patient has severe, oxygen-dependent COPD complicated by several exacerbations. She was hospitalized 72 hours ago with abrupt onset of chest pain and dyspnea. Chest radiography confirmed the presence of a large left-sided pneumothorax and a thoracotomy tube was placed. She had 90% expansion of the lung following thoracostomy.

On physical examination, the patient is frail appearing but comfortable. Vital signs are normal. Oxygen saturation is 96% breathing 3 L/min of oxygen through nasal cannula. Pulmonary examination reveals diminished but present breath sounds bilaterally. A left thoracostomy tube is in place.

Chest radiograph demonstrates resolution of pneumothorax with a thoracostomy tube in place.

Which of the following is the most appropriate management?

(A) Clamp thoracostomy tube
(B) Place thoracostomy tube to high suction
(C) Pleurodesis
(D) Remove thoracostomy tube

Item 57

A 66-year-old man with a history of COPD is evaluated during a routine visit. He is able to walk one flight of stairs and one block before he develops dyspnea. He was last treated for two acute exacerbations of COPD within the last year, one of which required hospitalization. He recently completed a pulmonary rehabilitation program. His medical history is significant for hypertension and a 60-pack-year smoking history. He quit smoking 5 years ago. Current medications are hydrochlorothiazide, glycopyrrolate/formoterol, and albuterol.

On physical examination, vital signs are normal; oxygen saturation is 94% on ambient air. Pulmonary examination reveals a prolonged expiratory phase. The cardiac and remainder of the physical examination are unremarkable.

Spirometry today shows a postbronchodilator FEV$_1$ of 35% of predicted. Chest radiograph at the time of his last exacerbation shows hyperinflation and no other findings. An electrocardiogram is normal.

Which of the following patient characteristics places him at highest risk for a recurrent acute exacerbation?

(A) Enrollment in a pulmonary rehabilitation program
(B) Hypertension
(C) Previous COPD exacerbations and FEV$_1$ level
(D) Smoking history and use of COPD medications

Item 58

A 70-year-old man is hospitalized for a 4-week history of dyspnea, orthopnea, and daytime sleepiness. He was diagnosed with amyotrophic lateral sclerosis 6 months ago. His only medication is riluzole.

On physical examination, blood pressure is 128/73 mm Hg, pulse rate is 90/min, and respiration rate is 28/min. Oxygen saturation is 87% breathing ambient air. He has right-hand atrophy, decreased mobility, and fasciculations. Lung examination reveals abdominal paradox with breathing, use of accessory breathing muscles, and shallow tachypnea. He is awake, alert, and interactive, but dozes off easily. His speech is clear with no secretions. He is able to move all extremities and shows no cranial nerve abnormality.

On arterial blood gas testing, pH is 7.30, P$_{CO_2}$ is 76 mm Hg (10.1 kPa), P$_{O_2}$ is 50 mm Hg (6.65 kPa), and bicarbonate is 36 mEq/L (36 mmol/L) on room air. The calculated alveolar-arterial oxygen gradient is normal.

Chest radiograph reveals bilateral basal opacities consistent with atelectasis and shallow inspiration.

H **Which of the following is the most appropriate treatment?**

CONT.

(A) Invasive mechanical ventilation

(B) Noninvasive ventilation with bilevel positive airway pressure

(C) Noninvasive ventilation with continuous positive airway pressure

(D) Oxygen administration through nasal cannula

H ## Item 59

A 60-year-old man is evaluated in the emergency department for headache, nausea, vomiting, and confusion lasting 4 hours. He ran out of his hypertensive medications a few days ago. Current medications are lisinopril, metoprolol succinate, hydrochlorothiazide, and aspirin.

On physical examination, blood pressure is 230/140 mm Hg and pulse rate is 100/min. All other vital signs are normal. He is too uncooperative to perform a mental status examination or funduscopic examination. The cardiovascular examination is positive for an S_4 but otherwise normal.

Laboratory studies reveal normal electrolytes; serum creatinine is 1.6 mg/dL (141.4 µmol/L). It was 1.2 mg/dL (106 µmol/L) at his last outpatient appointment.

Electrocardiogram shows left ventricular hypertrophy and sinus tachycardia. Chest radiograph is normal. CT scan of the brain shows no acute findings.

Which of the following is the most appropriate treatment?

(A) Intravenous hypertensive therapy to lower systolic blood pressure (SBP) to 160 mm Hg within the first 6 hours

(B) Intravenous hypertensive therapy to lower SBP to 120 mm Hg within the first hour

(C) Intravenous hypertensive therapy to lower SBP to 160 mm Hg within the first 48 hours

(D) Resume usual oral antihypertensive regimen and observe

H ## Item 60

A 30-year-old woman is evaluated in the emergency department after she was rescued from her home where her vinyl sofa caught fire. She is intubated and unconscious.

On physical examination, blood pressure is 108/78 mm Hg, pulse rate is 100/min, and respiration rate is 24/min. Oxygen saturation by pulse oximetry is 100% on mechanical ventilation using 50% oxygen. She is unresponsive. She has no visible burns on her skin, and her airway secretions are clear. Brainstem reflexes are all intact.

Laboratory studies:

Serum electrolytes:

Sodium	140 mEq/L (140 mmol/L)
Potassium	4.4 mEq/L (4.4 mmol/L)
Chloride	99 mEq/L (99 mmol/L)
Bicarbonate	13.1 mEq/L (13.1 mmol/L)

Arterial blood gas studies:

pH	7.29
Pco_2	28 mm Hg (3.7 kPa)
Po_2	233 mm Hg (31 kPa)
Carboxyhemoglobin	5%
Methemoglobin	2%
Lactate	11 mEq/L (1.2 mmol/L)

The oxygen is increased to 100%.

Which of the following is the most appropriate treatment?

(A) Hydroxocobalamin

(B) Hyperbaric oxygen therapy

(C) Methylene blue

(D) Sodium nitrite

Item 61

A 35-year-old man is evaluated for chronic cough productive of foul-smelling sputum. He has been treated with four courses of antibiotics in the last 12 months; several infections have been associated with *Pseudomonas* species. His symptoms have been present for many years and are also associated with chronic sinusitis. He was recently diagnosed with infertility.

On physical examination, all vital signs are normal. Oxygen saturation is 98% on ambient air. Clubbing is present. Pulmonary examination reveals rhonchi and wheezes in the upper lobes bilaterally.

Chest radiograph reveals bilateral upper-lobe bronchiectasis.

Laboratory studies reveal a negative sweat chloride test of 39 mEq/L (39 mmol/L).

Which of the following is the most appropriate management?

(A) Begin chronic ciprofloxacin therapy

(B) Begin tiotropium

(C) Repeat sweat chloride testing

(D) Test for α_1-antitrypsin deficiency

Item 62

A 62-year-old man undergoes routine follow-up evaluation. His medical history is significant for tobacco use (35-pack-year) and hypertension controlled with lisinopril. He quit smoking 3 months ago and does not have any cough, wheezing, or shortness of breath.

On physical examination, vital signs are normal. BMI is 31. Cardiopulmonary examination is normal.

Which of the following is the most appropriate test?

(A) 6-Minute walk test

(B) Chest radiograph

(C) Low-dose CT scan of the chest

(D) Office spirometry

(E) Urinary cotinine test

Item 63 **H**

A 22-year-old man is evaluated in the hospital for decreased responsiveness. He was hospitalized 4 days ago after a motor vehicle accident. He has multiple fractures and a chest contusion. He was intubated for respiratory distress in the emergency department and given morphine, propofol, and heparin. He is on volume-controlled continuous mandatory ventilation mode with an FIO_2 of 0.7.

On physical examination, temperature is 37.7 °C (99.9 °F), blood pressure is 124/65 mm Hg, pulse rate is 89/min, and respiration rate is 27/min. Oxygen saturation is 93% on mechanical ventilation. He is unresponsive to voice or pain, and his pupils are 3 mm and reactive; the neurological examination is otherwise nonfocal. He has external fixators in both lower extremities. There are bruises on the anterior chest wall. The remainder of the physical examination is noncontributory.

Which of the following is the most appropriate management?

(A) Change propofol to dexmedetomidine
(B) CT of the head
(C) Continuous electroencephalography
(D) Stop sedation and analgesia

Item 64

A 61-year-old man is evaluated in the emergency department after he collapsed on a hot and humid day. He was playing in a marching band and had to stand in the sun for 2 hours while wearing a heavy uniform. No other medical information is available.

On physical examination, temperature is 40 °C (104 °F), blood pressure is 90/45 mm Hg, pulse rate is 110/min, and respiration rate is 20/min. His face is flushed, he is somnolent, and although he is arousable, he is not coherent. There are no signs of trauma.

His clothing is removed.

Which of the following is the most appropriate treatment?

(A) Acetaminophen and a cooling blanket
(B) Continuous alcohol sponge bath with cooling fans
(C) Ice water immersion
(D) Intravenous dantrolene
(E) Sprayed water and cooling fans

Item 65

A 53-year-old man is evaluated in the emergency department after 4 days of cough, fever, chills, myalgia, and poor appetite. He currently has increased dyspnea and lightheadedness. His child was diagnosed with influenza 2 weeks ago.

On physical examination, temperature is 38.8 °C (101.8 °F), blood pressure is 82/40 mm Hg, pulse rate is 128/min, and respiration rate is 17/min. Oxygen saturation is 92% on ambient air. The cardiac examination reveals regular rhythm and tachycardia without an S_3 or jugular venous distention. Lungs are clear on auscultation and extremities are warm. The remainder of the examination is normal.

Laboratory studies:

Hemoglobin	10 g/dL (100 g/L)
Lactate	4.6 mEq/L (4.6 mmol/L)
Leukocyte count	18,000/µL (18 × 10⁹/L)
Arterial blood gases:	
pH	7.32
P_{CO_2}	32 mm Hg (4.3 kPa)
P_{O_2}	70 mm Hg (9.3 kPa)
Bicarbonate	16 mEq/L (16 mmol/L)

A chest radiograph shows basilar ground-glass opacities on the right. Electrocardiogram reveals sinus tachycardia but is otherwise normal.

Which of the following is the most appropriate initial treatment?

(A) 0.9% saline bolus
(B) Intravenous furosemide
(C) Norepinephrine
(D) Packed red blood cells

Item 66

A 19-year-old man is evaluated in the emergency department for cardiac arrest after he fell through the ice of a frozen lake. He was in the water for less than 10 minutes, but when he was pulled out onto the ice he was unresponsive and no pulse could be felt. Bystander cardiopulmonary resuscitation (CPR) was begun immediately and continued for 25 minutes until emergency medical services arrived. At the scene his rectal temperature was 27 °C (80.6 °F). He was intubated and bag ventilated and continued to receive CPR in the ambulance on the way to the emergency department.

On physical examination, temperature is 28 °C (82.4 °F). Oxygen saturation is 97% on mechanical ventilation with 65% oxygen. He is not responsive and shows no spontaneous movement or shivering. His heart rhythm on the monitor is ventricular fibrillation.

Which of the following is the most appropriate management?

(A) Continue CPR with active external rewarming
(B) Continue CPR with active internal (core) rewarming
(C) Continue CPR with passive external rewarming
(D) Discontinue CPR

Item 67

A 31-year-old man is evaluated near the end of a guided climb of a 3500-meter (11,482 feet) summit in the French Alps. He is confused and increasingly irritable. His only medication was prophylactic acetazolamide, which he discontinued due to bothersome nocturia.

On physical examination, pulse rate is 128/min and respiration rate is 22/min. In addition to confusion, his gait is ataxic. The neurological examination is otherwise nonfocal.

Supplemental oxygen is administered and arrangements are being made for descent.

Which of the following is the most appropriate additional treatment?

(A) Acetazolamide
(B) Dexamethasone
(C) Nifedipine
(D) Sildenafil

Item 68

A 42-year-old man was hospitalized 2 days ago with necrotizing fasciitis of the leg. He underwent extensive debridement and fasciotomy 2 hours earlier. He currently has severe pain in his leg wounds. He was well before this illness. Current medications are imipenem, clindamycin, vancomycin, and a morphine infusion.

On physical examination, blood pressure is 150/99 mm Hg, pulse rate is 110/min, and respiration rate is 24/min. He is awake, anxious, grimacing, and wriggling in bed. The remainder of the examination is noncontributory.

Which of the following is the most appropriate treatment?

(A) Add gabapentin
(B) Epidural for regional analgesia
(C) Intravenous bolus of morphine
(D) Replace morphine with intravenous fentanyl

Item 69

A 24-year-old woman is evaluated during a follow-up visit. She was initially evaluated 6 weeks ago after a fall at work and had a chest radiograph performed for evaluation of pleuritic chest pain. This symptom has since resolved. She has no other symptoms and takes no medications.

Upon physical examination, vital signs are normal. The remainder of the physical examination is normal.

Chest radiograph is shown.

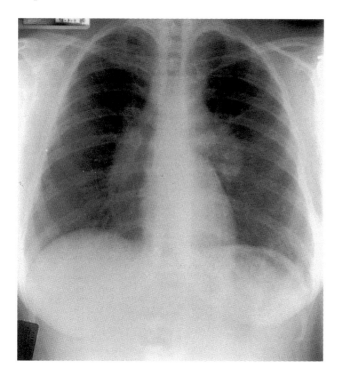

Which of the following is the most appropriate management?

(A) Endobronchial ultrasound and biopsy
(B) High-resolution CT scan of the chest
(C) Prednisone
(D) Observation

Item 70

A 34-year-old male is hospitalized for acute respiratory failure following a heroin overdose and aspiration. Current medications are piperacillin/tazobactam, propofol, heparin, and pantoprazole.

On physical examination, temperature is 37.7 °C (99.9 °F), blood pressure is 114/77 mm Hg, pulse rate is 74/min, and respiration rate is 16/min. His ideal body weight is 63 kg (138 lb). Ventilator settings are in the volume-controlled ventilation mode with tidal volume of 630 mL, a positive end-expiratory pressure (PEEP) of 8 cm H_2O, and F_{IO_2} of 0.5.

Arterial blood gas studies on an F_{IO_2} of 0.5 show a pH of 7.33, a P_{CO_2} of 46 mm Hg (6.1 kPa), and a P_{O_2} of 76 mm Hg (10.1 kPa).

Chest radiograph shows bilateral opacities.

Which of the following is the most appropriate next step?

(A) Decrease PEEP
(B) Increase PEEP
(C) Increase respiration rate
(D) Reduce tidal volume

Item 71

A 51-year-old man is evaluated for fever, hypotension, and confusion. He was admitted to the ICU 8 days ago for observation after complications resulting from an outpatient surgical procedure. He had experienced unexpected bleeding in the recovery room and had a central venous catheter inserted emergently for blood transfusion. On the first postoperative day he was weaned from mechanical ventilation, vomited once but recovered, and has been receiving supplemental oxygen through nasal cannula. Today he developed a fever, hypotension, and confusion. His hemoglobin has remained stable.

On physical examination, temperature is 38.6 °C (101.5 °F), blood pressure is 89/50 mm Hg, pulse rate is 101/min, and respiration rate is 23/min. Oxygen saturation is 100% on 2L/min of oxygen through nasal cannula. Lung examination reveals clear breath sounds.

Laboratory studies reveal a leukocyte count of 15,000/μL (15 × 10⁹/L) and a serum creatinine of 1.2 mg/dL (106.1 μmol/L).

An intravenous fluid bolus of 30 mL/kg of body weight is now infusing. Blood and respiratory cultures have been obtained and broad spectrum antibiotics are administered.

Which of the following is the most appropriate next step in management?

(A) Administer glucocorticoids
(B) Administer norepinephrine
(C) Obtain procalcitonin level
(D) Remove the central venous catheter

Item 72

A 31-year-old woman is evaluated for a 1-year history of daytime sleepiness. She falls asleep while watching TV, at the theater, and occasionally during a meal. She usually falls asleep between 10:00 PM and midnight and wakes during the workweek at 6:00 AM On weekends, she wakes at 9:00 AM. Her husband reports snoring but he hasn't observed breathing pauses. She has no cataplexy or symptoms of restless leg syndrome. She takes no medications.

On physical examination, vital signs are normal. BMI is 24.5. The physical examination, including inspection of nasal passages and oropharynx, is normal.

Which of the following is the most appropriate management?

(A) Actigraphy
(B) Modafinil
(C) Multiple sleep latency testing
(D) Polysomnography

Item 73

A 43-year-old man is evaluated in the emergency department for a 1-week history of cough, shortness of breath, chest pain, and night sweats. He has a 25-pack-year smoking history.

On physical examination, temperature is 38.8 °C (102 °F), blood pressure is 134/82 mm Hg, pulse rate is 142/min, and respiration rate is 30/min. Oxygen saturation is 88% breathing ambient air. There are decreased breath sounds at the right base and dullness to percussion. The remainder of the examination is noncontributory.

Laboratory studies reveal a leukocyte count of 29,000/µL (29.0×10^9/L).

Chest radiograph shows a large right pleural effusion with associated compressive atelectasis or consolidation, and consolidation in the right upper lobe.

The patient is prescribed broad-spectrum antibiotics and a diagnostic thoracentesis is performed that removes 100 mL of serous pleural fluid.

Pleural fluid studies:

pH	7.0
Lactate dehydrogenase	2310 U/L
Total protein	5.2 g/dL (52 g/L)
Glucose	42 mg/dL (2.3 mmol/L)
Gram stain	Negative

Which of the following is the most likely diagnosis?

(A) Complicated parapneumonic effusion
(B) Empyema
(C) Malignant effusion
(D) Uncomplicated parapneumonic effusion

Item 74

A 55-year-old woman is evaluated during a routine visit. She was previously diagnosed with spirometry-confirmed mild COPD for which she was prescribed a short-acting bronchodilator. She has a 20-pack-year history of cigarette smoking, but she quit 5 years ago. She is currently asymptomatic and has never received an influenza vaccination or pneumococcal vaccination. Her only medication is an albuterol inhaler.

On physical examination, vital signs are normal; oxygen saturation is 95% on ambient air. Lungs are clear to auscultation. The remainder of the physical examination is unremarkable.

Which of the following vaccinations should the patient receive at this time?

(A) High-dose influenza
(B) Pneumococcal polysaccharide (PPSV23) and standard influenza
(C) PPSV23 and pneumococcal conjugate (PCV13) and standard influenza
(D) PPSV23 and PCV13

Item 75

A 48-year-old woman is evaluated for recurrent pulmonary embolism. Her first episode was 18 months ago; she was treated with warfarin for 3 months. She was hospitalized 9 months ago for pulmonary embolism and has been treated with warfarin since then. She reports progressive exertional dyspnea. She has no chest pain, cough, hemoptysis, or wheezing. Her only medication is warfarin.

On physical examination, blood pressure is 108/68 mm Hg, pulse rate is 90/min, and respiration rate is 16/min. Oxygen saturation is 90% breathing ambient air. BMI is 36. The cardiovascular examination shows jugular venous distention, a prominent jugular venous a wave, and widened split S_2 with a prominent pulmonic component. Lung examination is unremarkable.

INR is 2.8.

Echocardiography reveals a normal left ventricle and dilated right ventricle with reduced function. Ventilation-perfusion scan shows multiple mismatched defects. Right heart catheterization reveals a mean pulmonary arterial pressure of 58 mm Hg and a normal pulmonary capillary wedge pressure. Pulmonary angiography is remarkable for pulmonary artery webs, intimal irregularities, and abrupt narrowing of the major pulmonary arteries.

Which of the following is the definitive treatment?

(A) Apixaban
(B) Inferior vena cava filter
(C) Nifedipine
(D) Pulmonary thromboendarterectomy

Item 76

A 65-year-old woman is evaluated for discontinuation of mechanical ventilation. She was placed on mechanical ventilation 5 days ago for respiratory failure secondary to an exacerbation of COPD. Ventilator settings are in the volume-controlled continuous mandatory ventilation mode, with a set respiration rate of 10/min, a tidal volume of 370 mL, an FIO_2 of 0.35, and a positive end-expiratory pressure of 5 cm H_2O. Current medications are albuterol/ipratropium, levofloxacin, prednisone, and fentanyl.

On physical examination, vital signs are normal. She is sleepy but arousable and can follow simple commands. Lung examination reveals distant breath sounds. The remainder of the examination is unremarkable.

Arterial blood gas studies show a pH of 7.46, PCO_2 of 47 mm Hg (6.25 kPa), and a PO_2 of 62 mm Hg (8.25 kPa). Other laboratory studies, including a leukocyte count, are normal.

Chest radiograph demonstrates hyperinflation but no infiltrates or evidence of heart failure.

Which of the following is the most appropriate test or evaluation to perform next?

(A) 30-Minute spontaneous breathing trial
(B) Cuff leak test
(C) Glasgow Coma Scale
(D) Measure negative inspiratory force

Item 77

A 48-year-old woman is hospitalized for a 2-week history of cough, sputum production, fever, and dyspnea.

On physical examination, temperature is 39.6 °C (103.3 °F), blood pressure is 110/63 mm Hg, pulse rate is 122/min, and respiration rate is 36/min. Oxygen saturation is 88% breathing ambient air. Lung examination reveals diminished breath sounds over the left base. Cardiac examination is notable only for tachycardia.

Chest radiograph reveals a small loculated effusion on the left.

A diagnostic thoracentesis is performed, which results in incomplete removal of the effusion.

Pleural fluid analysis:

pH	6.8
Lactate dehydrogenase	3289 U/L
Total protein	3.7 g/dL (37 g/L)
Glucose	9 mg/dL (0.5 mmol/L)
Gram stain	Gram-positive cocci in chains

Appropriate intravenous antibiotics are initiated.

Which of the following is the most appropriate intrapleural treatment of the effusion?

(A) Antibiotics
(B) Streptokinase
(C) Tissue plasminogen activator-deoxyribonuclease
(D) No additional therapy required

Item 78

A 67-year-old woman is evaluated for history of rhinorrhea, pharyngitis, nonproductive cough, and associated intermittent dyspnea. Her symptoms began 12 weeks ago associated with low-grade fevers, rhinorrhea, and pharyngitis. The fever, rhinorrhea, and pharyngitis resolved but her other symptoms persist. She has no chest pain, palpitations, edema, fever, chills, or orthopnea, and she has never smoked. Her medical history is significant for hypertension treated with an angiotensin receptor blocker.

On physical examination vital signs are normal. Cardiac examination, including jugular venous pressure, is normal. Lung examination is normal.

Laboratory studies, including complete blood count, are normal.

Chest radiograph and spirometry are normal.

Which of the following is the most appropriate diagnostic test to perform next?

(A) Echocardiography
(B) Exhaled nitric oxide testing
(C) High-resolution chest CT scan

(D) Methacholine challenge testing
(E) Nasal swab for influenza polymerase chain reaction

Item 79

An 18-year-old woman is evaluated in the emergency department for lip swelling after eating at a neighborhood picnic. She has a history of peanut and tree nut allergies that have caused lip swelling, but she has never been hospitalized for a reaction. She currently takes no medications.

On physical examination, blood pressure is 100/64 mm Hg, pulse rate is 108/min, and respiration rate is 19/min. Oxygen saturation is 100% breathing ambient air. Bilateral lip swelling is evident that affects the upper lip more than the lower lip. She has no tongue swelling or stridor. Lungs are clear to auscultation. Urticaria is present on the hands and trunk.

Which of the following is the most appropriate immediate treatment?

(A) Diphenhydramine
(B) Epinephrine
(C) Intravenous fluid bolus
(D) Intravenous methylprednisolone

Item 80

A 62-year-old man was admitted 12 hours ago with severe acute respiratory distress syndrome (ARDS). Overnight, he developed fever and increasing respiratory distress, was intubated, and has had rapidly increasing ventilator requirements. Current ventilator settings are in the volume-controlled continuous mandatory ventilation mode, and he is receiving appropriate low tidal volume ventilation. Current medications are fentanyl, midazolam, heparin, piperacillin/tazobactam, and norepinephrine.

On physical examination, temperature is 38.4 °C (101.2 °F), blood pressure is 89/45 mm Hg, pulse rate is 110/min, and his spontaneous respiration rate is 35/min with a positive end-expiratory pressure of 16 cm H_2O and an FIO_2 of 1.0.

Arterial blood gases:

pH	7.3
PCO_2	51 mm Hg (6.8 kPa)
PO_2	55 mm Hg (7.3 kPa)
Bicarbonate	24 mEq/L (24 mmol/L)

Chest radiograph shows diffuse, bilateral infiltrates throughout the lung fields.

Which of the following is the most appropriate management?

(A) Perform a recruitment maneuver
(B) Start inhaled nitric oxide
(C) Transition the patient to high-frequency oscillator ventilation
(D) Ventilate the patient in the prone position

Item 81

A 42-year-old man is evaluated in the office for chronic cough. He first developed a cough 3 years ago. It is productive of clear to yellow sputum that is occasionally blood-tinged. He has taken antibiotics when his sputum production increases, after which his cough improves but never completely resolves. He has no dyspnea. He does not smoke cigarettes. He currently is taking no medications.

On physical examination, vital signs are normal. Oxygen saturation is 96% breathing ambient air. BMI is normal. Pulmonary examination reveals scattered inspiratory squeaks.

A chest radiograph shows ill-defined linear atelectasis and irregular peripheral opacities in the right and left lower lobes. A CT scan of the chest with contrast is shown below.

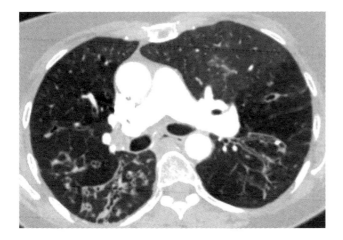

Which of the following is the most likely diagnosis?

(A) Bronchiectasis
(B) Centrilobular emphysema
(C) Chronic bronchitis
(D) Pulmonary Langerhans cell histiocytosis

Item 82

A 35-year-old woman is evaluated in the emergency department for a 3-week history of worsening cough and dyspnea. She works as a sand mover operator at a hydraulic fracturing site and she notes that there is a large amount of dust that often clogs her respirator. She is otherwise healthy and has no history of fever, chills, sweats, or sick contacts. She has no current medications.

On physical examination, pulse rate is 110/min and respiration rate is 26/min. Other vital signs are normal. Oxygen saturation is 92% breathing ambient air. Lung examination reveals inspiratory crackles bilaterally. Cardiovascular examination is normal.

Chest radiograph shows patchy bilateral opacities with areas of consolidation in the lower lobes.

Bronchoalveolar lavage shows fluid with milky white return but no organisms; bacterial cultures are negative.

Which of the following is the most likely diagnosis?

(A) Acute interstitial pneumonia
(B) Acute silicosis
(C) Asbestosis
(D) Cryptogenic organizing pneumonia

Item 83

A 66-year-old woman is evaluated for difficult weaning from mechanical ventilation. She was hospitalized 8 days ago with septic shock due to pneumococcal pneumonia and bacteremia. She required mechanical ventilation and was treated with glucocorticoids and neuromuscular blockers. Pneumonia and sepsis have resolved, but she is unable to be weaned from ventilation. Current medications are fentanyl and heparin.

On physical examination, temperature is 37.3 °C (99.1 °F), blood pressure is 133/88 mm Hg, pulse rate is 70/min, and respiration rate is 14/min. Oxygen saturation is 100% on an F_{IO_2} of 0.35. She is awake and obeys commands but displays generalized weakness; she has decreased grip strength, distal lower extremity sensory loss, decreased tendon reflexes, and cannot raise her arms or legs.

Laboratory studies, including the complete blood count, metabolic profile, and electrolytes, are normal.

Which of the following is the most appropriate next step in the evaluation?

(A) Cervical spine MRI
(B) Electrodiagnostic testing
(C) Medical Research Council muscle scale
(D) Muscle biopsy

Item 84

A 36-year-old woman is evaluated for dry cough and progressive dyspnea that limits her ability to exercise. She initially presented 8 weeks ago with cough, fever, sputum production, and dyspnea. A chest radiograph at that time revealed left-lower-lobe opacities; she was diagnosed with pneumonia and treated with azithromycin but had little improvement in her symptoms. Her fever and sputum production have resolved. She is a nonsmoker.

On physical examination, vital signs are normal. Lungs are clear to auscultation.

Repeat chest radiograph reveals patchy opacities bilaterally and several nodular densities that are peripherally predominant in different locations than previous radiographs. High-resolution CT scan of the chest shows extensive ground-glass changes bilaterally with several areas of nodular consolidation that are peripherally predominant and along bronchovascular bundles.

Which of the following is the most likely diagnosis?

(A) Acute HIV infection
(B) Community-acquired pneumonia
(C) Cryptogenic organizing pneumonia
(D) Idiopathic pulmonary fibrosis

Item 85

A 56-year-old man is evaluated in the ICU for hypotension. He was admitted 3 hours ago for acute onset dyspnea. A CT angiogram performed upon admission showed a large, central pulmonary embolism. Treatment was started with subcutaneous low-molecular-weight heparin, and he was transferred to the ICU for monitoring. An hour later he became hypotensive.

H CONT.

On physical examination, blood pressure is 78/54 mm Hg, pulse rate is 120/min, and respiration rate is 28/min. Oxygen saturation is 93% on 4 L/min of oxygen through nasal cannula. Lungs are clear on auscultation. Cardiac examination reveals a grade 2/6 systolic murmur above the left lower sternal border. The second heart sound is persistently split.

Which of the following is the most appropriate treatment?

(A) Add recombinant tissue plasminogen activator (rtPA)
(B) Change to apixaban
(C) Change to intravenous unfractionated heparin infusion
(D) Continue low-molecular-weight heparin

H **Item 86**

A 67-year-old woman is admitted to the ICU for abdominal distention, vomiting, and hypotension. She had a colectomy 3 weeks ago to treat recurrent diverticular bleeding, and postoperatively she had prolonged anorexia and nausea. She was discharged to an extended care facility on enteral nutrition through a small-bore nasogastric tube.

On physical examination, temperature is 36.8 °C (98.2 °F), blood pressure is 100/60 mm Hg, pulse rate is 109/min, and respiration rate is 19/min. BMI is 19. Preoperative BMI was 25. She has temporal wasting, colectomy wound with areas of dehiscence, lower extremity edema, decreased bowel sounds, and distended tympanitic abdomen.

Blood glucose is 65 mg/dL (3.6 mmol/L), albumin is 2.4 g/dL (24 g/L), creatinine is 0.6 mg/dL (53 µmol/L), and blood urea nitrogen is 6 mg/dL (2.14 mmol/L).

Radiograph and CT scan of the abdomen show dilated loops of small bowel. The nasogastric tube is in the proximal jejunum.

Intravenous fluid resuscitation is initiated and surgical consultation is obtained.

Which of the following is the most appropriate nutritional management?

(A) Maintain current enteral nutrition
(B) Measure gastric residual volume
(C) Start metoclopramide
(D) Switch to parenteral nutrition

Item 87

A 56-year-old woman is evaluated following screening for lung cancer with low-dose chest CT scan. She has a 35-pack-year history of cigarette smoking and continues to smoke. She has no symptoms.

On physical examination, vital signs and the remainder of the physical examination are normal.

Low-dose chest CT scan demonstrates diffuse centrilobular micronodules that are predominant in the midlung and upper lung. There is no evidence of septal line thickening, traction bronchiectasis, honeycombing, ground-glass opacities, or mediastinal or hilar lymphadenopathy.

Which of the following is the most likely diagnosis?

(A) Desquamative interstitial pneumonia
(B) Idiopathic pulmonary fibrosis

(C) Pulmonary Langerhans cell histiocytosis
(D) Respiratory bronchiolitis-associated interstitial lung disease

Item 88

A 73-year-old man is evaluated for a 3-month history of chronic productive cough, intermittent hemoptysis, night sweats, and 4.5 kg (10 lb) unintentional weight loss. He previously worked as a miner and has a history of chronic silicosis. He also has a 40-pack-year history of smoking, but quit 10 years ago.

On physical examination, vital signs are normal. He is thin and appears ill with temporal muscle wasting. Lung examination reveals bilateral upper-lobe crackles. Cardiac examination is unremarkable.

Chest radiograph reveals bilateral upper-lobe fibrosis with volume loss of the upper lobes and evidence of cavitation, traction of the hila upwards bilaterally, and bilateral calcified hilar lymphadenopathy.

Which of the following is the most appropriate management?

(A) Aspergillus IgG antibody test
(B) Bronchoscopy with transbronchial biopsy
(C) High-resolution CT scan of the chest
(D) Sputum sample for acid-fast bacillus

Item 89

A 32-year-old woman is evaluated for a 2-month history of gradually worsening dyspnea on exertion. She has difficulty climbing one flight of stairs, but has no wheezing or cough. She was hospitalized 6 months ago for a cholecystectomy complicated by sepsis, with a 2-week ICU stay requiring mechanical ventilation, but she recovered without difficulty. She uses an albuterol inhaler as needed, but this does not provide significant relief.

On physical examination, vital signs are normal. Oxygen saturation is 97% breathing ambient air. Cardiopulmonary examination is normal.

Chest radiograph is normal; spirometry is performed, and a flow-volume loop is shown.

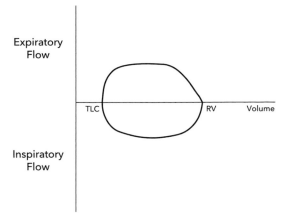

Which of the following is the most likely diagnosis?

(A) Asthma

(B) COPD

(C) Fixed upper airway obstruction

(D) Normal lung function

Item 90

A 24-year-old woman is evaluated for recent onset of exertional dyspnea and chest tightness occurring three to four times weekly. She has a history of asthma since childhood that was previously well controlled with albuterol and budesonide. She is 14 weeks pregnant, and she stopped taking her medications 4 weeks ago out of concern for effects on the fetus. She has no other medical problems.

On physical examination, vital signs are normal. Oxygen saturation is 97% breathing ambient air. Chest examination shows good air movement with occasional expiratory wheezing. The remainder of the examination is normal.

Spirometry demonstrates mild airflow obstruction.

Which of the following is the most appropriate management?

(A) Begin fluticasone/salmeterol

(B) Begin low-dose prednisone

(C) Monitor serial peak flow measurements

(D) Restart previous medications

Item 91

A 78-year-old man is evaluated for an 8-month history of nonproductive cough and dyspnea on exertion, particularly when going up an incline. He has a 40-pack-year smoking history but quit 15 years ago. His sister had pulmonary fibrosis.

On physical examination, vital signs are normal. Clubbing is present. Lung examination reveals inspiratory crackles at the bases. Cardiac examination is normal. Pulmonary function testing shows an FVC of 75% of predicted and an FEV_1/FVC ratio of 0.85.

Chest radiograph demonstrates small lung volumes and interstitial opacities at the bases.

Which of the following is the most appropriate diagnostic test to perform next?

(A) Contrast-enhanced chest CT scan

(B) High-resolution chest CT scan

(C) Low-dose chest CT scan

(D) PET/CT imaging

Item 92

A 62-year-old man is evaluated for a 2-month history of nonproductive cough, progressive dyspnea, and fatigue. He reports a 6.8-kg (15-lb) weight loss during this time. He has a 30-pack-year history of smoking. He worked in a navy ship yard 32 years ago. His history is otherwise unremarkable.

On physical examination, vital signs are normal. Oxygen saturation is 94% breathing ambient air. Lung examination findings are consistent with a right pleural effusion. The remainder of the examination is normal. A complete blood count and metabolic profile are normal.

Chest radiograph shows a large right pleural effusion.

Thoracentesis is performed and removes 1200 mL of serosanguineous fluid.

Pleural fluid analysis:

Cytology	Negative
Glucose	89 mg/dL (4.9 mmol/L)
Lactate dehydrogenase	200 U/L
pH	7.36
Total protein	3.8 g/dL (38 g/L)

Laboratory studies:

Serum lactate dehydrogenase	235 U/L
Serum total protein	6.2 g/dL (62 g/L)

The patient returns 2 weeks later with a recurrent pleural effusion. CT scan of his chest demonstrates a moderate right pleural effusion with no parenchymal or pleural abnormalities noted. Thoracentesis is repeated; pleural fluid analysis is similar to the initial analysis, and cytology is again negative.

Which of the following is the most appropriate next step?

(A) Closed pleural biopsy

(B) Measure pleural fluid triglycerides

(C) Resend a pleural fluid specimen for cytology

(D) Thoracoscopy and pleural biopsy

Item 93

A 63-year-old man is evaluated for symptoms of gradually increasing dyspnea on exertion. Symptoms began about 2 years ago with activities such as golfing, and recently he notes dyspnea and occasional nonproductive cough with stair climbing in his home. He has no palpitations, chest pressure, wheezing, orthopnea, or systemic symptoms. History is significant for hypertension, 30-pack-year tobacco use (quit smoking 1 year ago), and obesity. He currently takes chlorthalidone.

On physical examination, vital signs are normal. Oxygen saturation is 92% on ambient air. BMI is 31. Pulmonary examination demonstrates basilar inspiratory crackles; cardiac examination is normal. The remainder of the examination is unremarkable.

Laboratory studies, including a basic metabolic panel and complete blood count, are normal.

Pulmonary function testing reveals an FEV_1 of 70% of predicted, an FVC of 65% of predicted, an FEV_1/FVC ratio of 0.78%, and a DLco of 63% of predicted. Total lung capacity is 70% of predicted.

Chest radiograph demonstrates diffuse interstitial reticulonodular infiltrates.

Which of the following is the most appropriate test to perform next?

(A) Bronchoscopy with transbronchial lung biopsy

(B) Cardiopulmonary exercise test

(C) High-resolution CT scan of the chest

(D) Methacholine challenge testing

Item 94

A 42-year-old man is evaluated for a 1-year history of disruptive snoring. His wife has not observed gasping, choking, or pauses in breathing. His normal sleep schedule is 10:30 PM to 6:30 AM. He awakens feeling refreshed and has no daytime sleepiness.

On physical examination, vital signs are normal. BMI is 34.6. He has a low-lying soft palate, his neck is 43 cm (17 in) in circumference, and he has patent nasal passages.

Which of the following is the most appropriate management?

(A) Home sleep testing
(B) Polysomnography
(C) Radiofrequency ablation of soft palate
(D) Weight loss program

Item 95

A 58-year-old woman is evaluated for 6 months of progressive dyspnea and cough. She was treated for breast cancer 10 years ago with a radical mastectomy on the left side, lymph node dissection, chemotherapy, and radiation. Her functional status is limited only by the dyspnea.

On physical examination, vital signs are normal. Oxygen saturation is 94% breathing ambient air. Lung examination is consistent with a left-side pleural effusion. The remainder of the physical examination is normal.

Chest radiograph shows moderate left-sided pleural effusion.

Thoracentesis is performed removing 1100 mL of serosanguineous fluid, providing significant relief of her symptoms. Cytology is positive for adenocarcinoma. The patient initiates therapy for metastatic breast cancer. During the next 2 weeks the patient requires repeated thoracentesis to remove large quantities of pleural fluid. Each thoracentesis provides significant relief of dyspnea for about 2 to 3 days.

Which of the following is the most appropriate management of the pleural effusions?

(A) Indwelling pleural catheter placement
(B) Pleurectomy
(C) Serial thoracentesis
(D) Talc pleurodesis

Item 96

A 19-year-old man is brought to the emergency department after he attended a party with friends. He is anxious and tremulous. He has a history of depression. His only medication is fluoxetine.

On physical examination, he is alert and oriented. Temperature is 38.9 °C (102 °F), blood pressure is 136/79 mm Hg, pulse rate is 112/min, and respiration rate is 20/min. Oxygen saturation is 98% breathing ambient air. Physical examination is notable for slow, continuous, horizontal eye movements, tremor of extremities, hyperreflexia, and sustained ankle clonus and spontaneous myoclonus. The physical examination is otherwise normal.

Urine toxicology screening is pending.

Which of the following is the most likely diagnosis?

(A) Anticholinergic toxicity
(B) Malignant hyperthermia
(C) Neuroleptic malignant syndrome
(D) Serotonin syndrome

Item 97

A 62-year-old woman with alcoholic cirrhosis is evaluated for hypovolemic shock. She was hospitalized 24 hours ago with upper gastrointestinal bleeding. She underwent upper endoscopy, and a bleeding distal esophageal varix was controlled with epinephrine injection and banding. Gastric varices were also noted. Today she vomited 300 mL of bright red blood. Current medications are lactulose, rifaximin, pantoprazole, norfloxacin, and octreotide.

On physical examination, blood pressure is 79/54 mm Hg, pulse rate is 95/min, and respiration rate is 21/min. Oxygen saturation is 94% on 2 L/min of oxygen through nasal cannula. Ascites and splenomegaly are present.

Laboratory studies this morning reveal a hemoglobin level of 8 g/dL (80 g/L), platelet count of 74,000/µL (74 × 10^9/L), and an INR of 1.4.

Which of the following is the most appropriate immediate management?

(A) Packed red blood cell transfusion
(B) Recombinant factor VII infusion
(C) Transjugular intrahepatic portosystemic shunting
(D) Upper endoscopy

Item 98

A 45-year-old man is evaluated in the emergency department for alcohol intoxication, but the source and type of alcohol consumed are unknown. He has a history of heavy ethanol use and occasional isopropanol use.

On physical examination, vital signs are normal. Oxygen saturation is 97% on ambient air. He is somnolent but easily aroused.

Laboratory studies

Bicarbonate	24 mEq/L (24 mmol/L)
Blood urea nitrogen	14 mg/dL (5 mmol/L)
Chloride	106 mEq/L (106 mmol/L)
Creatinine	1.6 mg/dL (141.4 µmol/L)
Ethanol	Negative
Glucose	90 mg/dL (5 mmol/L)
Osmolality, plasma	315 mOsm/kg H$_2$O
Potassium	4.1 mEq/L (4.1 mmol/L)
Sodium	139 mEq/L (139 mmol/L)

In addition to monitoring for signs of alcohol withdrawal, which of the following is the most appropriate treatment?

(A) Fomepizole
(B) Hemodialysis
(C) Levetiracetam
(D) Supportive care

Item 99

A 63-year-old man is evaluated in follow-up for a lung mass found during evaluation for a persistent cough. He is a current smoker with a 60-pack-year smoking history. His medical history is otherwise unremarkable, and he takes no medications.

Upon physical examination, vital signs are normal. The remainder of the physical examination is normal.

Laboratory studies, including liver chemistry tests, sodium, and calcium, are normal.

Chest radiograph shows a 2-cm nodule in the right upper lobe that was not seen on previous imaging. CT and PET scans demonstrate PET positivity of the lung lesion and in the mediastinal lymph nodes.

Which of the following is the most appropriate diagnostic procedure to perform next?

(A) CT-guided needle biopsy
(B) Endobronchial ultrasound and mediastinal lymph node biopsy
(C) Sputum cytology
(D) Thoracoscopic lung biopsy with lymph node dissection

Item 100

A 38-year-old woman is evaluated in the emergency department for unresponsiveness. On arrival she was minimally responsive with miotic pupils and a respiration rate of 4/min, but 5 minutes after administration of two doses of intravenous naloxone, her respiration rate is 15/min, and she is awake, oriented, and able to converse. She does not remember what happened before her admission, but her history is significant for heroin use.

On physical examination, vital signs are normal. Oxygen saturation is 99% breathing ambient air. The physical examination is unremarkable save for miotic pupils and signs of "needle tracks" on the arms.

Which of the following is the most appropriate management?

(A) Administer regular doses of naloxone starting now
(B) Continue to observe for several hours
(C) Discharge now with outpatient follow-up
(D) Elective endotracheal tube placement now

Item 101

A 74-year-old woman is evaluated in the hospital for loss of consciousness 1 day after total hip replacement. She suddenly became unresponsive and hypotensive while sitting in bed. Before this event she was doing well and discharge planning was under way. She has a remote history of penicillin allergy manifesting as hives. She received one dose of prophylactic cefazolin at the time of surgery. Her only medications are oxycodone and low-molecular-weight heparin.

On physical examination, blood pressure is 76/48 mm Hg, pulse rate is 116/min, and respiration rate is 26/min. Oxygen saturation is 80% on a 100% oxygen nonrebreather mask. The skin is cool and mottled but without rash. Cardiac sounds are soft, without murmur, but with persistent splitting of the second heart sound. Jugular venous distention is noted. The lungs are clear bilaterally.

Which of the following is the most likely diagnosis?

(A) Anaphylactic shock
(B) Opiate overdose
(C) Pulmonary embolism
(D) Tension pneumothorax

Item 102

A 56-year-old woman is evaluated in follow-up after polysomnography documented an apnea-hypopnea index of 6, a mean oxyhemoglobin saturation of 86.4%, and 38% of sleep time with an oxygen saturation of less than 90% of predicted. She has type 2 diabetes mellitus and hypertension. Current medications are metformin and lisinopril.

On physical examination, vital signs are normal. Oxygen saturation is 91% breathing ambient air. BMI is 44. Other than +1 ankle edema, the remainder of the physical examination, including neurological examination, is unremarkable.

Laboratory studies reveal a hemoglobin level of 16.9 g/dL (169 g/L). Arterial blood gas studies show a pH of 7.36, a P_{CO_2} of 58 mm Hg (7.7 kPa), and a P_{O_2} of 59 mm Hg (7.8 kPa).

Chest radiograph demonstrates clear lung fields.

Which of the following is the most likely diagnosis?

(A) Amyotrophic lateral sclerosis
(B) Central sleep apnea
(C) Obesity hypoventilation syndrome
(D) Severe obstructive sleep apnea

Item 103

A 54-year-old woman is evaluated in the office for an exacerbation of bronchiectasis characterized by low-grade fever, cough, and voluminous purulent sputum production progressing during the past 5 days. Her last exacerbation was 3 months ago and was treated with antibiotics. The results of the sputum culture from that episode are not available.

On physical examination, temperature is 38.0 °C (100.4 °F) and respiration rate is 18/min. All other vital signs are normal. Oxygen saturation is 96% breathing ambient air. Pulmonary examination reveals scattered inspiratory squeaks but no wheezes or crackles.

A chest radiograph does not show any infiltrates.

Sputum Gram stain shows gram-negative bacilli and a culture is pending.

Which of the following is the most appropriate empiric treatment?

(A) Amoxicillin
(B) Azithromycin
(C) Azithromycin and prednisone
(D) Inhaled tobramycin
(E) Levofloxacin

Answers and Critiques

Item 1   Answer: A

Educational Objective: Treat an asthma exacerbation in the hospital.

This patient should be hospitalized for further management. She has an asthma exacerbation and factors that increase her risk of asthma-related death, including several recent exacerbations, history of intubation for asthma, history of anxiety, and poor compliance with her controller medications. She also has worrisome clinical signs, including tachycardia and diminished oxygen saturation, increased work of breathing and decreased air movement on chest examination. These physical findings suggest a severe degree of airflow obstruction and risk for impending respiratory failure; therefore, the most appropriate site of care is the hospital.

Management should include close monitoring of dyspnea, work of breathing, and vital signs; frequent bronchodilator treatment; and systemic glucocorticoids. Pulse oximetry may be falsely reassuring because patients maintain normal oxygen levels despite high work of breathing, and hypoxemia is a late sign of pending respiratory failure. In patients who are at high risk or have lack of symptom resolution with initial therapies, arterial blood gas assessment is vital and should initially reveal hyperventilation with a low arterial P_{CO_2}. Normalization of the arterial P_{CO_2} could be an early indicator of respiratory muscle fatigue and impending respiratory arrest.

Outpatient treatment with prednisone and the patient's other medications would not be appropriate for this high-risk patient with severe asthma.

KEY POINT

- Patients with asthma exacerbations who have signs that indicate a severe attack should be hospitalized.

Bibliography

Prasad Kerlin M. In the clinic. Asthma. Ann Intern Med. 2014;160:ITC3 2-15; quiz ITC3 16-9. [PMID: 24737276]

Item 2   Answer: C

Educational Objective: Recognize the role of NSAIDs in poor control of asthma.

Treatment with ibuprofen should be discontinued for this patient, and therapy with prednisone should be started. This patient is presenting with signs of aspirin-exacerbated respiratory disease, triggered by his use of ibuprofen. This condition refers to upper and lower respiratory tract reactions to ingestion of substances inhibiting cyclooxygenase-1, which includes aspirin and many NSAIDs. Also known as aspirin-exacerbated respiratory disease or Samter's triad, aspirin-sensitive asthma includes severe persistent asthma, aspirin sensitivity, and hyperplastic eosinophilic sinusitis with nasal polyposis. Asthma is worsened by exposure to aspirin or other NSAIDs, likely because of the inhibition of cyclooxygenase and the resulting increase in leukotriene synthesis. Ingestion of cyclooxygenase-1–inhibiting substances can sometimes cause life-threatening bronchospasm, but patients can also have less severe symptoms, which often cause them to not recognize these substances as a trigger. In addition, the sensitivity to aspirin and other NSAIDs develops over time, generally after the onset of rhinosinusitis. Treatment consists of avoidance of aspirin or other NSAIDs along with typical asthma management. For patients who require aspirin use (such as those with coronary artery disease), an aspirin desensitization procedure can be performed. Successful desensitization down-regulates leukotriene receptors and modifies interleukin sensitivity, which may relieve asthma symptoms in some patients. For this reason, the addition of a leukotriene inhibitor such as montelukast or zafirlukast to an asthma maintenance regimen is helpful for most patients to modify the leukotriene dysregulation thought to contribute to the syndrome; however, addition of a leukotriene inhibitor alone would not be the appropriate next step for this patient.

24-Hour esophageal pH monitoring is helpful to diagnose gastroesophageal reflux disease, but the patient has no symptoms of this; moreover, a trial of empiric proton pump inhibitor therapy would be indicated before invasive testing.

A nasal polypectomy may be helpful in the long-term management of this syndrome, but it is not the initial step.

KEY POINT

- Treatment of aspirin-exacerbated respiratory disease consists of symptom treatment with glucocorticoids and removal of the exposure; treatment can also include a leukotriene receptor antagonist.

Bibliography

Ledford DK, Wenzel SE, Lockey RF. Aspirin or other nonsteroidal inflammatory agent exacerbated asthma. J Allergy Clin Immunol Pract. 2014;2:653-7. [PMID: 25439353] doi:10.1016/j.jaip.2014.09.009

Item 3   Answer: B

Educational Objective: Treat chronic bronchitis and prevent frequent COPD exacerbations with roflumilast.

Roflumilast is the most appropriate treatment. It is used primarily as add-on therapy in severe COPD associated with chronic bronchitis and a history of recurrent exacerbations despite other therapies; it has been shown to improve lung function and reduce risk and frequency of exacerbations in these individuals. However, it is not a bronchodilator, is expensive, and has not been shown to be effective in other groups of patients with COPD. Common side effects include diarrhea, nausea, weight loss, and headache. Recently the FDA has raised concerns regarding psychiatric adverse events with roflumilast (anxiety, depression, insomnia). Roflumilast is contraindicated in patients with liver impairment and has significant drug interactions.

Oral glucocorticoids, such as prednisone, are reserved for limited periodic use in treating exacerbations of COPD and may provide some benefit in decreasing hospital readmission rates after exacerbation. Long-term oral glucocorticoid therapy has limited, if any, benefit in COPD and carries a high risk for other significant side effects (such as muscle weakness and decreased functional status) and is generally not recommended.

Methylxanthines such as theophylline have shown modest treatment benefit in COPD, likely due to a bronchodilating effect mediated by nonselective inhibition of phosphodiesterase. However, the potential toxicity of this class of drugs coupled with their reduced efficacy has led to increasingly limited use. Although they may be helpful in any classification of COPD, they tend to be used in selected patients with late-stage disease or for patients in whom other preferred therapies have proved ineffective for symptomatic relief; they may also be used when other medications are not available or affordable.

Clinical trials have demonstrated that chronic macrolide therapy is associated with a reduction in the rate of exacerbation in patients with moderate to severe COPD despite optimal maintenance inhaler therapy. Macrolide antibiotic therapy and roflumilast have not been directly compared in patients with frequent exacerbations of COPD and the choice among the two is informed by benefits and risks on an individual patient basis. Trimethoprim-sulfamethoxazole has not been shown to prevent exacerbations of COPD.

KEY POINT

- Roflumilast, a selective phosphodiesterase-4 inhibitor, is used as add-on therapy in severe COPD associated with chronic bronchitis and a history of recurrent exacerbations to reduce risk and frequency of exacerbations.

Bibliography

Chong J, Leung B, Poole P. Phosphodiesterase 4 inhibitors for chronic obstructive pulmonary disease. Cochrane Database Syst Rev. 2017;9:CD002309. [PMID: 28922692] doi:10.1002/14651858.CD002309.pub5

Item 4   Answer: B

Educational Objective: Evaluate a patient for obstructive sleep apnea.

The most appropriate next step is home sleep testing. This patient has signs (loud snoring, breathing pauses, gasping), symptoms (excessive daytime sleepiness, nocturia), and physical examination findings (BMI greater than 30, large neck size, crowded oropharynx, a low-lying soft palate) consistent with obstructive sleep apnea (OSA). Home sleep testing is

the preferred diagnostic test when there is a high likelihood of OSA and an absence of significant comorbidities such as cardiopulmonary or neuromuscular disease. If OSA is confirmed, daytime sleepiness represents a strong indication for treatment. Polysomnography performed in a sleep laboratory is the preferred diagnostic test for OSA in patients with underlying cardiopulmonary or neuromuscular disease who might require advanced positive airway pressure modes (such as bilevel positive airway pressure) or supplemental oxygen but would not be indicated for this patient who has no evidence of such comorbidities.

Objective testing should occur before treatment of OSA is prescribed. Auto-adjusting positive airway pressure generally follows home sleep testing that confirms OSA.

Occasionally, multiple sleep latency testing (MSLT) is used to provide an objective measure of sleepiness. MSLT requires a series of brief nap opportunities during the course of a full day in a sleep laboratory to determine the average time to fall asleep and is time and labor intensive; however, it is necessary to establish the diagnoses of narcolepsy and idiopathic hypersomnia. A mean sleep latency of less than 5 minutes is a clear indicator of pathologic sleepiness, whereas more than 15 minutes is considered normal. If these additional sleep disorders were suspected in a patient with obstructive sleep apnea, MSLT would occur only after positive airway pressure treatment has been optimized.

There is no established role for overnight pulse oximetry as a screening or diagnostic tool in OSA. With limited sensitivity and specificity in the symptomatic patient with a high pretest probability of OSA, overnight oximetry is not likely to add diagnostic information beyond home sleep testing, nor will it alter the decision to treat.

KEY POINT

- Home sleep testing is the first test indicated in a patient with a high probability of obstructive sleep apnea without underlying cardiopulmonary or neuromuscular disease.

Bibliography

Kapur VK, Auckley DH, Chowdhuri S, Kuhlmann DC, Mehra R, Ramar K, et al. Clinical practice guideline for diagnostic testing for adult obstructive sleep apnea: an American Academy of Sleep Medicine clinical practice guideline. J Clin Sleep Med. 2017;13:479-504. [PMID: 28162150] doi:10.5664/jcsm.6506

Item 5   Answer: A

Educational Objective: Evaluate a subsolid solitary pulmonary nodule.

The most appropriate management of the pulmonary nodule is to perform follow-up chest CT scanning at 6-12 months and then every 2 years for 5 years, as recommended by the Fleischner Society Guidelines. Nodules are classified as solid or subsolid. Subsolid nodules are either pure ground-glass nodules (no solid component) or part-solid nodules (both ground-glass and solid components). A ground-glass nodule is defined as a focal area of increased attenuation in the lung through which normal parenchymal structures can still be seen. The classification of nodules helps in the assessment of malignant potential (for example, adenocarcinoma is more likely to present as a subsolid and part-solid nodule) and guides appropriate follow-up. This patient has a solitary pure ground-glass subsolid nodule that is larger than 6 mm. Earlier guidelines recommended initial follow-up at 3 months, but this was changed to 6-12 months because earlier follow-up is unlikely to affect the outcome of these characteristically indolent lesions. The average doubling time of subsolid, cancerous nodules typically is 3-5 years. Therefore, longer initial and total follow-up intervals are recommended for subsolid nodules than for solid nodules.

Evaluation with a PET/CT scan would be recommended for a solid nodule that is greater than 8 mm in size. This test most commonly uses fluorodeoxyglucose (FDG) as a metabolic marker to identify rapidly dividing cells such as tumor cells and, to a lesser degree, any inflammatory lesion. A nodule that demonstrates no FDG uptake is unlikely to be malignant. PET/CT imaging can also be used for staging a cancer by determining the presence or absence of metastatic disease.

Tissue sampling would not be appropriate at this stage because the vast majority of these lesions are not malignant.

KEY POINT

- Subsolid lung nodules 6-8 mm in size should be initially followed up at 6-12 months and then every 2 years for 5 years because of the slow rate of growth if such masses are malignant.

Bibliography

MacMahon H, Naidich DP, Goo JM, Lee KS, Leung ANC, Mayo JR, et al. Guidelines for management of incidental pulmonary nodules detected on CT images: from the Fleischner Society 2017. Radiology. 2017;284:228-243. [PMID: 28240562] doi:10.1148/radiol.2017161659

Item 6   **Answer: A**

Educational Objective: Diagnose an acute exacerbation of idiopathic pulmonary fibrosis.

The most likely diagnosis is an acute exacerbation of idiopathic pulmonary fibrosis (IPF). The clinical course of an acute exacerbation is acute to subacute onset (typically shorter than 30 days) of worsening dyspnea, and the medical evaluation does not reveal another cause for dyspnea such as infection, heart failure, or pulmonary embolism. High-resolution CT scan shows new-onset diffuse bilateral ground-glass opacities. Patients may develop frank respiratory failure due to an exacerbation or stabilize at a new, worsened baseline. The proposed criteria for an acute IPF exacerbation have recently changed and now include the possibility of a "trigger" and, therefore, the history of a viral prodrome and presence of rhinovirus no longer exclude this diagnosis. Evidence-based treatment options are limited. The role for mechanical ventilation in this population is often futile if there is not a reversible cause and particularly if there is not a

path to lung transplantation. Glucocorticoids are often used in combination with broad spectrum antibiotics in the hopes of a clinical response. Many patients are now being treated for IPF with nintedanib or pirfenidone, although the value of continuing these antifibrotic therapies in the acute exacerbation phase of disease is currently unknown.

Heart failure does not fully explain the acute worsening of IPF because the B-type natriuretic peptide is low.

Hypersensitivity pneumonitis is the result of an immunologic response to repetitive inhalation of antigens and high-level exposure and will often be associated with fevers, flulike symptoms, cough, and shortness of breath, typically during a period of 48 hours. The most common sources of antigens are thermophilic actinomycetes, fungi, and bird droppings. High-resolution CT imaging of the chest shows findings of ground-glass opacities and centrilobular micronodules that are upper-lung and midlung predominant. The patient's history and radiological findings are not consistent with this diagnosis.

Nonspecific interstitial pneumonia (NSIP) is a disease that predominantly affects the lower lobes of the lung. Unlike IPF, NSIP tends to affect a younger patient population and is strongly associated with connective tissue disease. The ground glass opacities on this patient's CT scan indicate an acute exacerbation with a background of usual interstitial pneumonia and are not consistent with NSIP.

KEY POINT

- An acute exacerbation of idiopathic pulmonary fibrosis begins with an abrupt worsening during a few days to weeks in the absence of another cause for dyspnea such as infection, heart failure, or pulmonary embolism and is notable for new bilateral ground-glass opacities superimposed on findings consistent with usual interstitial pneumonia on CT scan.

Bibliography

Collard HR, Ryerson CJ, Corte TJ, Jenkins G, Kondoh Y, Lederer DJ, et al. Acute exacerbation of idiopathic pulmonary fibrosis. An international working group report. Am J Respir Crit Care Med. 2016;194:265-75. [PMID: 27299520] doi:10.1164/rccm.201604-0801CI

Item 7   **Answer: C**

Educational Objective: Diagnose a patient with vocal cord dysfunction.

The most appropriate management is laryngoscopy. This patient has symptoms suggestive of vocal cord dysfunction, which is caused by paradoxical adduction of the vocal cords during inspiration, leading to functional upper airway obstruction. The diagnosis is suggested by dysphonia midchest or throat tightness with exposure to particular triggers such as strong irritants or emotions; difficulty breathing in; and symptoms that only partially respond to asthma medications. Patients may also experience midchest tightness, dyspnea, cough, and dysphonia, and stridor may be detected as inspiratory monophonic wheezing. Vocal cord dysfunction

H **CONT.** is commonly misdiagnosed as asthma, leading to excessive health care use. Diagnosis is ideally made by visualization of the abnormal vocal cord adduction during laryngoscopy. It may also be diagnosed if spirometry happens to capture a flat inspiratory limb on the flow-volume loop. However, if patients are unable to tolerate laryngoscopy while symptomatic, empiric therapy should be started if there is a high clinical suspicion of vocal cord dysfunction. Treatment consists of speech therapy utilizing cognitive behavioral techniques.

Because disorders affecting the upper respiratory tract may affect the lower tract, sinus disorders may be associated with worsening control of asthma. Patients with frequent asthma exacerbations should be evaluated for occult sinus disease, as untreated upper airway inflammation may contribute to poor asthma control. However, CT scan of the sinuses is not appropriate because sinus disease cannot explain the patient's upper chest and throat tightness, dysphonia, inspiratory monophonic wheezing, or unresponsiveness to intensive asthma treatment.

Increasing the prednisone dose is not likely to improve the patient's symptoms, which are not likely or entirely due to airway inflammation and will expose the patient to more potential side effects of glucocorticoids.

Asthma has been associated with obstructive sleep apnea (OSA). In difficult-to-control asthma, OSA is a significant risk factor for frequent exacerbations. Treatment of OSA improves asthma symptoms. However, this patient has no obvious risk factors for OSA and OSA cannot explain the patient's upper chest and throat tightness, dysphonia, or inspiratory monophonic wheezing. Therefore polysomnography is not indicated.

KEY POINT

- The diagnosis of vocal cord dysfunction is suggested by midchest tightness with exposure to particular triggers such as strong irritants or emotions; difficulty breathing in; and symptoms that only partially respond to asthma medications.

Bibliography
Idrees M, FitzGerald JM. Vocal cord dysfunction in bronchial asthma. A review article. J Asthma. 2015;52:327-35. [PMID: 25365113] doi:10.3109/02770903.2014.982288

H **Item 8** **Answer:** **C**
Educational Objective: **Treat a patient on mechanical ventilation for delirium using nonpharmacologic interventions.**

Early mobilization with physical and occupational therapy and interruption of sedation should be used to decrease the duration of delirium. This patient has acute onset of cognitive dysfunction, impairment of attention, and fluctuating mental status, which are features of delirium. Increased or decreased psychomotor activity, disorganized thinking, disorientation, and perceptual disturbances are other supportive features. The use of a screening instrument (such as the Confusion Assessment Method) allows for improved recognition and diagnosis of delirium. Delirium contributes to length of ICU stay, morbidity, mortality, and post-intensive care cognitive impairment. A study of critically ill patients on mechanical ventilation demonstrated that an early physical and occupational therapy program reduced delirium by 2 days compared to controls.

Haloperidol is used to decrease hyperactive features of delirium. Currently, there is no strong evidence in favor of its use for treating delirium in critically ill patients.

Current guidelines for sedation in the ICU favor strategies that control pain, target lighter sedation, avoid benzodiazepines, and favor early mobility. The use of benzodiazepines is associated with an increased incidence of delirium, and would not be appropriate for this patient showing signs of delirium when compared with nonbenzodiazepine sedation strategies.

The practice of having all critically ill patients on mechanical ventilation receive continuous deep sedation is no longer followed, thus increasing the propofol dosage would not be appropriate. A practice-changing trial demonstrated that daily interruption of sedation decreased length of mechanical ventilation and stay in the ICU. Recent trials demonstrated that the use of a light sedation protocol had similar patient outcomes to daily interruption of sedation. Light levels of sedation using a protocol are associated with shorter length of mechanical ventilation and ICU stay.

KEY POINT

- Early mobilization with physical and occupational therapy and interruption of sedation should be used to prevent and treat delirium in critically ill patients.

Bibliography
Schweickert WD, Pohlman MC, Pohlman AS, et al: Early physical and occupational therapy in mechanically ventilated, critically ill patients: a randomised controlled trial. Lancet 2009; 373:1874-1882 PMID 19446324

Item 9 **Answer:** **D**
Educational Objective: **Identify mortality benefits of smoking cessation.**

Smoking cessation is the best way to prevent deaths and complications from lung cancer and other diseases. There is evidence of risk reduction within 5 years of quitting smoking. In addition, case-control studies have demonstrated an 80% to 90% relative risk reduction for lung cancer in former smokers who have been abstinent for 15 years.

Chest radiograph and sputum cytology are not recommended as screening tools for lung cancer. Several large-scale controlled clinical trials have been performed and none of them demonstrated a mortality benefit for screening with cytology or chest radiography.

Recently the national lung screening trial demonstrated that screening with low-dose CT (LDCT) reduced mortality in a high-risk population (based on age and smoking history) compared with screening by radiograph (relative risk reduction of 20%). However, smoking cessation is still more likely to save a life than LDCT. The U.S. Preventive Services Task Force does recommend annual screening for lung cancer with LDCT in adults age 55-80 years who have a 30-pack-year smoking history and currently smoke or have quit within the past 15 years. Candidates for screening should take part in shared decision making, which includes a discussion of benefits and risks. Ideally it should take place in the context of a multidisciplinary program to ensure that it is properly performed and downstream testing is managed appropriately. Active smokers engaged in lung cancer screening should be counseled and assessed for smoking cessation at every opportunity.

KEY POINT

- Smoking cessation is the best way to prevent deaths and complications from lung cancer and other diseases.

Bibliography

Aberle DR, Adams AM, Berg CD, Black WC, Clapp JD, Fagerstrom RM, et al; National Lung Screening Trial Research Team. Reduced lung-cancer mortality with low-dose computed tomographic screening. N Engl J Med. 2011;365:395-409. [PMID: 21714641] doi:10.1056/NEJMoa1102873

Item 10   Answer: E

Educational Objective: Prevent airway aspiration by establishing a secure airway in patients who are unable to protect their airway.

An endotracheal tube should be placed to establish a secure airway. This patient has upper gastrointestinal bleeding and several features of cirrhosis (telangiectasias, jaundice, ascites), and likely has an acute variceal bleed. Mortality in these patients is high and requires multidisciplinary management. Initial management of esophageal variceal bleeding includes placement of two large-bore intravenous lines, fluid resuscitation, and erythrocyte transfusion to a goal hemoglobin level of 7 g/dL (70 g/L) or greater. Up to 50% of patients with cirrhosis and gastrointestinal bleeding develop infections within 1 week, and prophylactic antimicrobial agents improve mortality rates. A splanchnic vasoconstrictor such as octreotide is recommended for 3 to 5 days. Upper endoscopy with band ligation should be performed urgently after the patient is stabilized, followed by addition of a nonselective β-blocker. For the 10% to 20% of patients with uncontrolled bleeding and those with early rebleeding, a transjugular intrahepatic portosystemic shunt (TIPS) should be placed. Early airway management to prevent aspiration is essential when a patient cannot protect the airway or is otherwise at risk for aspiration of blood or gastric contents. This patient has altered mental status and ongoing hemorrhage, both risk factors for airway aspiration.

A nonselective β-blocker is recommended as secondary prophylaxis against rebleeding after recovery from a variceal bleed, but it would not be warranted in the acute setting in this patient with hypotension.

Oxygen by nasal cannula is not indicated as the patient has adequate oxygenation; furthermore, additional oxygen though nasal cannula would not help establish a secure airway.

An upper endoscopy should be performed in this patient with presumed variceal hemorrhage, but only after his airway has been secured and he has been treated with standard pharmacotherapy (octreotide and antibiotics) and appropriately resuscitated to enable safe endoscopy.

Noninvasive bilevel positive airway pressure ventilation does not provide a secure airway and is contraindicated in patients with altered mental status or risk of vomiting because it can increase the risk of aspiration if the patient were to vomit into the mask.

KEY POINT

- In patients who cannot maintain a patent airway or protect the airway against aspiration, a secure airway should be established.

Bibliography

Long B, Koyfman A. The emergency medicine evaluation and management of the patient with cirrhosis. Am J Emerg Med. 2017 Dec 23. pii: S0735-6757(17)31049-5. doi: 10.1016/j.ajem.2017.12.047. [Epub ahead of print] [PMID:29290508]

Item 11   Answer: A

Educational Objective: Treat inadequately controlled mild persistent asthma by stepping up therapy.

This patient has mild persistent asthma (albuterol use more than twice weekly but no more than once per day, and FEV_1 greater than 80% predicted) and the most appropriate management is to begin low-dose inhaled glucocorticoids such as beclomethasone. An appropriate dosage would be 40 μg per puff with 1 inhalation twice daily. Patients with asthma who require a short-acting $β_2$-agonist more than twice per week for symptom control, rather than to prevent exercise-induced bronchospasm, are considered uncontrolled. The next step in treatment is the addition of low-dose inhaled glucocorticoids. An alternative would be to add montelukast but low-dose inhaled glucocorticoid therapy is preferred. Inhaler technique should be confirmed in all patients when beginning therapy and reviewed regularly.

When inhaled glucocorticoids alone do not achieve asthma control, the addition of a long-acting $β_2$-agonist (LABA) has proved to be effective as step-up therapy. Combination preparations that contain an inhaled glucocorticoid and a LABA are available, such as fluticasone/salmeterol. In addition to bronchodilation, LABAs appear to potentiate anti-inflammatory effects of inhaled glucocorticoids when taken together. However, beginning an inhaled glucocorticoid and a LABA combination is not appropriate, as this patient has mild persistent asthma and a combination inhaled glucocorticoid/LABA is indicated for moderate persistent asthma.

Anticholinergic agents dilate bronchial smooth muscle by decreasing the constrictive cholinergic tone in the airways. Although it is less effective than β_2-agonists, the short-acting agent ipratropium can be used as adjunctive quick-relief therapy during asthma exacerbations. However, this patient has poorly controlled asthma and it is appropriate to start controller therapy, such as an inhaled glucocorticoid, to reduce airway inflammation from asthma.

Leukotriene receptor antagonists (LTRAs), such as montelukast, are not considered preferred first-line controller therapy in any asthma population. LTRAs may have a particular role in aspirin-sensitive asthma and a protective role in exercise-induced asthma; however, low-dose inhaled glucocorticoids are preferred in this patient with uncontrolled mild persistent asthma.

KEY POINT

- Patients with mild persistent asthma uncontrolled with a short-acting β_2-agonist should be stepped up to a controller medication; low-dose inhaled glucocorticoids are preferred.

Bibliography

McCracken JL, Veeranki SP, Ameredes BT, Calhoun WJ. Diagnosis and management of asthma in adults: a review. JAMA. 2017;318:279-290. [PMID: 28719697] doi:10.1001/jama.2017.8372

Item 12   Answer: C

Educational Objective: Diagnose idiopathic pulmonary fibrosis.

The most likely diagnosis is idiopathic pulmonary fibrosis (IPF). Patients with IPF typically present with chronic shortness of breath on exertion and a dry cough. The prevalence of disease increases with increasing age and is rare in individuals younger than 50 years. Clubbing is common. A history of smoking is a risk factor for the development of IPF and is commonly seen in these patients. The finding of bilateral, peripheral, and basal predominant septal line thickening with honeycomb changes on CT scan is consistent with usual interstitial pneumonia pathologic pattern and can also be seen in connective tissue disease, asbestosis, and chronic hypersensitivity pneumonitis. However, the history is negative for symptoms suggestive of connective tissue disease and for significant environmental exposures. The exclusion of connective tissue diseases and environmental exposures combined with a definite usual interstitial pneumonia imaging pattern supports the diagnosis of IPF. Tobacco smoke is associated with the development of several diffuse parenchymal lung diseases (DPLDs), including IPF. There are also several disorders that generally develop only in individuals who are active smokers; these diseases are all subacute, evolving during weeks to months.

Desquamative interstitial pneumonia is due to extensive, diffuse macrophage filling of alveolar spaces and is accompanied by predominant cough and dyspnea symptoms and bilateral ground-glass opacities on chest imaging.

Hypersensitivity pneumonitis, in its chronic form, is the most common DPLD included in the differential diagnosis

for patients with IPF. When fibrosis occurs with chronic hypersensitivity pneumonitis, it is typically in the midlung and upper-lung zones and is associated with an environmental exposure, which was not elicited in this patient. Although many patients with chronic hypersensitivity pneumonitis may no longer have an exposure to a causative antigen, the typical age of onset, history, and basal predominant CT scan abnormalities favor a diagnosis of IPF rather than hypersensitivity pneumonitis.

Pulmonary Langerhans cell histiocytosis is characterized by thin-walled cysts with accompanying nodules and is often associated with pulmonary hypertension. All of these diseases are subacute, evolving during weeks to months and present in active smokers.

Respiratory bronchiolitis–associated interstitial lung disease is used to describe disease in active smokers who have imaging findings of centrilobular micronodules with a pathologic finding of respiratory bronchiolitis on biopsy.

KEY POINT

- Idiopathic pulmonary fibrosis typically occurs in older individuals with nonproductive cough and progressive dyspnea on exertion; the diagnosis is supported by findings of usual interstitial pneumonitis on a high-resolution CT scan of the chest.

Bibliography

Raghu G, Collard HR, Egan JJ, Martinez FJ, Behr J, Brown KK, et al; ATS/ERS/JRS/ALAT Committee on Idiopathic Pulmonary Fibrosis. An official ATS/ERS/JRS/ALAT statement: idiopathic pulmonary fibrosis: evidence-based guidelines for diagnosis and management. Am J Respir Crit Care Med. 2011;183:788-824. [PMID: 21471066] doi:10.1164/rccm.2009-040GL

Item 13   Answer: E

Educational Objective: Assess intravascular volume status.

No further testing is required. The physical examination has several features that suggest she has decreased intravascular volume and reduced systemic vascular resistance. The presence of warm and vasodilated skin, a very low diastolic pressure, absent jugular venous distention, and tachycardia all suggest severe vasodilation. There are several invasive and noninvasive devices available to aid the clinician to confirm the clinical diagnosis; however, none of them alone can provide a definite answer. Integrating the physical examination and basic vital signs remains the best clinical method to define intravascular volume status and the type of shock.

Central venous catheter measurement of venous pressure can provide information that helps confirm the diagnosis of low central venous pressure; however, it is invasive, subject to technical issues, and the presence of spontaneous breathing needs to be considered when obtaining readings. Studies have demonstrated that a single measurement does not help define intravascular volume status or volume responsiveness. Thus the value must be taken in the context of the history and physical exam.

CONT. Fullness of the vena cava as detected by ultrasonography is thought to correlate with increased right atrial pressure, whereas a collapsing inferior vena cava at the end of expiration suggests volume responsiveness. Volume responsiveness refers to an increase in cardiac output upon the administration of fluid. A common inference is that intravascular volume is high when the patient is not volume responsive; however, this would be a limited assumption as the response to volume also involves cardiac function and infusion volume. In addition, the presence of increased respiratory effort will make the measurements unreliable.

A pulmonary artery catheter will provide a plethora of information on the intravascular pressures (by inference, the volume status) and cardiac output of the patient. However, placing a pulmonary artery catheter in a patient with sepsis is invasive, does not improve management, increases complications, and has not demonstrated improved outcome.

Pulse pressure is the difference between systolic and diastolic arterial blood pressure during respiration induced by positive pressure ventilation. A low variation in pulse pressure is believed to be an indicator of unresponsiveness to a fluid challenge whereas a pulse pressure variation of at least 13% to 15% is associated with volume responsiveness. However, this measurement is only reliable in patients who are mechanically ventilated (and not spontaneously triggering the ventilator), receiving 8 mL/kg or more of tidal volume, and in sinus rhythm.

> **KEY POINT**
>
> - The most appropriate method to evaluate volume status remains the physical examination; several technologies can help confirm the assessment.

Bibliography

Teboul JL, Saugel B, Cecconi M, De Backer D, Hofer CK, Monnet X, et al. Less invasive hemodynamic monitoring in critically ill patients. Intensive Care Med. 2016;42:1350-9. [PMID: 27155605] doi:10.1007/s00134-016-4375-7

Item 14   Answer: C

Educational Objective: Diagnose small cell lung cancer.

The most likely diagnosis is small cell lung cancer (SCLC). SCLC is a neuroendocrine tumor that accounts for approximately 15% of all lung cancers and occurs predominantly in smokers.

This patient has signs and symptoms of hyponatremia and chest CT scan shows a large mediastinal right hilar mass and right-lower-lobe mass (arrows).

Imaging studies in SCLC commonly demonstrate a large hilar mass with bulky mediastinal lymphadenopathy; some patients may not have an obvious primary lesion. Signs and symptoms include cough, dyspnea, weight loss, and debility. Less commonly SCLC can present with endocrinologic or neurologic paraneoplastic syndromes. The

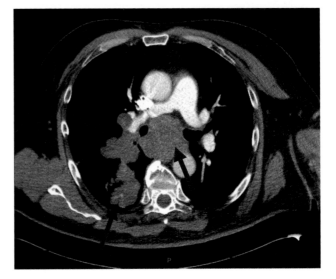

syndrome of inappropriate antidiuretic hormone secretion (SIADH) due to ectopic production of antidiuretic hormone (ADH) is most often due to a SCLC and is rarely seen with other lung tumors. It occurs in approximately 10% of patients and results in hyponatremia. The severity of symptoms is related to the degree of hyponatremia and rapidity of the decrease. They may include anorexia, nausea, and vomiting, but if the decrease is rapid, cerebral edema can occur and may result in irritability, restlessness, personality changes, confusion, coma, seizures, and respiratory arrest. SCLC is more aggressive than non-small cell lung cancer (NSCLC), is usually already disseminated at presentation, and requires prompt treatment; however, it is often initially more sensitive to chemotherapy and radiotherapy but typically relapses and becomes resistant to further treatment. Staging should not delay treatment.

NSCLC accounts for 80% of lung cancers, of which adenocarcinoma is the most common type, followed by squamous cell. Although NSCLC is in the differential diagnosis for this patient, hyponatremia and a large mediastinal mass are most consistent with SCLC.

Malignant pleural mesothelioma typically presents as a recurrent exudative pleural effusion with pleural thickening in a patient with exposure to asbestos. This patient did not present with a pleural effusion, which makes this diagnosis less likely.

> **KEY POINT**
>
> - Typical imaging findings in patients with small cell lung cancer (SCLC) include a large mediastinal mass; hyponatremia due to ectopic production of antidiuretic hormone is most often due to SCLC and is rarely seen with other lung tumors.

Bibliography

Jett JR, Schild SE, Kesler KA, Kalemkerian GP. Treatment of small cell lung cancer: diagnosis and management of lung cancer, 3rd ed: American College of Chest Physicians evidence-based clinical practice guidelines. Chest. 2013;143:e400S-e419S. [PMID: 23649448] doi:10.1378/chest. 12-2363

Item 15   **Answer: B**

Educational Objective: Evaluate an acute exacerbation of COPD.

An electrocardiogram should be obtained for this patient to evaluate other causes of her acute presentation, such as acute myocardial infarction, arrhythmia, and atrial fibrillation. The first steps in managing a patient with a presumed COPD exacerbation are to confirm the diagnosis. Studies helpful in the evaluation may include pulse oximetry to assess oxygenation or guide oxygen therapy; a chest radiograph to rule out an alternative diagnosis; a complete blood count to identify the presence of polycythemia, anemia, or leukocytosis; arterial blood gas studies; a biochemical panel to assess for electrolyte and glycemic abnormalities; and an electrocardiogram to evaluate tachycardia (as in this patient) and for other possible cardiac comorbidity. This patient has already had a chest radiograph and appropriate laboratory studies but an electrocardiogram is also indicated.

Patients with pulmonary embolism (PE) can present with symptoms similar to a COPD exacerbation. Because of this, pretest probability models such as the Wells criteria have been developed and validated to assist in clinical decision making. Patients who have a low pretest probability for PE using the Wells criteria, such as this patient, and who meet all Pulmonary Embolism Rule-Out Criteria do not need further testing to rule out PE. Physicians should obtain a D-dimer assay in patients with intermediate pretest probability for PE or for those with a low pretest probability for PE who do not meet all Pulmonary Embolism Rule-Out Criteria. In these patients, imaging studies should not be used for initial evaluation.

A sputum culture or Gram stain is not routinely used to assess COPD exacerbations as it rarely changes management. For patients with a confirmed COPD exacerbation with cough, increased sputum, and dyspnea, antibiotics are usually initiated regardless of the results of the sputum Gram stain or culture.

KEY POINT

- The first steps in managing a patient with a presumed COPD exacerbation are to confirm the diagnosis and to evaluate other causes of the acute presentation.

Bibliography
Holden V, Slack III D, McCurdy MT, Shah NG. Diagnosis and management of acute exacerbations of chronic obstructive pulmonary disease. Emerg Med Pract. 2017;19:1-24. [PMID: 28926214]

Item 16   **Answer: C**

Educational Objective: Identify the sequela of obstructive sleep apnea most responsive to therapy.

Excessive daytime sleepiness is the strongest indication for treatment of obstructive sleep apnea (OSA). Excessive daytime sleepiness is thought to result primarily from disruption of sleep architecture due to repetitive breathing events.

Randomized trials and meta-analyses of systematic reviews show that positive airway pressure therapy reduces the frequency of respiratory events during sleep and is associated with reduction in daytime sleepiness and improved sleep-related quality of life.

Observational studies that suggest benefit from positive airway pressure therapy on the natural history of atrial fibrillation is yet to be proved in randomized trials. There is a similar lack of proved benefit in other important conditions, such as cardiovascular death. In addition, a recent large multicenter trial failed to show mortality benefit afforded by positive airway pressure therapy in those with OSA and cardiovascular disease.

Trials assessing various measures of glucose homeostasis (fasting glucose, insulin resistance, hemoglobin A_{1c}) in patients with OSA treated with positive airway pressure have shown inconsistent results. This patient requires adjustment of his medication with the goal of reducing the hemoglobin A_{1c} level.

Positive airway pressure therapy has been shown to modestly reduce blood pressure in those with OSA, but the effects are not always consistent. Those with excessive daytime sleepiness tend to be more responsive to these effects than those who are not sleepy. Also, comparative efficacy trials in those with OSA have shown greater reductions in blood pressure with antihypertensive drug therapy than positive airway pressure. This patient's antihypertensive medications should be adjusted with the goal of achieving the target blood pressure level recommended by the American College of Cardiology/American Heart Association of less than 130/80 mm Hg.

KEY POINT

- Excessive daytime sleepiness is the strongest indication for treatment of obstructive sleep apnea.

Bibliography
McEvoy RD, Antic NA, Heeley E, Luo Y, Ou Q, Zhang X, et al; SAVE Investigators and Coordinators. CPAP for prevention of cardiovascular events in obstructive sleep apnea. N Engl J Med. 2016;375:919-31. [PMID: 27571048] doi:10.1056/NEJMoa1606599

Item 17   **Answer: B**

Educational Objective: Treat a patient with obesity hypoventilation syndrome and hypercarbic respiratory failure who does not improve quickly with noninvasive ventilation.

The most appropriate treatment is endotracheal intubation. This patient has developed acute on chronic hypercapnic respiratory failure in the setting of obesity hypoventilation syndrome. In a patient who is able to protect the airway, the initial management of acute hypercapnic respiratory failure due to obesity hypoventilation syndrome includes noninvasive positive pressure ventilation. Because he has an intact gag and cough reflex and is arousable, noninvasive positive pressure ventilation was an appropriate initial choice. However,

H
CONT.

when patients cannot protect their airway, do not tolerate bilevel positive airway pressure, or do not improve quickly, such as this patient, early intubation should be considered.

Respiratory stimulants such as acetazolamide have been considered adjunctive therapies of last resort for patients who chronically continue to have hypoventilation despite BPAP therapy and weight loss. Acetazolamide, by blocking carbon dioxide conversion to bicarbonate, can lower pH in the brain and theoretically increases central ventilatory drive. This patient already demonstrates significant acidemia with inadequate central respiratory drive. In addition, randomized trials demonstrating efficacy are lacking. Thus, acetazolamide is not recommended for either acute or chronic hypercapnic respiratory failure.

Although many patients with morbid obesity demonstrate features of obstruction or air trapping on pulmonary function testing, only a fraction have true reversible obstructive airways disease pathology. This patient has no clear evidence of obstruction on examination or chest radiograph and no history of asthma or other obstructive airways pathology. Therefore, prednisone use in this setting is not indicated.

Theophylline is a bronchodilator as well as a direct respiratory stimulant. Its use in obesity-hypoventilation syndrome has never been studied and thus is not recommended for treatment of this or other hypercapnic states.

KEY POINT

- Early intubation is indicated for patients with obesity hypoventilation syndrome and hypercapnic respiratory failure who do not improve with noninvasive positive pressure ventilation.

Bibliography

Manthous CA, Mokhlesi B. Avoiding management errors in patients with obesity hypoventilation syndrome. Ann Am Thorac Soc. 2016;13:109-14. [PMID: 26512908] doi:10.1513/AnnalsATS.201508-562OT

Item 18   Answer: A

Educational Objective: Diagnose a patient with α_1-antitrypsin deficiency.

An α_1-antitrypsin level should be obtained. This patient is younger than the usual age of presentation of COPD, and he does not have a significant smoking history. In this situation it is prudent to rule out other causes of dyspnea, especially in a patient where a diagnosis of COPD is unexpected. White patients experiencing symptoms of COPD and who are younger than 45 years of age or have a strong family history of COPD should be tested for α_1-antitrypsin deficiency. Several guidelines even recommend that all patients with COPD regardless of age should be tested for α_1-antitrypsin deficiency after weighing the risks and benefits of testing. Patients with this disorder are often misdiagnosed with asthma for many years. They may have a modest smoking history and basilar emphysema (although they may present with any pattern of emphysema), and they may have concurrent liver disease.

Patients with α_1-antitrypsin deficiency who never smoke may develop symptoms later in life. If the diagnosis of α_1-antitrypsin deficiency is confirmed, α_1-antitrypsin augmentation therapy may slow disease progression, although data on its efficacy are limited.

Nitric oxide promotes dilation of bronchial blood vessels and airways. The fractional exhaled nitric oxide (FENO) is a noninvasive test most commonly used in patients with severe airflow obstruction when other techniques are difficult to perform (for example, assessing airflow in a child or mentally impaired adult). High levels of FENO are typically associated with asthma and other inflammatory airway conditions. Measurement of FENO is not indicated as the next diagnostic test in this patient with a history strongly suspicious for α_1-antitrypsin deficiency.

High-resolution CT (HRCT) is indicated if diffuse parenchymal lung disease is suspected. HRCT can help narrow the differential diagnosis based on the distribution of the lung parenchymal abnormalities and the presence or absence of associated findings. Diffuse parenchymal lung disease should be suspected in the presence of restrictive or combined obstructive/restrictive diseases. HRCT is also diagnostically definitive for bronchiectasis, but this condition is typically characterized by cough and voluminous, often purulent, sputum production, which is not present in this patient.

A vascular endothelial growth factor-D level can help in the diagnosis of lymphangioleiomyomatosis (LAM). However, LAM is a cystic lung disease that mostly affects young women, so testing would not be indicated for this patient.

KEY POINT

- Measurement of α_1-antitrypsin level is indicated for white patients experiencing symptoms of COPD and who are younger than 45 years of age or have a strong family history of COPD.

Bibliography

American Thoracic Society. American Thoracic Society/European Respiratory Society statement: standards for the diagnosis and management of individuals with alpha-1 antitrypsin deficiency. Am J Respir Crit Care Med. 2003;168:818-900. [PMID: 14522813]

Item 19   Answer: C

Educational Objective: Treat a patient for side effects of positive airway pressure therapy.

The most appropriate treatment is heated humidification. A common complication of positive airway pressure therapy is desiccation of the nasopharyngeal mucosa by the forced air, often resulting in throat irritation and nasal congestion. In-line heated humidification, available on all positive airway pressure machines, is a simple intervention to mitigate mucosal irritation. Patients can control the temperature and degree of humidity. Although there is conflicting evidence that in-line humidification improves adherence to positive airway pressure therapy, it does mitigate upper airway symptoms.

Bilevel positive airway pressure is indicated for hypoventilation syndromes caused by severe COPD or neuromuscular weakness. There is no evidence that bilevel positive airway pressure is superior to continuous positive airway pressure for the treatment of obstructive sleep apnea without hypoventilation. This patient does not suffer from a hypoventilation syndrome, and he is improving on current therapy; therefore, a change in therapy is not indicated. Finally, bilevel positive airway pressure without humidification will not relieve his upper airway symptoms.

The role of hypnotics in promoting positive airway pressure adherence is controversial and not generally recommended. One study showed nightly eszopiclone (a benzodiazepine receptor agonist) administered to unselected patients during the first 2 weeks of continuous positive airway pressure treatment improved adherence as long as 6 months later. Its continued use beyond initiation of positive airway pressure treatment has not been studied and the risk of side effects may outweigh its benefit. Finally, eszopiclone will not relieve this patient's throat irritation or nasal congestion.

Topical nasal steroids are often prescribed to reduce these side effects of nasal congestion and rhinorrhea, but evidence supporting their effectiveness in reducing upper airway symptoms is sparse. A recent randomized clinical study failed to show a reduction in nasal symptoms or improved adherence to therapy in patients treated with nasal fluticasone compared to placebo.

KEY POINT

- In-line heated humidification is available on all positive airway pressure machines and is a simple intervention to mitigate mucosal irritation.

Bibliography

Sommer JU, Kraus M, Birk R, Schultz JD, Hörmann K, Stuck BA. Functional short- and long-term effects of nasal CPAP with and without humidification on the ciliary function of the nasal respiratory epithelium. Sleep Breath. 2014;18:85-93. [PMID: 23657665] doi:10.1007/s11325-013-0853-0

Item 20 Answer: C

Educational Objective: Treat a patient with eosinophilic asthma with mepolizumab.

The most appropriate treatment is initiation of a trial of mepolizumab therapy. This patient has signs and symptoms of severe persistent asthma that is uncontrolled (more than two exacerbations per year), despite treatment with a high-dose inhaled glucocorticoid, long-acting β_2-agonist, long-acting anticholinergic agent, leukotriene-receptor antagonist, and oral glucocorticoids, so her therapy should be stepped up. Biologic therapies that target atopic pathways of asthma are indicated in appropriate patients. Currently available agents are directed against either eosinophils or their products (IgE). Interleukin (IL-5) is a pro-eosinophilic cytokine that promotes eosinophil production and contributes to eosinophilic inflammation in the airways. Mepolizumab and

reslizumab are monoclonal antibodies to IL-5 and both agents reduce exacerbations of severe asthma in patients who have blood eosinophil counts of 150/µL or 300/µL, respectively, or higher. Mepolizumab is administered subcutaneously every 4 weeks, whereas reslizumab is an infusion. Although these agents are expensive, patients with uncontrolled eosinophilic asthma treated with mepolizumab have reduced emergency department visits and hospitalizations, and both agents have reduced the requirement for inhaled and oral glucocorticoids. Use of these agents is contraindicated during acute asthma exacerbations.

Treatment with doxycycline is not indicated because there are no signs or symptoms of bacterial infection.

Changing from one inhaled glucocorticoid/long-acting β_2-agonist to another would not be expected to have a significant effect, as the inhaled glucocorticoid dose is similar and there is no apparent difference in the efficacy of the various combinations.

Omalizumab, a humanized monoclonal antibody directed at IgE, was the first biologic agent approved by the FDA for use in asthma. Administered subcutaneously every 2 to 4 weeks, omalizumab is indicated in patients with moderate to severe persistent asthma with the following characteristics: (1) symptoms inadequately controlled with inhaled glucocorticoids, (2) evidence of allergies to perennial aeroallergens, and (3) serum IgE levels between 30 and 700 U/mL (30-700 kU/L) (normal range, 0-90 U/mL [0-90 kU/L]). Omalizumab has been shown to reduce exacerbations and emergency department visits; it is not indicated for use in patients other than those meeting these treatment parameters.

KEY POINT

- In patients with moderate to severe uncontrolled asthma with the eosinophilic phenotype, treatment with mepolizumab can reduce emergency department visits, hospitalizations, and requirements for inhaled and oral glucocorticoids.

Bibliography

Israel E, Reddel HK. Severe and difficult-to-treat asthma in adults. N Engl J Med. 2017;377:965-976. [PMID: 28877019] doi:10.1056/NEJMra1608969

Item 21 Answer: D

Educational Objective: Treat severe carbon monoxide poisoning with hyperbaric oxygen therapy.

This patient should receive hyperbaric oxygen therapy. Inhaled carbon monoxide has a much higher affinity for hemoglobin binding sites than oxygen and readily forms carboxyhemoglobin, which is an ineffective oxygen transporter and results in reduced tissue oxygen content. Symptoms of carbon monoxide poisoning vary and include headache, confusion, nausea, vomiting, and, in severe cases, loss of consciousness. It is important to understand that carboxyhemoglobin does not lower oxygen saturation measured by standard pulse oximetry or reduce arterial P_{O_2} determined by blood gas analysis.

Co-oximetry, which measures carboxyhemoglobin levels, is used to make the diagnosis. She has severe carbon monoxide poisoning due to unvented combustion in a small, enclosed area. Cited indications for hyperbaric oxygen therapy include loss of consciousness, ischemic cardiac changes, neurological deficits, significant metabolic acidosis, or carboxyhemoglobin level greater than 25%. A carboxyhemoglobin level of 50% is critical and needs to be reduced as quickly as possible. Breathing 100% oxygen at normal atmospheric pressure, this patient will clear the carboxyhemoglobin with a half-life of 90 minutes, but hyperbaric oxygen therapy will lower the half-life to 30 minutes. Also, there is considerable risk of delayed neurocognitive impairment following a severe exposure such as this, and hyperbaric oxygen is believed to lower the risk of this long-term complication, although the strength of this evidence is disputed.

Maintaining the current ventilator settings of 50% oxygen or decreasing the oxygen to 30% will not clear the carboxyhemoglobin as rapidly as hyperbaric oxygen. If hyperbaric oxygen therapy is unavailable, or if the toxicity is less severe, administration of 100% oxygen is the most appropriate therapy. However, this patient has mental status changes and the carboxyhemoglobin level is 50%; hyperbaric treatment is clearly indicated.

Carbon monoxide poisoning resulting from smoke inhalation should prompt consideration of concomitant inhaled cyanide poisoning. Hydroxocobalamin effectively binds intracellular cyanide to form cyanocobalamin, which poses no harm. However, this patient's carbon monoxide poisoning is due to combustion of propane in an enclosed space, not a house fire; therefore, hydroxocobalamin is not indicated.

KEY POINT

- Cited indications for hyperbaric oxygen therapy include loss of consciousness, ischemic cardiac changes, neurological deficits, significant metabolic acidosis, or carboxyhemoglobin level greater than 25%.

Bibliography

Hampson NB, Piantadosi CA, Thom SR, Weaver LK. Practice recommendations in the diagnosis, management, and prevention of carbon monoxide poisoning. Am J Respir Crit Care Med. 2012;186:1095-101. [PMID: 23087025] doi:10.1164/rccm.201207-1284CI

Item 22   Answer: A

Educational Objective: Evaluate a patient who has an acute exacerbation of COPD with arterial blood gas analysis.

Arterial blood gas analysis is the most appropriate test for this patient with a COPD exacerbation. An exacerbation is considered mild when a change in the clinical condition is noted but no change in medication is necessary; moderate when medication changes are made; and severe if emergency department evaluation or hospitalization is required. A severe exacerbation can also be diagnosed if the patient has two of the three following symptoms: increased dyspnea, increased sputum volume, or increased sputum purulence. Studies helpful in the evaluation of a severe exacerbation may include pulse oximetry to assess oxygenation or guide oxygen therapy; a chest radiograph to rule out an alternative diagnosis; a complete blood count to identify the presence of polycythemia, anemia, or leukocytosis; a biochemical panel to assess for electrolyte and glycemic abnormalities; an electrocardiogram to evaluate for a possible cardiac comorbidity; and arterial blood gas analysis. Arterial blood gas analysis is recommended for patients with a severe exacerbation of COPD to assess for hypercapnia and hypoxemia. This information is helpful in determining site of care and the need for additional therapy such as noninvasive mechanical ventilation.

The patient has no signs or symptoms of heart failure or other cardiac disease to explain his presentation. Therefore, B-type natriuretic peptide measurement and echocardiogram are unlikely to change management at this time.

According to best practice advice from the Clinical Guidelines Committee of the American College of Physicians, patients who have a low pretest probability for pulmonary embolism (PE) using a validated clinical prediction rule (such as the Wells criteria for prediction of PE) and who meet all Pulmonary Embolism Rule-Out Criteria do not need further testing to rule out PE. Using the Wells criteria, this patient is a low risk for PE (0 points) and scores 2 points on the Pulmonary Embolism Rule-Out Criteria (fails to meet 2 criteria: age younger than 50 years and oxygen saturation greater than 94%). Additional evaluation for PE in this patient might include a D-dimer measurement as an initial test, but not an imaging study.

KEY POINT

- Arterial blood gas analysis is recommended for patients with a severe exacerbation of COPD to assess for hypercapnia and hypoxemia.

Bibliography

Qureshi H, Sharafkhaneh A, Hanania NA. Chronic obstructive pulmonary disease exacerbations: latest evidence and clinical implications. Ther Adv Chronic Dis. 2014;5:212-27. [PMID: 25177479] doi:10.1177/2040622314532862

Item 23   Answer: C

Educational Objective: Evaluate suspected pulmonary arterial hypertension with transthoracic echocardiography.

The next most appropriate initial test is transthoracic echocardiography. Pulmonary hypertension is easily overlooked because early signs and symptoms, such as exertional dyspnea and fatigue, are nonspecific. As the disorder progresses, right ventricular impairment may be heralded by exertional chest pain, syncope, and peripheral edema. Findings on physical examination depend on the severity of disease. The cardiovascular examination may show jugular venous distention, a prominent jugular venous a wave, parasternal heave, a widened split S_2 with a prominent pulmonic component, or murmurs of tricuspid regurgitation as the right ventricle dilates. Transthoracic echocardiography is a useful initial tool in the evaluation of suspected pulmonary hypertension as it allows an estimation of pulmonary artery pressures and right heart function as well as an assessment of the left heart. Because echocardiography may underestimate true pulmonary artery pressures, the evaluation should not end with an unrevealing echocardiogram if the index of suspicion for pulmonary hypertension is high. In such cases, right heart catheterization may be confirmatory. Once pulmonary hypertension is confirmed, further testing, guided by clinical history, helps determine identifiable causes. Left heart catheterization can assess coronary flow and left ventricular function. Diagnostic tests for respiratory diseases might include pulmonary function tests, chest imaging, ventilation-perfusion ($\dot{V}/\dot{Q}$) scanning, and overnight pulse oximetry.

High-resolution CT scanning of the chest allows a detailed assessment of the lung parenchyma and is useful in the evaluation of suspected interstitial lung diseases, but is unlikely to be helpful as an initial test in a patient with an unremarkable lung examination and clear lung fields on chest radiograph.

Pulmonary function testing is an important diagnostic test for suspected airways disease such as asthma, COPD, or interstitial lung disease. However, this patient has no symptoms or physical examination findings indicative of either obstructive or restrictive disease. In the patient with isolated pulmonary hypertension, pulmonary function tests demonstrate a reduction in diffusing capacity, which is a nonspecific finding.

$\dot{V}/\dot{Q}$ scanning is the diagnostic test of choice for suspected chronic thromboembolic pulmonary hypertension (CTEPH). Although CTEPH hasn't yet been excluded in this patient, $\dot{V}/\dot{Q}$ scanning would typically be performed after transthoracic echocardiography to first establish the presence of pulmonary hypertension.

KEY POINT

- Transthoracic echocardiography can estimate pulmonary artery pressures and is the preferred initial test if pulmonary hypertension is suspected.

Bibliography
Vonk Noordegraaf A, Groeneveldt JA, Bogaard HJ. Pulmonary hypertension. Eur Respir Rev. 2016;25:4-11. [PMID: 26929415] doi:10.1183/16000617.0096-2015

Item 24   Answer: E

Educational Objective: Manage obesity-related asthma with a supervised weight loss program.

This patient should be referred to a supervised weight loss program. He has poorly controlled asthma despite maximal medical therapy and in the absence of other factors known to exacerbate asthma (environmental triggers, uncontrolled gastroesophageal reflux disease, sinus disease, or obstructive sleep apnea). Obesity is associated with poor asthma control,

and the incidence of asthma is 1.47 times greater in obese patients than nonobese patients. Weight loss in patients with obesity-related asthma improves asthma control, lung function, and quality of life; reduces asthma medication use; and should be considered an essential part of the treatment plan.

Addition of beclomethasone is not appropriate because this patient is already on adequate inhaled therapy and glucocorticoids; increasing the inhaled steroid dose is unlikely to be beneficial.

Between attacks and exacerbations of asthma, spirometry can be normal in patients with suspected but undiagnosed asthma. Therefore, a bronchial challenge test, such as a methacholine challenge, may be helpful for diagnosis if positive or make the diagnosis less likely if negative. Methacholine challenge testing is not necessary in this patient because spirometry confirms reversible airflow obstruction (with a 12% or greater improvement in FEV_1 or FVC of 200 mL after administration of a bronchodilator), supporting a diagnosis of asthma.

Mepolizumab is a monoclonal antibody to IL-5 that has been shown to reduce asthma exacerbations in patients with difficult-to-control asthma and elevated blood eosinophil counts. This patient's eosinophil count was normal; therefore, add-on therapy with mepolizumab is not indicated.

Although omalizumab can reduce hospitalizations when added to standard therapy, it is a monoclonal antibody used for treatment of allergic asthma, and it targets elevated levels of IgE. Because this patient does not have a history of allergies and his IgE level is normal, treatment with omalizumab would not be appropriate.

KEY POINT

- Weight loss in patients with obesity-related asthma improves asthma control, lung function, and quality of life; reduces asthma medication use; and should be considered an essential part of the treatment plan.

Bibliography
Pakhale S, Baron J, Dent R, Vandemheen K, Aaron SD. Effects of weight loss on airway responsiveness in obese adults with asthma: Does weight loss lead to reversibility of asthma? Chest. 2015;147:1582-1590. [PMID: 25763936] doi:10.1378/chest.14-3105

Item 25   Answer: C

Educational Objective: Treat heart failure in a patient with a Cheyne-Stokes breathing pattern.

Diuresis with furosemide is the most appropriate treatment option. This patient has central sleep apnea with Cheyne-Stokes breathing in the setting of decompensated heart failure, a state of ventilatory instability. Cheyne-Stokes breathing is an abnormal respiratory pattern characterized by cyclic crescendo-decrescendo respiratory effort during sleep (and sometimes during wakefulness), in the absence of upper airway obstruction. Apnea accompanying the decrescendo effort defines central sleep apnea. The degree of central sleep apnea tends to correlate with left ventricular dysfunction.

This patient has evidence on examination of volume overload (crackles and wheezing on lung exam, jugular venous distention, peripheral edema). Optimizing medical management of heart failure and improving fluid balance should precede other therapies for sleep apnea.

Adaptive servo-ventilation is a form of positive airway pressure therapy initially designed as a treatment of Cheyne-Stokes breathing. However, a large multicenter trial unexpectedly showed increased mortality in a subset of patients with systolic heart failure (left ventricular ejection fraction less than 45%) and central sleep apnea treated with adaptive servo-ventilation.

Auto-adjusting positive airway pressure is not an initial treatment for central sleep apnea. It is used to treat obstructive sleep apnea, where proprietary algorithms deliver varying pressure sufficient to prevent upper airway closure.

Supplemental oxygen is sometimes used in advanced heart failure where impaired gas exchange results in hypoxemia. This patient has preserved oxyhemoglobin saturation. Small trials have studied the use of nocturnal supplemental oxygen in the setting of central sleep apnea, with variable results. Such treatment would be premature before optimization of fluid status.

KEY POINT

- Initial treatment of central sleep apnea should target modifiable risk factors; medical optimization of heart failure has been shown to improve central sleep apnea and Cheyne-Stokes breathing and should precede other therapies for sleep apnea.

Bibliography

Hernandez AB, Patil SP. Pathophysiology of central sleep apneas. Sleep Breath. 2016;20:467-82. [PMID: 26782104] doi:10.1007/s11325-015-1290-z

Item 26   Answer: B

Educational Objective: Treat asthma-COPD overlap syndrome.

The most appropriate treatment is a combination inhaled glucocorticoid and a long-acting β_2-agonist. This patient has progressive symptoms, spirometry showing diminished FEV_1 that partially reversed with bronchodilation, and eosinophilia. Several diagnostic terms have been used to describe patients with both asthma and COPD, most including the word *overlap*, but there is no universally agreed upon term or defining diagnostic features for this condition. Given her progression of symptoms, her short-acting inhaler therapy should be augmented. Although a long-acting β_2-agonist is indicated in symptomatic patients with COPD and an FEV_1 of less than 60% of predicted, this may not be the best treatment for a patient with asthma. Patients with asthma are at increased risk of mortality when a long-acting bronchodilator is prescribed without a controller medication. Experts recommend that patients who have an asthma-COPD overlap syndrome who are receiving a long-acting bronchodilator should

ideally also be prescribed an inhaled glucocorticoid. Combination therapy seems to mitigate the excess risk of mortality observed in patients with asthma treated with long-acting β_2-agonist monotherapy. Therefore, the patient should be started on a combination therapy of an inhaled glucocorticoid and a long-acting β_2-agonist.

Chronic macrolide therapy can reduce the incidence of acute exacerbations but this patient has not had any exacerbations to warrant starting a macrolide.

Using a long-acting β_2-agonist or a long-acting muscarinic agent/long-acting β_2-agonist combination inhaler is likely not indicated for this patient with asthma-COPD overlap syndrome based on current guidelines. Long-acting bronchodilators should only be used in combination with inhaled glucocorticoids in patients with a history of asthma. Using long-acting bronchodilators alone has been linked to increased risk of asthma-related deaths.

KEY POINT

- Patients with a history of asthma-COPD overlap syndrome should not be prescribed a long-acting β_2-agonist without concurrent therapy with an inhaled glucocorticoid because of the increased risk of mortality in patients with asthma who are prescribed long-acting β_2-agonist monotherapy.

Bibliography

GINA/GOLD Joint Report. 2015 asthma, COPD and asthma-COPD overlap syndrome (ACOS) [Internet] Bethesda: Global Initiative for Asthma; 2016. Available from: http://ginasthma.org/asthma-copd-and-asthma-copdoverlap-syndrome-acos/. Accessed May 1, 2018.

Item 27   Answer: C

Educational Objective: Diagnose pneumothorax in a patient with lung disease in the setting of air travel.

The most likely diagnosis is pneumothorax. An estimated 12% of in-flight medical emergencies involve a respiratory complaint. Commercial airline cabins are partially pressurized, typically to the equivalent of approximately 1400 to 2500 meters (4000 to 8000 feet) above sea level, limiting exposure to extreme hypobaric conditions. The risk of pneumothorax is therefore mitigated but it is most likely to occur at cruising altitude in patients with bullous lung disease, particularly those with a recent exacerbation of airways disease who are, therefore, more prone to air trapping. Pain is typically pleuritic; dyspnea may be present, depending upon the volume of trapped air. If tension physiology develops (hypotension, shock, altered mental status), needle thoracostomy using the on-board equipment can be life-saving. Descending to a lower altitude may also be beneficial, because cabin pressure is inversely related to the altitude of the aircraft.

Descending aortic dissection typically presents with acute, severe back pain. Although chest pain can occur, it is less common. Radiation of pain to the abdomen can occur with disruption of blood flow to the abdominal viscera. Hypertension is the most important risk factor and is present in more than half of patients with descending aortic dissection. Pulse deficits are common. However, this patient does not have a history of hypertension and has normal peripheral pulses, making a diagnosis of descending aortic dissection unlikely.

Pneumocystis jirovecii pneumonia is unlikely to present in this manner. Although systemic glucocorticoids increase the risk for opportunistic lung infections such as *P. jirovecii* pneumonia, the risk is minimal during the course of a typical prednisone burst and taper used for a COPD exacerbation. In general, those taking prednisone dosage equivalents of at least 20 mg/day for more than 3 weeks should receive *P. jirovecii* pneumonia prophylaxis.

Air travel increases the risk of venous thromboembolism, though the risk is higher during relative immobilization on long flights and in those with other risk factors, such as cancer. The risk of pulmonary embolism does not really increase until the flight distance becomes greater than 5000 km (3000 miles). It is unlikely that a flight duration of only 90 minutes would heighten thrombotic risk in this patient.

KEY POINT

- During air travel, pneumothorax is most likely to occur at cruising altitude in patients with bullous lung disease, particularly those with a recent exacerbation of airways disease who are, therefore, more prone to air trapping.

Bibliography

Nable JV, Tupe CL, Gehle BD, Brady WJ. In-flight medical emergencies during commercial travel. N Engl J Med. 2015;373:939-45. [PMID: 26332548] doi:10.1056/NEJMra1409213

Item 28   Answer: B

Educational Objective: Evaluate a patient with upper-lobe emphysema and significant exercise limitations for lung volume reduction surgery.

Evaluation for lung volume reduction surgery is the most appropriate management for this patient with upper-lobe emphysema, significant exercise limitation, and poor quality of life. Lung volume reduction surgery excises areas of emphysematous lung, improves the mechanical efficiency of respiratory muscles, and increases the elastic recoil of the lungs to improve expiratory flow and reduce exacerbations. The National Emphysema Treatment Trial (NETT) demonstrated that carefully selected patients with upper-lobe predominant emphysema and significant exercise limitation despite participation in a pulmonary rehabilitation program had improved quality of life and survival with lung volume reduction surgery. Symptomatic improvement with the surgery appears to be durable.

Roflumilast is an oral selective phosphodiesterase-4 inhibitor. It is used primarily as add-on therapy in severe COPD associated with chronic bronchitis and a history of recurrent exacerbations despite other therapies; it has been shown to relieve symptoms and reduce risk and frequency of exacerbations in these individuals. However, it is not a bronchodilator, is expensive, and has not been shown to be effective in other groups of patients with COPD. It is not indicated in the treatment of primary emphysema and has not been shown to decrease exertional dyspnea and would not benefit this patient.

Although patients with chronic lung conditions can develop pulmonary hypertension, this patient had an unremarkable echocardiogram and has no evidence of pulmonary hypertension on examination. Therefore, proceeding with a right heart catheterization is unnecessary and unlikely to change management at this time.

This patient has already participated in a pulmonary rehabilitation program. Although it is helpful for patients to continue exercise, restarting a formal pulmonary rehabilitation program is unlikely to provide him with any more significant symptomatic improvement.

KEY POINT

- Lung volume reduction surgery improves quality of life and survival for patients with upper-lobe predominant emphysema and significant exercise limitations.

Bibliography

Ginsburg ME, Thomashow BM, Bulman WA, Jellen PA, Whippo BA, Chiuzan C, et al. The safety, efficacy, and durability of lung-volume reduction surgery: a 10-year experience. J Thorac Cardiovasc Surg. 2016;151:717-724.e1. [PMID: 26670190] doi:10.1016/j.jtcvs.2015.10.095

Item 29   Answer: D

Educational Objective: Diagnose COPD with spirometry.

This patient's symptoms are consistent with a possible diagnosis of COPD and spirometry should be performed. Spirometric evaluation is required for the clinical diagnosis of COPD. Spirometry is warranted in any patient presenting with dyspnea, chronic cough, or sputum production. Screening for COPD with spirometry should not be performed in asymptomatic patients. For diagnosis of COPD, spirometry should be performed both before and after administration of an inhaled bronchodilator. A postbronchodilator FEV_1/FVC of less than 0.70 is diagnostic of airflow obstruction that is not completely reversible with bronchodilator therapy and is consistent with a diagnosis of COPD.

Diagnostic testing for structural heart disease should be based on a thorough history and physical examination. New murmurs or a change in examination findings or symptoms in a patient with known structural heart disease should prompt further evaluation. The patient's examination is not consistent with pulmonary hypertension, heart failure, or valvular disease. Therefore, an echocardiogram is unlikely to be helpful.

In patients with a previous history of coronary artery disease and worsening cardiac symptoms, stress testing is helpful to assess for possible recurrent or progressive disease. Given this patient's cough, which would be an unusual presentation of heart disease in the absence of volume overload, a diagnosis of COPD is much more likely and should be investigated further. A cardiac stress test could be considered if his evaluation is otherwise unremarkable.

Although interstitial lung disease can present with similar symptoms, the absence of pulmonary crackles and normal chest radiograph do not support this diagnosis. Therefore, a high-resolution chest CT is currently not indicated.

> **KEY POINT**
>
> - A postbronchodilator FEV_1/FVC of less than 0.70 is diagnostic of airflow obstruction and is consistent with the diagnosis of COPD.

Bibliography

Qaseem A, Wilt TJ, Weinberger SE, Hanania NA, Criner G, van der Molen T, et al; American College of Physicians. Diagnosis and management of stable chronic obstructive pulmonary disease: a clinical practice guideline update from the American College of Physicians, American College of Chest Physicians, American Thoracic Society, and European Respiratory Society. Ann Intern Med. 2011;155:179-91. [PMID: 21810710] doi:10.7326/0003-4819-155-3-201108020-00008

Item 30   Answer: D

Educational Objective: Manage a patient with progressive idiopathic pulmonary fibrosis with palliative care.

This patient should receive palliative care including morphine for the symptom of dyspnea. Idiopathic pulmonary fibrosis (IPF) is the most common idiopathic interstitial pneumonia. It occurs predominantly in older individuals. Prognosis is poor, and individuals diagnosed with IPF have an estimated average survival of 3 to 5 years. The most common cause of death in IPF is respiratory failure. Patients with IPF may experience an acute exacerbation of IPF, diagnosed when the chest radiograph shows new alveolar infiltrates and medical evaluation does not reveal another cause for dyspnea such as infection, heart failure, or pulmonary embolism. Despite maximal supportive care during the past 5 days, this patient has progressed and is now on the brink of respiratory failure. Lung transplantation has been shown to provide a survival advantage in select patients with IPF. This patient gives a history consistent with severe and prolonged deconditioning associated with chronic respiratory failure. She now presents with frank respiratory failure and rapid progression of IPF with an unclear trigger. Consideration for transplant typically includes a full assessment of the patient for evidence of additional organ disease and education regarding the risks and benefits of the procedure. This is best accomplished long before the development of an acute exacerbation. Because of this patient's age, functional status, and lack of previous assessment by a transplant center, lung transplantation is not a viable option for her. At this time, she remains awake and alert and is able to participate in her end-of-life decision making. Patients with this presentation and functional status do not typically respond favorably to intubation and mechanical ventilation and, as such, recommending palliative medicines and comfort measures is most appropriate.

Although high-dose glucocorticoids are often used for acute exacerbation, their efficacy remains unknown. This patient has already been treated with glucocorticoids without apparent improvement; this indicates that administration of additional glucocorticoids is not likely to be of benefit.

Albuterol is a bronchial vasodilator. Unfortunately, the limitation in patients with IPF that results in hypoxemia and dyspnea is at the level of the interstitium, and bronchial dilators have little effect on these symptoms.

For individuals who develop severe respiratory distress that has no underlying reversible cause, supportive mechanical ventilation is of little long-term benefit. Therefore, the most recent evidence-based consensus statement recommends against mechanical ventilation for individuals with acute respiratory failure due to either progression or an acute exacerbation of IPF. In these circumstances, the focus should be on palliation of the patient's underlying dyspnea.

> **KEY POINT**
>
> - For individuals with idiopathic pulmonary fibrosis who develop severe respiratory distress that has no underlying reversible cause, supportive mechanical ventilation is of little long-term benefit; in these circumstances, the focus should be on palliation of the patient's underlying dyspnea.

Bibliography

Raghu G, Collard HR, Egan JJ, Martinez FJ, Behr J, Brown KK, et al; ATS/ERS/JRS/ALAT Committee on Idiopathic Pulmonary Fibrosis. An official ATS/ERS/JRS/ALAT statement: idiopathic pulmonary fibrosis: evidence-based guidelines for diagnosis and management. Am J Respir Crit Care Med. 2011;183:788-824. [PMID: 21471066] doi:10.1164/rccm.2009-040GL

Item 31   Answer: C

Educational Objective: Evaluate a patient with diffuse cutaneous systemic sclerosis for diffuse parenchymal lung disease.

This patient should receive a high-resolution CT (HRCT) scan of the chest. She has a history of diffuse cutaneous systemic sclerosis and has a chronic cough and dyspnea concerning for the possibility of scleroderma-associated interstitial lung disease. The most common cause of death from scleroderma is no longer kidney disease but progressive respiratory failure due to diffuse parenchymal lung disease. Among patients with the scleroderma spectrum disorders, patients with diffuse cutaneous systemic sclerosis and anti-Scl antibodies have the highest risk of interstitial lung disease. The most common pathologic finding in such patients is nonspecific interstitial pneumonia (NSIP). This patient has physiologic evidence of parenchymal lung disease with a mild restrictive defect and exercise-induced oxygen desaturation. Chest radiography can often miss mild disease and in these cases more advanced imaging is required. HRCT findings associated with NSIP include peripheral and basal predominant ground-glass opacities (cellular form) that spare the subpleural areas, basal predominant septal line thickening, and traction bronchiectasis in the fibrotic form.

Results of a 6-minute walk test (6MWT) are helpful to assess disability and prognosis in chronic lung conditions. During a 6MWT, oxygen saturation, heart rate, dyspnea and fatigue level, and distance walked in 6 minutes are recorded. The 6MWT is routinely used before, during, and after pulmonary rehabilitation programs. It would not be helpful in this patient with probable interstitial lung disease.

Cardiopulmonary exercise testing is routinely performed to assess prognosis in patients being evaluated for transplantation. Patients with low oxygen consumption or a high ratio of ventilation-to-carbon dioxide production have a poor 1-year prognosis. It may also be helpful in detecting deconditioning as a cause of dyspnea of unclear cause. It would not be appropriate in this patient with known restrictive lung disease.

Patients with a pulmonary nodule or other findings suggestive of malignancy may require PET/CT. This test most commonly uses fluorodeoxyglucose as a metabolic marker to identify rapidly dividing cells such as tumor cells and, to a lesser degree, any inflammatory lesion. It has no role in the evaluation on this patient with probable interstitial lung disease.

> **KEY POINT**
>
> - Patients with diffuse cutaneous systemic sclerosis are at high risk for the development of diffuse parenchymal lung disease, which is the leading cause of death in these patients.

Bibliography

Suliman S, Al Harash A, Roberts WN, Perez RL, Roman J. Scleroderma-related interstitial lung disease. Respir Med Case Rep. 2017;22:109-112. [PMID: 28761806] doi:10.1016/j.rmcr.2017.07.007

Item 32   Answer: D

Educational Objective: Diagnose cough-variant asthma.

The most appropriate management is to perform methacholine challenge testing. This patient has a chronic cough with no cause identified by history or physical examination, and a normal chest radiograph. In such patients who are not taking ACE inhibitors and are not exposed to environmental irritants or tobacco smoke, the most common causes are asthma, gastroesophageal reflux disease (GERD), and rhinosinusitis. Cough-variant asthma refers to asthma in which the predominant manifestation is cough, without other typical asthma symptoms such as wheezing, breathlessness, and chest tightness. Although most patients with asthma have obstructive physiology on pulmonary function testing, in those patients with normal spirometry, methacholine challenge testing is indicated to evaluate for bronchial hyperreactivity, which supports a diagnosis of asthma. Bronchial challenge testing uses a controlled inhaled stimulus to induce bronchospasm in association with spirometry; a positive test is indicated by a drop in the measured FEV_1. Methacholine is a commonly used agent that induces cholinergic bronchospasm at low

concentrations in patients with asthma; levels of exhaled nitric oxide may also be elevated. Positive methacholine testing is not specific enough to diagnose asthma; therefore, patients with cough and a positive methacholine challenge must also respond clinically to treatment with asthma therapies to be considered to have cough-variant asthma.

Although an empiric trial of asthma treatment with budesonide and albuterol could be considered, expert consensus indicates that it is preferable to first establish a diagnosis to avoid making an incorrect diagnosis and prescribing unnecessary or incorrect treatment.

Esophageal manometry and 24-hour pH testing would not be appropriate because the patient has no symptoms of GERD. Current guidelines suggest an empiric trial of diet and lifestyle modification for cough due to GERD before invasive testing for the disease.

A high-resolution CT scan of the chest would be indicated in some patients with chronic cough to evaluate for interstitial lung disorders or bronchiectasis, but the chest radiograph and physical examination findings are normal and the more common condition of asthma should be excluded first.

> **KEY POINT**
>
> - Cough-variant asthma refers to asthma in which the predominant manifestation is cough, and without other typical asthma symptoms; the diagnosis is supported by abnormal spirometry or methacholine challenge testing if spirometry is normal.

Bibliography

Kahrilas PJ, Altman KW, Chang AB, Field SK, Harding SM, Lane AP, et al; CHEST Expert Cough Panel. Chronic cough due to gastroesophageal reflux in adults: CHEST Guideline and Expert Panel Report. Chest. 2016;150:1341-1360. [PMID: 27614002] doi:10.1016/j.chest.2016.08.1458

Item 33   Answer: B   H

Educational Objective: Treat a patient with shock using a peripheral wide-bore catheter.

The most appropriate treatment is to insert a peripheral wide-bore central venous catheter. This patient is in shock with several possible causes. Flow of fluid through a catheter is inversely proportional to catheter length and proportional to the radius of the catheter to the fourth power. Therefore, the highest flow rates may be achieved through shorter, large-bore catheters. Peripheral intravenous (IV) catheters are shorter and larger than catheters used for central access or peripherally inserted central catheters and can deliver high volumes of fluid rapidly. For this reason, use of larger, shorter peripheral catheters is preferred for fluid resuscitation in patients requiring emergent treatment. However, peripheral IV catheters can sometimes be difficult to insert in patients in shock, and intraosseous ports and central venous catheters are the alternatives.

Intraosseous ports provide rapid access, but this patient has osteoporosis, which is a contraindication to this method.

CONT.
When used, an initial dose of lidocaine is needed before infusing because pain levels are very high with initial flushes and infusion.

Subcutaneous intravenous ports are long and small bore, which makes them useful for blood draws and small-volume infusion administration but not for rapid, large-volume fluid resuscitation.

A triple-lumen central catheter is an acceptable alternative when no other intravenous access can be obtained; however, it takes longer to insert compared to a peripheral wide-bore central venous catheter. When used, care should be taken to choose wider-bore catheters to overcome the flow restriction from longer lengths.

KEY POINT

- Peripheral wide-bore venous catheters are the preferred method for rapid intravenous administration of large amounts of fluids.

Bibliography

Khoyratty SI, Gajendragadkar PR, Polisetty K, Ward S, Skinner T, Gajendragadkar PR. Flow rates through intravenous access devices: an in vitro study. J Clin Anesth. 2016;31:101-5. [PMID: 27185686] doi:10.1016/j.jclinane.2016.01.048

Item 34   Answer: B

Educational Objective: Diagnose pulmonary embolism as a potential trigger for acute COPD exacerbations.

This patient should undergo CT pulmonary angiography. Some COPD exacerbations thought to be of unknown cause may actually be due to other medical conditions, including a pulmonary embolism (PE). A meta-analysis suggests that the prevalence of PE in patients hospitalized for an acute COPD exacerbation is as high as 25%. Testing for PE is indicated for patients who are not responding to typical therapy for acute exacerbations unless the pretest probability for PE is unlikely. Other important entities in the differential diagnosis with high risk for mortality include heart failure and pneumonia. These entities are less likely in this patient because of the absence of fever, crackles, edema, normal chest radiograph, and normal B-type natriuretic peptide level.

Spirometry usually does not change management during an acute exacerbation. In addition, the patient may not be able to complete the testing given his symptoms and the increased work of breathing.

Evaluation for influenza may be useful in patients who present with compatible symptoms, including fever, headache, myalgia, pharyngeal irritation, and respiratory symptoms (nonproductive cough and nasal discharge), particularly during an influenza outbreak. During a confirmed local influenza outbreak, infection can be reliably diagnosed on the basis of clinical criteria alone. When confirmation is needed, polymerase chain reaction testing can be performed. Testing for influenza in this patient is not necessary in the absence of influenza symptoms.

Similarly, a sputum culture is usually not indicated as it infrequently changes management of COPD. An antibiotic is often added because infections are the most common triggers for an acute exacerbation.

KEY POINT

- Patients who are not responding to typical therapy for COPD exacerbations should be carefully evaluated for heart failure, pneumonia, and pulmonary embolism.

Bibliography

Aleva FE, Voets LWLM, Simons SO, de Mast Q, van der Ven AJAM, Heijdra YF. Prevalence and localization of pulmonary embolism in unexplained acute exacerbations of COPD: a systematic review and meta-analysis. Chest. 2017;151:544-554. [PMID: 27522956] doi:10.1016/j.chest.2016.07.034

Item 35   Answer: C

Educational Objective: Evaluate a solitary pulmonary nodule in a patient at high risk for malignancy.

Definitive treatment is recommended for this patient and, therefore, a surgical wedge resection is appropriate. She has several risk factors for malignancy, including age, size of the nodule, upper-lobe location of the nodule, smoking history, and history of malignancy. In addition, the PET/CT scan showed fludeoxyglucose avidity, confirming the high probability of malignancy but without evidence of distant metastasis. As with subcentimeter nodules, the availability of previous imaging of the chest to assess the stability or growth of these lesions is helpful. An enlarging or new pulmonary nodule warrants more aggressive evaluation with tissue diagnosis or excision depending on the nodule's pretest probability of malignancy. The first step when evaluating a solid pulmonary nodule that is larger than 8 mm is to estimate the probability of malignancy. This can be done either clinically or using quantitative models and should place the patient in one of three categories: low probability (less than 5%), intermediate probability (5% to 65%), or high probability (greater than 65%). This is most useful when nodules are 8-30 mm. If the lesion is larger than 30 mm, the likelihood of malignancy is so high that it typically is resected; in contrast, when the lesion is smaller than 8 mm, the likelihood of malignancy is low and the patient should undergo routine radiological surveillance with serial CT scans.

Biopsy of the nodule or a transthoracic approach is preferred when the probability of malignancy is intermediate (5% to 65%) and would not be appropriate for this patient with a hypermetabolic nodule on PET/CT scan suggesting a high probability of malignancy. Furthermore, the sampling procedure is chosen according to size and location of the nodule, availability, and local expertise. Typically, peripheral nodules are sampled using CT-guided transthoracic needle aspiration, and more central lesions are sampled using bronchoscopic techniques. This lesion is described as peripheral.

Radiologic surveillance with serial CT scans is preferred if the probability of malignancy is low (less than 5%).

This patient's lung nodule is highly suspicious for malignancy on CT/PET scan so sampling with CT-guided transthoracic needle aspiration is not indicated.

KEY POINT

- Patients with a solid indeterminate lung nodule larger than 8 mm and high probability of malignancy should be staged using a PET/CT scan followed by definitive management.

Bibliography

Gould MK, Donington J, Lynch WR, Mazzone PJ, Midthun DE, Naidich DP, et al. Evaluation of individuals with pulmonary nodules: When is it lung cancer? Diagnosis and management of lung cancer, 3rd ed: American College of Chest Physicians evidence-based clinical practice guidelines. Chest. 2013;143:e93S-e120S. [PMID: 23649456] doi:10.1378/chest.12-2351

Item 36   Answer: A

Educational Objective: Diagnose a patient with asbestosis.

The most likely diagnosis is asbestosis. Asbestosis refers to the pneumoconiosis caused by inhalation of asbestos fibers. Asbestos is a silicate mineral fiber previously used as an insulating material that is a major cause of lung disease. Workers in construction, naval shipyards, and the automotive service industries are particularly at risk for asbestosis, with duration and extent of exposure being the key risk factors for the development of disease. Although asbestos use in the United States has been virtually eliminated since its peak in the 1980s, asbestos-related diseases will persist well into this century owing to the long latency period between exposure and disease development (15 to 35 years). Parietal pleural plaques are the most common finding and differentiate asbestos-induced parenchymal disease from other interstitial lung diseases. Diffuse parenchymal lung disease (DPLD) due to asbestos is related to the extent of the fiber burden. The most common symptom is exertional dyspnea; cough and sputum production are unusual unless the patient is a cigarette smoker. The CT scan imaging of pleural plaques and DPLD combined with the exposure history is adequate to make the diagnosis of asbestosis.

Chronic forms of hypersensitivity pneumonitis are believed to be associated with more chronic low-level exposures to inhaled antigen. This patient's hobby is wood working and wood dust is a potential source of antigen exposure. Patients with chronic hypersensitivity pneumonitis will ultimately present with cough, dyspnea, malaise, and weight loss. High-resolution CT findings include centrilobular micronodules in upper-lung and midlung distribution, as well as evidence of septal line thickening and fibrosis. Pleural plaques are not found. This patient's symptoms and CT findings are not compatible with this diagnosis.

Although this patient has some CT scan findings consistent with idiopathic pulmonary fibrosis, that diagnosis

can only be made in a patient who does not have another plausible cause for fibrosis. In addition, the finding of pleural plaques makes idiopathic pulmonary fibrosis unlikely.

Respiratory bronchiolitis–associated DPLD is a disease in active smokers who have imaging findings of centrilobular micronodules. The patient's negative smoking history and presence of pleural plaques on imaging excludes this diagnosis.

KEY POINT

- Parietal plaques are the most common radiologic finding in patients with asbestos exposure and are the features that differentiate asbestosis from other interstitial lung diseases.

Bibliography

Fishwick D, Barber CM. Non-malignant asbestos-related diseases: a clinical view. Clin Med (Lond). 2014;14:68-71. [PMID: 24532750] doi:10.7861/clinmedicine.14-1-68

Item 37   Answer: B

Educational Objective: Treat a patient for an acute asthma exacerbation with magnesium sulfate.

The most appropriate treatment is a single dose of magnesium sulfate. This patient is experiencing an acute asthma exacerbation. Treatment of acute asthma exacerbations can be difficult and requires prompt, aggressive management. The cornerstone of therapy in severe acute asthma exacerbation includes early administration of several doses of a short-acting β_2-agonist (SABA), a short-acting muscarinic antagonist (SAMA), and oral or intravenous glucocorticoids. In patients with a moderate to severe asthma exacerbation, combination therapy with a SAMA/SABA has been shown to reduce hospitalizations and improve lung function compared to SABA alone. Although use of a SAMA is not FDA-approved for treatment of an acute asthma exacerbation, several trials have demonstrated efficacy in both children and adults, and its use is supported by guidelines. Magnesium sulfate administration should also be considered early in the course of severe asthma exacerbation given its ability to relax bronchial smooth muscle tissue. A 2014 systematic review concluded that a single intravenous infusion of 1.2 g or 2 g of magnesium sulfate over 15 to 30 minutes reduces hospital admissions and improves lung function in adults with acute asthma who have not responded sufficiently to oxygen, nebulized SABAs and intravenous glucocorticoids.

Despite the theoretical bronchodilatory effect of intravenous ketamine, two randomized controlled trials have failed to demonstrate added bronchodilator effects when ketamine was compared to conventional management of asthma exacerbation.

Adjunct therapies such as a long-acting β_2-agonist, montelukast sodium, and theophylline have not demonstrated therapeutic benefit when used in the treatment of an acute asthma exacerbation and are not appropriate choices

CONT.

for this patient. However, their efficacy as long-term options in the outpatient setting should be considered in the overall treatment of asthma once the patient has been stabilized and is ready for hospital discharge.

> **KEY POINT**
> - Intravenous magnesium sulfate reduces hospital admissions and improves lung function in adults with acute asthma who have not responded sufficiently to oxygen, nebulized short-acting β_2-agonists, and intravenous glucocorticoids.

Bibliography

Albertson TE, Sutter ME, Chan AL. The acute management of asthma. Clin Rev Allergy Immunol. 2015;48:114-25. [PMID: 25213370] doi:10.1007/s12016-014-8448-5

Item 38   Answer: B

Educational Objective: Treat septic shock that persists after adequate fluid resuscitation using glucocorticoids.

Hydrocortisone is the most appropriate treatment. There is controversy about the role of glucocorticoids in the treatment of septic shock, but the Surviving Sepsis Guidelines published in 2016 recommend that if glucocorticoids are used, they should be used in refractory shock with persistent hypotension after adequate fluid resuscitation and after vasopressor medications have been titrated to high dose, and that the dose should be no more than 200 mg of hydrocortisone in 24 hours.

It is unlikely that substituting norepinephrine with another catecholamine vasopressor (dopamine) will lead to increased blood pressure. Dopamine also has a higher risk of inducing cardiac arrhythmias, and in this elderly patient who already has sinus tachycardia and frequent ectopic beats, dopamine would be an inappropriate substitution. Dopamine might best be reserved for selected patients with hypoperfusion and relative bradycardia.

Vasopressin levels in septic shock have been reported to be lower than anticipated for a shock state. Low doses of vasopressin may be effective in raising blood pressure in shock refractory to other vasopressors. Guidelines suggest adding vasopressin (up to 0.03 U/min) to norepinephrine with the intent of raising blood pressure to target or to decrease norepinephrine dosage. Vasopressin is not titrated like other pressors. Higher doses of vasopressin lead to ischemic complications, which more than offset any hemodynamic benefit.

Guidelines currently recommend against the use of intravenous (IV) immunoglobulins in patients with sepsis or septic shock. The most recent systematic review and meta-analysis differentiated between standard polyclonal IV immunoglobulins and M-enriched polyclonal immunoglobulin. Studies included in the review had low to moderate certainty of results based on risk of bias and heterogeneity. After excluding low-quality trials, no survival benefit was discernable with either immune globulin preparation.

> **KEY POINT**
> - Glucocorticoids are indicated in patients with sepsis who have not achieved hemodynamic stability from intravenous fluid administration and vasopressor therapies.

Bibliography

Rhodes A, Evans LE, Alhazzani W, Levy MM, Antonelli M, Ferrer R, et al. Surviving Sepsis Campaign: international guidelines for management of sepsis and septic shock: 2016. Intensive Care Med. 2017;43:304-377. [PMID: 28101605] doi:10.1007/s00134-017-4683-6

Item 39   Answer: C

Educational Objective: Diagnose malignant pleural mesothelioma.

The most likely diagnosis is malignant pleural mesothelioma. Asbestos exposure is the primary risk factor for mesothelioma, which has a latency period of 20 to 40 years, and this patient likely has a history of asbestos exposure from working as a brake mechanic. Occupational exposure to asbestos is most common in miners, electricians, plumbers, brake mechanics, shipyard workers, home remodelers, and selected military personnel. Patients most commonly present with symptoms of chest pain and a slowly enlarging pleural effusion. Chest imaging typically shows a unilateral pleural effusion, but patients can also present with pleural thickening, calcification, nodules, or masses. If malignant pleural mesothelioma is suspected, a thoracentesis should be performed, including pleural fluid cytology. Additional evaluation includes a chest CT scan to determine the extent of disease and evaluate for pleural lesions. Confirmation of the diagnosis requires pleural biopsy. Video-assisted thoracoscopic biopsy or open thoracotomy is required when the diagnosis remains uncertain, as diagnosis of mesothelioma cannot be made using cytology alone.

Empyema often presents with unilateral loculated exudative pleural effusion; however, the patient would not have a 6-month history of symptoms in the absence of fever and with a normal complete blood count. Finally, the pleural fluid characteristics are not consistent with empyema (typically pleural fluid pH less than 7.2, purulent effusion, or positive Gram stain).

Although cough, dyspnea, and pleural effusion could occur in patients with heart failure, the lack of physical examination findings consistent with volume overload and findings of a serosanguineous exudative effusion on thoracentesis would not be consistent with a diagnosis of heart failure (transudative effusion).

Rheumatoid pleuritis would also present with an exudative pleural effusion, but the patient has no other signs or symptoms of rheumatoid arthritis.

> **KEY POINT**
> - Asbestos exposure is the primary risk factor for malignant pleural mesothelioma, and patients most commonly present with symptoms of chest pain and a slowly enlarging pleural effusion.

Bibliography

Scherpereel A, Astoul P, Baas P, Berghmans T, Clayson H, de Vuyst P, et al; European Respiratory Society/European Society of Thoracic Surgeons Task Force. Guidelines of the European Respiratory Society and the European Society of Thoracic Surgeons for the management of malignant pleural mesothelioma. Eur Respir J. 2010;35:479-95. [PMID: 19717482] doi:10.1183/09031936.00063109

Item 40   Answer: C

Educational Objective: Treat a patient with newly diagnosed mild COPD.

The most appropriate treatment is a short-acting bronchodilator. Two commonly used, evidence-based treatment schemes are available to guide therapy. The American College of Physicians, American College of Chest Physicians, American Thoracic Society, and European Respiratory Society classification and treatment scheme for stable COPD recommends an inhaled short-acting bronchodilator (anticholinergic or β₂-agonist) for patients with an FEV₁ between 60% and 80% of predicted. The Global Strategy for Diagnosis, Management and Prevention of COPD (GOLD) classification model allows for therapy for COPD based on spirometry, risk, and symptoms. According to the GOLD classification scheme, this patient is in group A (low risk, few symptoms, documented mild airflow obstruction with one or no exacerbations per year). Like the previous guideline, GOLD recommends a short-acting bronchodilator or a combination of short-acting bronchodilators.

Roflumilast is a phosphodiesterase-4 (PDE-4) inhibitor used as add-on therapy to reduce exacerbations in patients with severe COPD associated with chronic bronchitis and a history of recurrent exacerbations despite other therapies. Inhibition of PDE-4 decreases inflammation, which may be helpful in a limited number of patients with COPD in whom inflammation is a significant factor. Roflumilast has minimal bronchodilator activity and should always be used with at least one long-acting bronchodilator. This patient has no indication for roflumilast therapy and it should not be used as monotherapy.

If the patient's symptoms and airflow obstruction progress, both guidelines recommend the addition of a long-acting bronchodilator (either a long-acting β₂-agonist or long-acting muscarinic agent). If symptoms persist, either an inhaled glucocorticoid or long-acting muscarinic agent can be added to the regimen.

Because this patient has mild disease with minimal symptoms, it is not necessary to start an inhaled glucocorticoid at this time. Short prednisone bursts are used to treat patients with acute exacerbations but are not indicated for the management of mild chronic symptoms related to COPD.

KEY POINT

- Patients whose symptoms and spirometry are consistent with mild COPD can begin treatment with a short-acting bronchodilator as needed.

Bibliography

Qaseem A, Wilt TJ, Weinberger SE, Hanania NA, Criner G, van der Molen T, et al; American College of Physicians. Diagnosis and management of stable chronic obstructive pulmonary disease: a clinical practice guideline update from the American College of Physicians, American College of Chest Physicians, American Thoracic Society, and European Respiratory Society. Ann Intern Med. 2011;155:179-91. [PMID: 21810710] doi:10.7326/0003-4819-155-3-201108020-00008

Item 41   Answer: A

Educational Objective: Treat a patient with chronic hypoventilation due to neuromuscular disease with noninvasive ventilation.

Bilevel positive airway pressure is the most appropriate next step in management. This patient has chronic hypoventilation due to amyotrophic lateral sclerosis (ALS), as indicated by the elevated arterial Pco₂ and a compensatory metabolic alkalosis, resulting in a normal pH on blood gas testing. ALS is marked by hypoventilation during sleep and may be exacerbated by acute illness and anesthesia. Bilevel positive airway pressure therapy augments ventilation by providing pressure support, improves quality of life, and may prolong survival in patients with ALS. Ventilatory support should be started in the presence of respiratory symptoms or hypercarbia. It also is essential to discuss prognosis and establish goals of care with patients and families, thereby avoiding unnecessary diagnostic and therapeutic measures.

Continuous positive airway pressure is designed to maintain upper airway patency in obstructive sleep apnea (OSA) and would not be appropriate ventilatory support in the setting of chronic respiratory failure due to hypoventilation.

Hypoglossal nerve stimulation is a treatment of OSA that activates the tongue muscles to increase upper airway caliber and prevent collapse. It has no effect on the respiratory pump muscles weakened by ALS.

Supplemental oxygen should generally not be prescribed for patients with hypoventilation due to neuromuscular disease without adjunctive ventilatory support because supplemental oxygen may further impair ventilation in patients with respiratory muscle weakness.

Tracheostomy may be appropriate for some patients with advanced respiratory failure due to neuromuscular disease, particularly those who experience difficulty in managing secretions or who require support during the waking hours. However, this patient is not yet affected by those issues, and noninvasive therapy should be the initial choice.

KEY POINT

- Assisted breathing devices, such as bilevel positive airway pressure, can be prescribed to support gas exchange in patients with neuromuscular disorders and may prolong survival in amyotrophic lateral sclerosis.

Bibliography

Radunovic A, Annane D, Rafiq MK, Brassington R, Mustfa N. Mechanical ventilation for amyotrophic lateral sclerosis/motor neuron disease. Cochrane Database Syst Rev. 2017;10:CD004427. [PMID: 28982219] doi:10.1002/14651858.CD004427.pub4

H **Item 42** **Answer:** **C**

Educational Objective: Prevent recurrent spontaneous pneumothorax with smoking cessation.

Smoking cessation is the most effective measure to prevent recurrent pneumothorax. This patient has a primary spontaneous pneumothorax (PSP) (air in the pleural space in someone without underlying lung disease). Cigarette smoking is a significant risk factor for PSP, likely because of airway inflammation. The lifetime risk of pneumothorax for men who are lifelong heavy smokers is 12%, compared to 0.1% for men who have never smoked. Because of the strong association between smoking and occurrence of PSP, smoking cessation may help prevent recurrence. Other risk factors for PSP are family history of PSP and thoracic endometriosis. PSP usually develops when the patient is at rest, and presenting patients are typically in their early 20s. Symptoms include the sudden onset of dyspnea and pleuritic chest pain. Recurrence is estimated at 23% to 50% during the first 5 years. Interventions to prevent recurrence includes chemical and mechanical pleurodesis, which are recommended after the second occurrence of PSP on the ipsilateral side, or first occurrence if the patient has a high-risk occupation such as deep sea diver or airplane pilot.

Air travel should be discouraged until resolution of the pneumothorax, but it is not in itself a risk factor for developing a pneumothorax.

There is no association between mountain climbing and development of a pneumothorax.

There is no association between the onset of pneumothorax and physical activity, with the occurrence being as likely when the patient is sedentary as when active.

KEY POINT

- Patients with a primary spontaneous pneumothorax should be encouraged to stop smoking to prevent recurrence.

Bibliography

MacDuff A, Arnold A, Harvey J; BTS Pleural Disease Guideline Group. Management of spontaneous pneumothorax: British Thoracic Society Pleural Disease Guideline 2010. Thorax. 2010;65 Suppl 2:ii18-31. [PMID: 20696690] doi:10.1136/thx.2010.136986

Item 43 **Answer:** **D**

Educational Objective: Diagnose an adult with cystic fibrosis.

The most likely underlying diagnosis is cystic fibrosis. This patient has acute symptoms of increased cough, sputum production, fever, chills, wheezing, dyspnea, clubbing, and a chest radiograph (shown) with bilateral upper-lobe predominant bronchiectasis with mucoid impaction (arrows), as well as a history of chronic pulmonary and gastrointestinal disease. This constellation of signs and symptoms is most consistent with an acute exacerbation of bronchiectasis in a patient with cystic fibrosis.

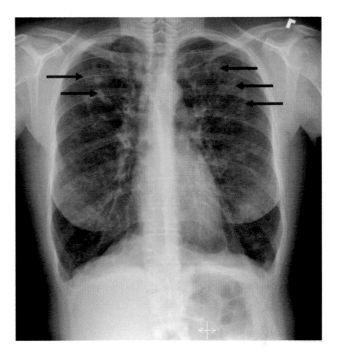

Common variable immunodeficiency involves B- and T-cell abnormalities and results in clinically significant immune dysregulation. The primary manifestation is hypogammaglobulinemia, and adults present with recurrent respiratory infections. The gastrointestinal tract is frequently involved with malabsorption or chronic diarrhea. The diagnosis is made by confirming low levels of total IgG and IgA or IgM, as well as by a poor antibody response to vaccines. The patient's normal serum immunoglobulin levels exclude this diagnosis.

The most common of the early complement disorders is $C2$ deficiency; $C6$ deficiency is the most common of the late complement disorders. Patients lacking one of the early components usually present with a rheumatologic disorder. Those with late complement component deficiencies usually present with recurrent, invasive meningococcal or gonococcal infections. The patient's history and findings are not consistent with either early or late complement component deficiency.

Although the patient has obstruction on pulmonary function testing, her age and history of chronic sinus and gastrointestinal disease make a diagnosis of COPD less likely than cystic fibrosis.

KEY POINT

- Conditions suggesting the diagnosis of cystic fibrosis in adults include chronic asthma-like symptoms, chronic sinusitis, nasal polyposis, recurrent pancreatitis, infertility, and bronchiectasis.

Bibliography

Nick JA, Nichols DP. Diagnosis of adult patients with cystic fibrosis. Clin Chest Med. 2016;37:47-57. [PMID: 26857767] doi:10.1016/j.ccm.2015.11.006

Item 44   Answer: A

Educational Objective: Treat a patient with an acute exacerbation of COPD.

The most appropriate treatment of the COPD exacerbation in this patient is azithromycin and prednisone. Exacerbations are marked by increased breathlessness and are usually accompanied by increased cough and sputum production. The degree of exacerbation is considered mild when a change in the clinical condition is noted but no change in medication is necessary. An exacerbation is considered moderate when medication changes are made. A severe exacerbation results in hospitalization. Short-acting bronchodilator therapy is a mainstay of therapy for treating COPD exacerbation. Glucocorticoids, such as prednisone, have been shown to reduce recovery time, improve lung function and arterial hypoxemia, decrease risk of early relapse, decrease treatment failure, and decrease length of hospital stay. Guidelines recommend 40 mg of prednisone or an oral equivalent for 5 to 7 days. The most recent Global Initiative for Chronic Obstructive Lung Disease report recommends that antibiotics should be considered in patients with moderate or severe COPD and symptoms of increased dyspnea, increased sputum, and sputum purulence. Recent studies in patients with moderate COPD have demonstrated improved patient outcomes. Commonly used regimens include an advanced macrolide (such as azithromycin), a cephalosporin, or doxycycline.

This patient's COPD appears to be well-controlled at baseline, so the addition of an inhaled glucocorticoid such as mometasone is not indicated for long-term COPD management. An inhaled glucocorticoid is not an effective treatment of an exacerbation of COPD.

Noninvasive positive pressure ventilation (NIPPV) has a significant role in the management of patients with very severe COPD during an acute exacerbation and may be helpful to avoid intubation. NIPPV is strongly recommended in patients with acute COPD exacerbations who have respiratory acidosis. This patient does not have an indication for NIPPV.

Although roflumilast has been shown to decrease the frequency of recurrent exacerbations, there is no role for this agent in the treatment of an acute exacerbation. As this is a first exacerbation of COPD, chronic roflumilast therapy is not indicated.

KEY POINT

- An exacerbation of COPD is defined as a sustained worsening of symptoms, typically cough, dyspnea, and sputum production; standard treatment of moderate to severe exacerbations includes antibiotics and oral glucocorticoids.

Bibliography

Holden V, Slack III D, McCurdy MT, Shah NG. Diagnosis and management of acute exacerbations of chronic obstructive pulmonary disease. Emerg Med Pract. 2017;19:1-24. [PMID: 28926214]

Item 45   Answer: D

Educational Objective: Treat pulmonary hypertension secondary to chronic hypoxemia.

The most appropriate treatment is supplemental oxygen. The clinical assessment and echocardiographic findings are consistent with pulmonary hypertension in the setting of advanced COPD (Group 3 pulmonary hypertension [PH]). The mainstay of treatment of Group 3 PH targets the underlying lung disease. This patient is on maximal inhaler therapy for COPD. Hypoxemia during daytime rest and, in the setting of cor pulmonale or secondary polycythemia, hypoxemia during sleep, is an indication for supplemental oxygen, which has proved benefit in pulmonary hemodynamics and survival in this population.

Bilevel positive airway pressure is indicated in patients with hypercapnia in the setting of COPD. Furthermore, in patients with overlap of COPD and sleep disordered breathing, continuous positive airway pressure has been shown to increase quality of life and prolong survival. The arterial blood gas study shows this patient to be normocapnic, and polysomnography demonstrates hypoxemia but no sleep apnea. Therefore, positive airway pressure therapy is not indicated.

A short course of prednisone is indicated in acute exacerbations of COPD, which typically present with acute dyspnea, cough, and sputum production. The more insidious course of this patient's symptoms is not consistent with an acute exacerbation of COPD, and there is no role for systemic glucocorticoids in patients with PH due to COPD.

Therapy with a vasodilator such as sildenafil is generally not indicated in patients with pulmonary hypertension related to lung disease or hypoxemia. Such drugs may cause harm by worsening ventilation-perfusion matching and further impairing gas exchange.

KEY POINT

- Patients with pulmonary hypertension secondary to lung disease and associated hypoxemia should be treated with supplemental oxygen.

Bibliography

Continuous or nocturnal oxygen therapy in hypoxemic chronic obstructive lung disease: a clinical trial. Nocturnal Oxygen Therapy Trial Group. Ann Intern Med. 1980;93:391-8. [PMID: 6776858]

Item 46   Answer: A

Educational Objective: Treat pulmonary arterial hypertension.

The most appropriate treatment is bosentan. This patient has pulmonary hypertension most consistent with Group 1 (pulmonary arterial hypertension [PAH]), based upon the right heart catheterization demonstrating high pulmonary arterial pressures in the absence of left-sided heart failure, lung disease, and venous thromboembolic disease. Before administering advanced therapy for patients with PAH, vasoreactivity testing with nitric oxide is performed to identify those who may respond to calcium channel blockers (CCBs). CCBs are desirable therapy because they are less expensive and have fewer side effects than other forms of advanced therapy. Failure to achieve a favorable hemodynamic response with nitric oxide predicts unresponsiveness to CCBs and the need for other advanced therapy. The endothelin receptor antagonist bosentan is one of many oral pulmonary vasoactive drugs that is indicated in PAH in patients with negative vasoreactivity testing, such as this patient, some of which have been shown to increase exercise capacity and improve echocardiographic parameters.

CCBs such as diltiazem may be used in the setting of PAH when a response to a vasodilator such as nitric oxide is demonstrated during right heart catheterization. When a response is not found, CCBs are not indicated.

β-Blockers such as metoprolol do not have a proved role specific to PAH, though they might be used as an adjunct agent for supraventricular tachyarrhythmias that are common in this population.

Pirfenidone is an antifibrotic agent indicated for the treatment of idiopathic pulmonary fibrosis. Pulmonary hypertension is frequently observed in patients with idiopathic pulmonary fibrosis, but pirfenidone would not be indicated for a patient with PAH without idiopathic pulmonary fibrosis.

KEY POINT

- Before administering advance therapy for patients with pulmonary arterial hypertension (PAH), particularly idiopathic PAH, vasoreactivity testing directs agent selection by identifying those who may respond to calcium channel blockers.

Bibliography

Galiè N, Humbert M, Vachiery JL, Gibbs S, Lang I, Torbicki A, et al. 2015 ESC/ERS Guidelines for the diagnosis and treatment of pulmonary hypertension: The Joint Task Force for the Diagnosis and Treatment of Pulmonary Hypertension of the European Society of Cardiology (ESC) and the European Respiratory Society (ERS): Endorsed by: Association for European Paediatric and Congenital Cardiology (AEPC), International Society for Heart and Lung Transplantation (ISHLT). Eur Respir J. 2015;46:903-75. [PMID: 26318161] doi:10.1183/13993003.01032-2015

Item 47   Answer: C

Educational Objective: Evaluate a patient for occupational exposure using a Material Safety Data Sheet.

The most appropriate management is to review the employer Material Safety Data Sheet (MSDS). This patient is concerned that an occupational exposure is causing new respiratory symptoms and potentially may worsen her asthma control. When an occupational lung disease is being considered, clinicians should request the MSDS, which details chemical properties and known health risks associated with substances within the workplace. The U.S. Occupational Safety and Health Administration (OSHA) requires that this information is available upon request for employees who work with potentially harmful materials. Establishing a clear causal link between this patient's symptoms of asthma and an occupa-

tional exposure is essential in diagnosis and management. Her history suggests a temporal relationship between the introduction of the new chemical and her cough. In addition, she feels the need to use her albuterol inhaler after exposure. Examples of known respiratory irritants include chlorine gas and sulfur dioxide, which are triggers of bronchospasm. Toluene diisocyanate is associated with allergic sensitization, cough, and bronchospasm that can develop weeks or months after initial exposure. Additional evaluation for occupational illness can include peak flow meter measurements before and after exposure, bronchoprovocation testing after prolonged time away from work and return to work, and, in select cases, specific inhalational challenges.

A chest CT scan is usually not needed for the evaluation of a patient with suspected occupational asthma. Exceptions to this rule include patients with abnormal chest radiography or suspected hypersensitivity pneumonitis. This patient has a normal lung examination, normal spirometry, and no symptoms compatible with acute hypersensitivity pneumonitis (fevers, flulike symptoms, cough, and shortness of breath). This patient has no indication for advanced imaging.

Although several commercial entities offer testing of hair samples for toxic chemicals, this testing is expensive, unlikely to be covered by insurance, and of questionable validity. It is, therefore, not recommended in the assessment of occupational exposure by primary care internists.

Supporting a patient's request to transfer work areas related to a health concern should be based on sound clinical assessment and judgment. A clinician's initial assessment should establish the presence of an occupational illness by assessing exposures, including known chemicals in the workplace, and establishing a temporal relationship between the introduction of the new chemical and symptoms.

KEY POINT

- When an occupational lung disease is being considered, clinicians should request a Material Safety Data Sheet detailing chemical properties and known health risks associated with substances within the workplace.

Bibliography

Friedman-Jimenez G, Harrison D, Luo H. Occupational asthma and work-exacerbated asthma. Semin Respir Crit Care Med. 2015;36:388-407. [PMID: 26024347] doi:10.1055/s-0035-1550157

Item 48   Answer: A

Educational Objective: Evaluate a patient with an anterior mediastinal mass and symptoms of myasthenia gravis.

An acetylcholine receptor (AChR) antibody test should be ordered. The mediastinum can be divided into three separate compartments (anterior, middle, and posterior), which can help narrow the differential diagnosis of a mediastinal mass. Each compartment normally contains separate and distinct anatomic structures that can lead to development of a mass. Patients may be asymptomatic and are often diagnosed after obtaining a chest radiograph for another reason, whereas others present with symptoms related to compression of adjacent structures. For example, they may present with dyspnea if the airway is compressed from a nearby mass or with upper extremity edema if vascular structures are compressed.

This patient has an anterior mediastinal mass (arrow) and neurologic symptoms. Masses in this location are usually remembered as the "terrible T's": thymoma, teratoma/germ cell tumor, "terrible" lymphoma, and thyroid. Additional considerations include thoracic aneurysm. Thymomas are the most common cause of an anterior mediastinal mass. Patients usually present as middle-age adults and may develop paraneoplastic syndromes. For example, myasthenia gravis can develop in 30% to 50% of patients with a thymoma. In comparison, only 10% to 15% of patients with myasthenia gravis have a thymoma. The second most common cause is lymphoma; these patients are typically younger at the time of presentation. Other less common paraneoplastic syndromes include pure red blood cell aplasia, nonthymic cancers, and acquired hypogammaglobulinemia.

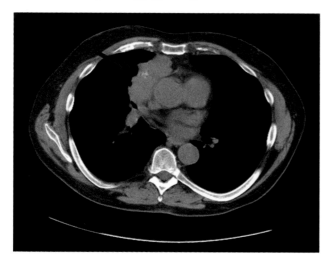

Myasthenia gravis is an autoimmune disorder of the neuromuscular junction that is characterized by fatigable (or fluctuating) muscular weakness. Common symptoms are ptosis and diplopia, which this patient has. Diagnosis of myasthenia gravis is based on clinical findings, detection of disease-specific antibodies (acetylcholine receptor antibodies in 90% of patients and anti–muscle-specific kinase [MuSK] antibodies in another 5% [with 5% of patients remaining antibody negative]), and electromyography findings (such as a characteristic decremental response to repetitive stimulation). Thymectomy should be performed in all patients with thymoma.

α-Fetoprotein and β-human chorionic gonadotropin are commonly elevated in germ cell tumors, which are also part of the differential diagnosis of an anterior mediastinal mass. However, this patient also has symptoms of myasthenia gravis, which is not associated with germ cell tumors.

Lactate dehydrogenase is commonly elevated in lymphoma and seminomas but is not as specific as other tumor markers and will not help determine the cause of this patient's symptoms.

Bibliography

Strollo DC, Rosado de Christenson ML, Jett JR. Primary mediastinal tumors. Part 1: tumors of the anterior mediastinum. Chest. 1997;112:511-22. [PMID: 9266892]

Item 49   Answer: B

Educational Objective: Treat pneumonia in a patient with inhalational injury.

Administration of empiric intravenous antibiotics for presumed pneumonia is the most appropriate treatment. This patient suffered an inhalational injury as a result of her exposure to a house fire. Common acute complications of inhalational injury include systemic toxicity from carbon monoxide and hydrogen cyanide, upper airway obstruction from pharyngeal edema, mucosal sloughing, bronchial cast formation, bronchoconstriction, pneumonia, acute respiratory distress syndrome, and pulmonary edema. The most common complication following smoke inhalation injuries is pneumonia. Inhalational injury increases the risk for respiratory infections, especially from *Staphylococcus* and *Pseudomonas* species, because of several mechanisms, including impaired pulmonary macrophage activity, direct injury to the airway cilia and tracheobronchial mucosal epithelium, and impaired surfactant production. Although the patient is only borderline febrile, her increasing leukocyte count and the presence of a focal consolidation in her left lower lobe on chest radiograph increase the index of suspicion for pneumonia.

Acute cyanide poisoning primarily occurs through fire and occupational exposures. Although no reliable test for cyanide poisoning exists, patients suspected of cyanide poisoning should receive hydroxocobalamin. Because this patient's inhalational exposure occurred 3 weeks ago, it is unlikely that her acute respiratory failure is due to cyanide poisoning. Thus, hydroxocobalamin is not indicated.

Tracheobronchial stenosis is an infrequent but real complication of inhalational injury. However, it most commonly occurs several months postexposure. The patient's recent normal airway inspection also suggests stenosis is a less likely cause of her respiratory decline. Other long-term complications following smoke inhalation include vocal cord fixation, airway polyps, persistent dysphonia, bronchiolitis obliterans, and bronchiectasis.

Common indications for thoracostomy tube placement include empyema or pneumothorax. Although pneumothorax should be considered in a patient with acute respiratory failure, there is no pneumothorax on this patient's radiograph. A thoracentesis is indicated for any new unexplained pleural effusion. Observation and initiation of therapy without diagnostic thoracentesis is reasonable in the setting of a small parapneumonic effusion, as is seen in the left base of

CONT.

this patient's radiograph. If an empyema or other small fluid collection requires evaluation, the initial investigation with needle thoracentesis is generally indicated before consideration of thoracostomy tube placement.

> **KEY POINT**
>
> - Secondary respiratory infections are common in patients with inhalational injuries, especially from *Staphylococcus* and *Pseudomonas* species, and are a major cause of morbidity and mortality.

Bibliography

Walker PF, Buehner MF, Wood LA, Boyer NL, Driscoll IR, Lundy JB, et al. Diagnosis and management of inhalation injury: an updated review. Crit Care. 2015;19:351. [PMID: 26507130] doi:10.1186/s13054-015-1077-4

Item 50   Answer: D

Educational Objective: Treat a patient at risk for alcohol withdrawal who has overdosed on benzodiazepines.

This patient should be kept on mechanical ventilation and monitored for signs of agitation. He shows signs of benzodiazepine overdose, combined with alcohol abuse. His airway is secure, and he is easily supported with mechanical ventilation, which can continue until he has metabolized the drug and his mental status has improved. Because of his history of alcohol abuse, he is at risk for alcohol withdrawal. Alcohol withdrawal occurs with chronic heavy alcohol use within hours to days after alcohol cessation. Early withdrawal symptoms occur within a few hours of abstinence and include agitation, anxiety, tremulousness, headache, and symptoms of autonomic hyperactivity (fever, diaphoresis, tachycardia, hypertension). Generalized tonic-clonic seizures may occur usually within 6 to 24 hours and should be treated with benzodiazepines because if left untreated, up to one third of patients may progress to delirium tremens.

Flumazenil, a γ-aminobutyric acid (GABA)–receptor antagonist, is the antidote for benzodiazepine toxicity, but reversing the benzodiazepine he took could put him at risk for seizures, especially if he is a chronic user. The short half-life of flumazenil makes it challenging to use in patients requiring sustained reversal of long-acting benzodiazepines, and given the overall low risk of benzodiazepine overdose, it is safer to allow his body to metabolize the benzodiazepine and eliminate it along with the alcohol.

Fomepizole inhibits alcohol dehydrogenase. It is used to block the metabolism of ethylene glycol and methanol into toxic metabolites when either of these alcohols is ingested. There is no reason to suspect either agent, especially in a patient with normal blood pH and a normal anion gap. Administration would therefore not be appropriate.

Dialysis would not be appropriate because there is no acute indication for this invasive and costly intervention. In principle, hemodialysis is indicated for drug intoxications when the clearance of the drug by hemodialysis is significantly shorter than metabolic clearance and the patient is deteriorating or when measured drug concentrations are

predictive of a poor outcome without hemodialysis. Dialysis will remove alcohols effectively, but the patient is stable and does not require an invasive intervention.

> **KEY POINT**
>
> - Treatment for benzodiazepine overdose is supportive with assurance of adequate ventilation; flumazenil is generally not recommended for benzodiazepine overdose as it can precipitate seizures in chronic users and its short half-life makes it difficult to sustain reversal of long-acting benzodiazepines.

Bibliography

An H, Godwin J. Flumazenil in benzodiazepine overdose. CMAJ. 2016;188:E537. [PMID: 27920113]

Item 51   Answer: A

Educational Objective: Treat hypersensitivity pneumonitis.

This patient has acute hypersensitivity pneumonitis and should be counseled not to return to work. The acute form of hypersensitivity pneumonitis presents within 48 hours of a high-level exposure and will often be associated with fever, flu-like symptoms, cough, and shortness of breath. Radiographic imaging can demonstrate bilateral hazy opacities, whereas high-resolution CT imaging of the chest shows findings of ground-glass opacities and centrilobular micronodules that are upper- and midlung predominant. Symptoms typically wane within 24 to 48 hours after removal from the exposure. Recurrence of symptoms with exposure to the respiratory antigen is the hallmark of this disorder, and careful attention to the history will help identify the cause. Primary treatment of acute hypersensitivity pneumonitis is removal from the offending antigen. Studies indicate that pulmonary function can continue to gradually recover, with initial improvements in oxygen exchange followed by increased FVC and improved chest radiograph findings.

Although treatment of acute hypersensitivity pneumonitis with systemic glucocorticoids is appropriate for those with more severe disease, patient response is variable, and prolonged use is associated with significant side effects. There are no data to support the use of inhaled glucocorticoids for acute hypersensitivity pneumonitis and, again, the primary treatment is to remove the offending agent.

Idiopathic pulmonary fibrosis (IPF) is the most common idiopathic interstitial pneumonia. It occurs predominantly in older individuals; the diagnosis of IPF is rare in those younger than 50 years of age. Gradual onset of dyspnea and cough during months to years is typical. Pirfenidone is a novel therapeutic agent that regulates transforming growth factor β (TGF-β) and tumor necrosis factor α (TNF-α) activity through an unknown mechanism that is used in the treatment of idiopathic pulmonary fibrosis. Similarly, nintedanib is a tyrosine kinase inhibitor known to block pathways that lead to activation of the fibroblast. Although these therapies are an important step forward in the management of IPF, they are not curative. This patient does not have IPF and treatment with pirfenidone is not indicated.

Lymphangioleiomyomatosis is a rare disorder that occurs sporadically in women or in association with tuberous sclerosis. It manifests as a diffuse cystic lung disease due to infiltration of smooth muscle cells into the pulmonary parenchyma. Genetic mutations within the cells lead to activation of the mechanistic target of rapamycin (mTOR) pathway. Diagnosis is based on imaging studies with diffuse thin-walled cysts as well as spontaneous pneumothorax and angiomyolipomas. Treatment is inhibition of the mTOR with sirolimus. Such treatment is not indicated in this patient with hypersensitivity pneumonitis.

> **KEY POINT**
>
> • Removal of the offending antigen is the most appropriate treatment of acute hypersensitivity pneumonitis.

Bibliography

Vasakova M, Morell F, Walsh S, Leslie K, Raghu G. Hypersensitivity pneumonitis: perspectives in diagnosis and management. Am J Respir Crit Care Med. 2017;196:680-689. [PMID: 28598197] doi:10.1164/rccm.201611-2201PP

Item 52   Answer: B

Educational Objective: **Treat a patient with a macrolide antibiotic to reduce frequent COPD exacerbations.**

The most appropriate guideline-recommended (grade 2A) treatment of this patient with severe COPD and frequent exacerbations is chronic macrolide therapy. Macrolide antibiotics have inflammatory and antimicrobial effects and may reduce the frequency of exacerbations when used long-term by patients with severe COPD. Several clinical trials to assess prophylactic use and benefit have demonstrated a reduction in the rate of exacerbation in patients with moderate to severe COPD with one or more moderate or severe exacerbations in the previous year despite optimal maintenance inhaler therapy. The duration and exact dosage of macrolide therapy are unknown. The primary concerns with long-term macrolide therapy are development of antibiotic resistance, including macrolide-resistant strains of nontuberculous mycobacteria. In addition, hearing loss and potentially fatal arrhythmias due to prolongation of the QT interval have occurred in association with azithromycin.

The long-term use of systemic glucocorticoids is avoided in the chronic management of COPD due to lack of demonstrated benefit and recognized increased risk of significant side effects such as diabetes, hypertension, muscle weakness, and decreased functional status.

The use of supplemental oxygen in patients with COPD and hypoxemia has been shown to improve quality of life and mortality in patients who have resting hypoxemia with an arterial P_{O_2} of 55 mm Hg (7.31 kPa) or lower, or oxygen saturation on pulse oximetry (Sp_{O_2}) of 88% or lower. This patient's Sp_{O_2} is above 88% at rest and on exertion on her current level of supplemental oxygen. Increasing this further has not been shown to decrease the rate of acute exacerbations.

Mucolytics such as nebulized hypertonic saline and airway clearance maneuvers may provide some symptomatic relief in patients with significant sputum production, but this patient does not have cough or sputum production. Moreover, these interventions have not been shown to decrease the rate of acute exacerbations in patients with COPD.

> **KEY POINT**
>
> • In patients with severe COPD and frequent exacerbations, chronic macrolide therapy has been shown to decrease COPD exacerbations.

Bibliography

Criner GJ, Bourbeau J, Diekemper RL, Ouellette DR, Goodridge D, Hernandez P, et al. Prevention of acute exacerbations of COPD: American College of Chest Physicians and Canadian Thoracic Society Guideline. Chest. 2015;147:894-942. [PMID: 25321320] doi:10.1378/chest.14-1676

Item 53   Answer: C

Educational Objective: **Treat a patient with acute hypoxemic respiratory failure with invasive mechanical ventilation.**

The most appropriate treatment is intubation and mechanical ventilation. This patient has dyspnea, severe hypoxemia, bilateral opacities on chest radiograph, and acute hypoxemic respiratory failure after aspiration, all of which are diagnostic for acute respiratory distress syndrome (ARDS). ARDS is associated with heterogeneous but often widespread damage to the alveolar epithelium and vascular endothelium, as well as surfactant dysfunction leading to alveolar instability and collapse. The changes can severely reduce lung compliance, making adequate ventilation difficult and further worsening hypoxia. Most patients with ARDS require intubation and mechanical ventilation to ensure adequate delivery of high levels of inspired oxygen and positive end-expiratory pressure to stabilize alveoli.

Continuing oxygen through a face mask would not be appropriate. Although the patient is maintaining appropriate oxygen saturation, the presence of anxiety, diaphoresis, tachycardia, tachypnea, hypercapnia, and hypoxemia signal impending respiratory failure that should be treated with intubation and mechanical ventilation.

High-flow humidified nasal cannula devices decrease the work of breathing, provide heated and humidified air, provide a reliable F_{IO_2}, and decrease dead space. Their initial application should occur in the critical care setting with close monitoring for tolerance and effectiveness. A recent trial demonstrated that in patients with acute hypoxemic respiratory failure, the use of high flow nasal cannula led to decreased mortality compared to continuing face mask oxygen or noninvasive face mask ventilation; however, the study excluded patients with hypercapnia, such as this

CONT.

patient. This patient shows features of respiratory muscle fatigue, including rapid breathing, diaphoresis, use of accessory muscles of respiration, and an elevated arterial P_{CO_2}, all indications for mechanical ventilation.

Noninvasive positive pressure ventilation (NIPPV) is the delivery of positive airway pressure using a cushioned face mask or helmet or without the use of an invasive connection directly in a patient's airway. In patients with hypoxemic respiratory failure, the use of NIPPV is controversial. Select patients may benefit from short-duration NIPPV to avoid intubation and associated complications but some studies have demonstrated increased mortality, likely due to delay in the implementation of appropriate invasive mechanical ventilation. This patient with deteriorating ventilation should be intubated and mechanically ventilated.

KEY POINT

- Most patients with acute respiratory distress syndrome require intubation and mechanical ventilation to ensure adequate delivery of high levels of inspired oxygen and positive end-expiratory pressure to stabilize alveoli.

Bibliography
Wilson JG, Matthay MA. Mechanical ventilation in acute hypoxemic respiratory failure: a review of new strategies for the practicing hospitalist. J Hosp Med. 2014;9:469-75. [PMID: 24733692] doi:10.1002/jhm.2192

Item 54   Answer: D

Educational Objective: Diagnose pulmonary arterial hypertension in a patient with limited cutaneous systemic sclerosis and CREST syndrome.

The most likely diagnosis is pulmonary arterial hypertension. Pulmonary involvement is frequent (greater than 70%) in patients with systemic sclerosis and can be symptomatic and disabling. The two principal clinical manifestations are interstitial lung disease and pulmonary vascular disease. Pulmonary vascular disease leading to pulmonary arterial hypertension may occur secondary to interstitial lung disease (typically in diffuse cutaneous systemic sclerosis) or as an isolated process (typically in limited cutaneous systemic sclerosis). This patient has several features of limited cutaneous systemic sclerosis with CREST syndrome (a condition defined by calcinosis cutis, Raynaud phenomenon, esophageal dysmotility, sclerodactyly, and telangiectasias). Patients are usually asymptomatic in early disease but later develop dyspnea on exertion and diminished exercise tolerance. Severe disease can lead to right-sided heart failure. Chest imaging is often normal and pulmonary function tests demonstrate a reduced D_{LCO} with normal lung volumes.

Organizing pneumonia is a patchy process that involves proliferation of granulation tissue within alveolar ducts, alveolar spaces, and surrounding areas of chronic inflammation. There are many known causes of this pattern, including acute infections and autoimmune disorders such as rheumatoid arthritis. The term *cryptogenic organizing pneumonia*

(COP) is reserved for individuals who have this pattern but do not have a clear associated cause. Patients with COP will typically present with symptoms during 6 to 8 weeks that mimic community-acquired pneumonia. Evaluation typically demonstrates bilateral diffuse alveolar opacities on chest radiograph with normal lung volumes. This patient's presentation is not consistent with cryptogenic organizing pneumonia.

Lymphangioleiomyomatosis is a multisystem disease that almost exclusively affects young women. Pulmonary complications are prominent and include diffuse pulmonary cysts, pneumothorax, chylous pleural effusions, and obstructive airways disease. Lymphangioleiomyomatosis would be very unlikely in a patient with an unremarkable chest radiograph.

Lymphoid interstitial pneumonia is an interstitial lung disease characterized by lymphocytic infiltration of the pulmonary interstitium. It is observed in patients with Sjögren's syndrome and viral infections, especially HIV. Patients with lymphoid interstitial pneumonia often have crackles on the pulmonary examination, interstitial infiltrates on chest radiography, and decreased lung volumes and diffusing capacity on pulmonary function testing.

KEY POINT

- Pulmonary arterial hypertension is commonly associated with connective tissue diseases, such as limited cutaneous systemic sclerosis.

Bibliography
Kato M, Atsumi T. Pulmonary arterial hypertension associated with connective tissue diseases: A review focusing on distinctive clinical aspects. Eur J Clin Invest. 2018;48. [PMID: 29285766] doi:10.1111/eci.12876

Item 55   Answer: A

Educational Objective: Treat sepsis with immediate fluid resuscitation.

The most appropriate management is an intravenous fluid bolus of 30 mL/kg of body weight. Successful treatment of severe sepsis and septic shock depends on the rapid institution of hemodynamic support, empiric treatment of infection, and infection control. Crystalloid infusion (normal [0.9%] saline or lactated Ringer solution) to support circulating intravascular volume should be administered to all patients with severe sepsis and septic shock. The 2016 update to the Surviving Sepsis Guidelines recommends using an initial bolus of 30 mL/kg of body weight.

The 2018 American Diabetes Association Standards for Care recommend that insulin therapy be initiated for treatment of persistent hyperglycemia starting at a threshold of 180 mg/dL (10.0 mmol/L). Once insulin therapy is started, a target glucose range of 140 to 180 mg/dL (7.8–10.0 mmol/L) is recommended for most critically ill and noncritically ill patients. This patient's plasma glucose is not so high that it is an emergency; therefore, administration of insulin is a lower priority than treatment of shock.

CONT.

This patient may have also have developed a paraspinous abscess (fever, new-onset back pain, difficulty urinating). This patient may need spine imaging but the more urgent priority is his hemodynamic instability, which requires fluid resuscitation before he can undergo any diagnostic imaging study.

Before this patient can be evaluated for surgical source control, he needs to be resuscitated. He is not showing signs of necrotizing fasciitis, which would be a surgical emergency, but even if he were suspected of this diagnosis, he would need aggressive fluid resuscitation while arrangements were made for urgent surgical debridement.

KEY POINT

- Patients with hypoperfusion due to sepsis should be managed with aggressive crystalloid fluid resuscitation using an initial bolus of 30 mL/kg of body weight.

Bibliography

Rhodes A, Evans LE, Alhazzani W, Levy MM, Antonelli M, Ferrer R, et al. Surviving Sepsis Campaign: international guidelines for management of sepsis and septic shock: 2016. Intensive Care Med. 2017;43:304-377. [PMID: 28101605] doi:10.1007/s00134-017-4683-6

Item 56 Answer: C

Educational Objective: Treat secondary spontaneous pneumothorax with chemical pleurodesis.

The most appropriate management of this patient with severe COPD and secondary pneumothorax is pleurodesis. Pneumothorax (air in the pleural space) can occur spontaneously, as a result of trauma, or iatrogenically. Spontaneous pneumothorax is further characterized as a primary spontaneous pneumothorax (PSP) in a person without underlying lung disease or a secondary spontaneous pneumothorax (SSP) in a person with underlying lung disease. Patients presenting with SSP are at higher risk for persistent air leak, further expansion of the pneumothorax, or pneumothorax recurrence due to their underlying lung disease. Intervention to prevent recurrence includes both chemical and mechanical pleurodesis, which is recommended in all patients with SSP and after the second occurrence of a PSP. In patients with SSP the cause of persistent air leak following pneumothorax is usually subpleural bullae or cysts. Additional interventions are required to close the leak. For patients who are surgical candidates, video-assisted thoracoscopic surgery (VATS) is recommended to locate and staple or resect blebs followed by mechanical pleurodesis. Patients who cannot tolerate surgery are treated with blood patch or chemical pleurodesis. These procedures are designed to seal the leak and prevent recurrence of pneumothorax. A blood patch is performed by injecting a quantity of the patient's blood into the thoracostomy tube. Chemical pleurodesis is performed by instilling tetracycline or one of its derivatives or specialized talc powder through the thoracostomy tube. Success rate for chemical pleurodesis ranges from 60% to 90% but it is not as effective as mechanical pleurodesis using VATS.

Clamping or removing the thoracostomy tube would not be appropriate because the patient has a secondary spontaneous pneumothorax and the likelihood of recurrence is high.

Placing the thoracostomy tube to high suction would not be appropriate because high levels of suction can increase the risk for reexpansion and pulmonary edema; in addition, the pneumothorax has resolved so no additional suction is needed.

KEY POINT

- Recurrence prevention with pleurodesis is recommended after the first occurrence of secondary spontaneous pneumothorax.

Bibliography

MacDuff A, Arnold A, Harvey J; BTS Pleural Disease Guideline Group. Management of spontaneous pneumothorax: British Thoracic Society Pleural Disease Guideline 2010. Thorax. 2010;65 Suppl 2:ii18-31. [PMID: 20696690] doi:10.1136/thx.2010.136986

Item 57 Answer: C

Educational Objective: Identify risk factors of acute exacerbations of COPD.

The patient's previous COPD exacerbations and FEV_1 of 35% of predicted are most associated with high risk for recurrent acute exacerbations of COPD. In the Evaluation of COPD Longitudinally to Identify Predictive Surrogate Endpoints (ECLIPSE) prospective study, the best predictor of exacerbations was a history of exacerbations, regardless of COPD severity. In this study the number of exacerbations in the previous 12 months, degree of airflow obstruction, and number of hospitalizations for an exacerbation refined the risk estimate. A history of 0 or 1 exacerbation, FEV_1 of 50% or better, and no hospitalizations predicts a low risk of future exacerbations, whereas more than 1 exacerbation, FEV_1 less than 50% predicted, and hospitalization predicts a high future risk of exacerbation. Exacerbations of COPD can be prevented by optimizing treatment with appropriate interventions based on risk classification and overall disease management; this includes immunizations and lifestyle changes such as maintaining physical activity and addressing anxiety and depression.

Pulmonary rehabilitation is recommended for all symptomatic patients with an FEV_1 of less than 50% of predicted and specifically for those hospitalized with an acute exacerbation of COPD. Use of such a program is not causally linked with an increased risk of COPD exacerbation.

Several comorbidities are associated with an increased risk of acute exacerbation, including heart failure, ischemic heart disease, diabetes, kidney failure, and hepatic failure. However, hypertension has not been associated with an increased risk of acute COPD exacerbations.

Current tobacco use is an independent risk factor for the development of COPD. However, past tobacco use and significant pack-year history are not associated with an

Answers and Critiques

increased risk for acute exacerbation. Discontinuing maintenance COPD mediations is associated with COPD exacerbations, whereas the use of such medications is not.

> **KEY POINT**
>
> - Patients with COPD who have had two or more acute exacerbations within the last year, who have an FEV_1 of less than 50% of predicted, or who have ever been hospitalized for an acute exacerbation are considered to be at high risk for recurrent acute exacerbations.

Bibliography

Hurst JR, Vestbo J, Anzueto A, Locantore N, Müllerova H, Tal-Singer R, et al; Evaluation of COPD Longitudinally to Identify Predictive Surrogate Endpoints (ECLIPSE) Investigators. Susceptibility to exacerbation in chronic obstructive pulmonary disease. N Engl J Med. 2010;363:1128-38. [PMID: 20843247] doi:10.1056/NEJMoa0909883

Item 58   Answer: B

Educational Objective: Treat a patient with neurologic disease and hypercapnic respiratory failure with bilevel positive airway pressure.

The use of bilevel positive airway pressure (BPAP) ventilation is the most appropriate treatment. This patient has features consistent with chronic hypercapnic respiratory failure secondary to neuromuscular disease. He has dyspnea and, more characteristically, orthopnea. The patient has chronic respiratory acidosis with a normal alveolar-arterial (A-a) oxygen gradient. BPAP delivers both inspiratory positive airway pressure and expiratory positive airway pressure and improves survival and quality of life of patients with neuromuscular disease. The settings generate a pressure difference that augments the patient's own respiratory muscle activity, leading to an increase in the size of each breath. The Pco_2 level will decrease due to the increase in minute ventilation and efficiency of breathing.

Invasive mechanical ventilation (mechanical ventilation with airway intubation or tracheostomy) is a therapeutic option in the setting of acute hypercapnic respiratory failure due to neuromuscular disease. However, the patient is awake, has excellent bulbar control (swallows and gags), and has a chronic disease that responds well to noninvasive ventilation.

Continuous positive airway pressure (CPAP) delivers positive airway pressure at a level that remains constant throughout the respiratory cycle preventing upper airway collapse or narrowing during sleep. No additional pressure above the level of CPAP is provided and patients must initiate every breath. CPAP does not increase minute ventilation, and it is not helpful in patients with hypercapnic respiratory failure due to neuromuscular disorders.

The patient has a normal A-a oxygen gradient and hypercapnia, which confirm that the hypoxemia is secondary to hypoventilation rather than a ventilation-perfusion mismatch or shunt; therefore, oxygen administration should not be needed once his Pco_2 improves. More importantly,

the administration of oxygen in the absence of supportive ventilation should be avoided in patients with neuromuscular disease and chronic hypercapnic respiratory failure; it has been associated with acute hypercapnia, in some cases leading to death.

> **KEY POINT**
>
> - Bilevel positive airway pressure ventilation improves survival and quality of life in patients with neuromuscular disease.

Bibliography

Gregoretti C, Pisani L, Cortegiani A, Ranieri VM. Noninvasive ventilation in critically ill patients. Crit Care Clin. 2015;31:435-57. [PMID: 26118914] doi:10.1016/j.ccc.2015.03.002

Item 59   Answer: A

Educational Objective: Treat a patient with hypertensive encephalopathy.

The appropriate treatment is intravenous hypertensive therapy to lower the systolic blood pressure (SBP) to 160 mm Hg within the first 6 hours. Appropriate intravenous agents could include fenoldopam, nicardipine, or nitroprusside. Hypertensive emergency refers to elevation of SBP greater than 180 mm Hg, diastolic blood pressure (DBP) greater than 120 mm Hg, or both, that is associated with end-organ damage. Patients with hypertensive emergency require rapid, tightly controlled reductions in blood pressure that avoid overcorrection. Management typically occurs in an ICU with continuous arterial blood pressure monitoring and continuous infusion of antihypertensive agents. According to the 2017 American College of Cardiology/American Heart Association hypertension guidelines, for adults with a compelling condition (aortic dissection, severe preeclampsia or eclampsia, or pheochromocytoma crisis), SBP should be reduced to less than 140 mm Hg during the first hour and to less than 120 mm Hg in aortic dissection. For adults without a compelling condition, such as this patient, SBP should be reduced by no more than 25% within the first hour; then, if stable, to 160 mm Hg within the next 2 to 6 hours; and then cautiously to normal during the following 24 to 48 hours.

Because autoregulation of tissue perfusion is disturbed in hypertensive emergencies, reducing blood pressure too rapidly can result in ischemic organ damage. Therefore, targeting a blood pressure of 120/80 mm Hg during the first hour of treatment is inappropriate because it could result in further worsening of kidney injury, encephalopathy, or both.

Conversely, lowering the SBP to 160 mm Hg during 48 hours is likely too slow and not in keeping with current guidelines.

This patient's normal medication combined with observation is not aggressive enough. Eventually he will need a stable outpatient hypertension regimen with education on the importance of adherence to that regimen, but not in this acute setting.

- For adults with a hypertensive emergency and without a compelling condition (such as aortic dissection) systolic blood pressure should be reduced by no more than 25% within the first hour; then, if stable, to 160 mm Hg within the next 2 to 6 hours; and then cautiously to normal during the following 24 to 48 hours.

Bibliography

Whelton PK, Carey RM, Aronow WS, Casey DE Jr, Collins KJ, Dennison Himmelfarb C, et al. 2017 ACC/AHA/AAPA/ABC/ACPM/AGS/APhA/ASH/ASPC/NMA/PCNA guideline for the prevention, detection, evaluation, and management of high blood pressure in adults: a report of the American College of Cardiology/American Heart Association Task Force on Clinical Practice Guidelines. Hypertension. 2017. [PMID: 29133356] doi:10.1161/HYP.0000000000000065

Item 60   Answer: A

Educational Objective: Treat a patient for cyanide poisoning as a coexposure to carbon monoxide poisoning after a house fire.

This patient should be treated with intravenous hydroxocobalamin, which is the preferred antidote for cyanide poisoning. Cyanide toxicity is common in victims of house fires, with up to 90% of rescued victims having elevated cyanide levels and 35% having significantly elevated levels, which is higher than the rate of carbon monoxide poisoning among such victims. Cyanide disrupts oxidative phosphorylation, forcing cells to convert to anaerobic metabolism despite adequate oxygen supply. The result in severe cases is multiorgan failure with coma, seizures, and cardiovascular symptoms, including hypotension, bradycardia, heart block, and ventricular arrhythmias. Early manifestations are nonspecific. Diagnostic clues include lactic acidosis and inappropriately elevated central venous oxyhemoglobin saturation, which manifests as bright red venous blood. Cyanide levels are not readily available and because toxicity is rapidly fatal, prompt empiric treatment is imperative in suspected cases. Hydroxocobalamin avidly binds to cyanide to produce cyanocobalamin, which is soluble, nontoxic, and readily excreted. In addition, ongoing exposure, such as contaminated clothing, should also be eliminated. Hydroxocobalamin can affect accuracy of lab results for methemoglobin, lactate, and other tests, so it is important to obtain blood for these tests before administering the antidote, if possible.

Carbon monoxide is removed by competitive binding of oxygen to hemoglobin. The initial treatment is administration of 100% oxygen, which reduces the half-life of carboxyhemoglobin from 5 hours to 90 minutes. Hyperbaric oxygen therapy yields an even higher alveolar P_{O_2}, thereby reducing the half-life to 30 minutes while substantially increasing the amount of oxygen directly dissolved in blood. However, hyperbaric oxygen therapy would not be appropriate because this patient's carboxyhemoglobin level is not high enough to suggest severe carbon monoxide poisoning.

Hyperbaric oxygen is usually recommended for levels of 25% to 40% or higher, or for victims with lower levels who are pregnant.

Methylene blue would be recommended for toxic levels of methemoglobin, usually 20% to 30% or higher, but it is not indicated for this patient.

Although sodium nitrite is an antidote for cyanide poisoning, it is contraindicated in victims of smoke inhalation because it works by inducing methemoglobinemia, which would further impair oxygen delivery by additive or synergistic effects on oxygen binding and delivery in cases of carbon monoxide toxicity.

Sodium thiosulfate is also used as an antidote for cyanide toxicity and is safer than sodium nitrite, but has a slower onset of action. It is considered second-line therapy after hydroxocobalamin, but the two agents can be given to the same patient, possibly with synergistic effect. However, they should not be administered simultaneously or through the same intravenous catheter.

- Hydroxocobalamin effectively removes cyanide from the mitochondrial respiration system and is the preferred antidote for cyanide poisoning.

Bibliography

Hamad E, Babu K, Bebarta VS. Case files of the University of Massachusetts Toxicology Fellowship: Does this smoke inhalation victim require treatment with cyanide antidote? J Med Toxicol. 2016;12:192-8. [PMID: 26831054] doi:10.1007/s13181-016-0533-0

Item 61   Answer: C

Educational Objective: Manage a patient with clinical signs of cystic fibrosis and a negative sweat chloride test.

The most appropriate next step is to repeat the sweat chloride testing. Diagnosis of cystic fibrosis (CF) is based on a combination of CF-compatible clinical findings in conjunction with either biochemical (sweat testing, nasal potential difference) or genetic (*CFTR* mutations) techniques. Genetic counseling should always occur before any genetic test is performed. The essential components of counseling include informing the patient of the test purpose, implications of diagnosis, and alternative testing options. Ultimately, the decision of whether or not to be tested rests with the patient. Use of the sweat test has been the mainstay of laboratory confirmation. Negative sweat chloride testing does not exclude the diagnosis of CF. This patient has many findings suggestive of CF upper-lobe predominant bronchiectasis, chronic sinus disease, colonization with *Pseudomonas*, clubbing, and infertility. Therefore, the index of suspicion for CF, as well as ciliary dyskinesia disorders, is extremely high for this patient. Because sweat chloride testing can give variable results, it is appropriate to repeat the testing and, if still negative, refer the patient to a center with expertise in CF or genetic testing.

Chronic oral macrolide antibiotics and inhaled antibiotic therapy are beneficial in patients with a confirmed diagnosis of CF. However, individuals with bronchiectasis are often exposed to several courses of antibiotics, and resistance to quinolones is common. Therefore, initiation of chronic ciprofloxacin therapy is not indicated.

In a recent phase 3 trial, tiotropium was well tolerated in patients with CF, but lung function improvements compared with placebo were not statistically significant and such treatment is not generally recommended.

Patients with α_1-antitrypsin deficiency can present with lung disease and liver disease. A characteristic radiographic finding of the emphysema associated with α_1-antitrypsin deficiency is bullous changes most prominent at the bases, which are not present in this patient. Additionally, α_1-antitrypsin deficiency cannot account for the patient's sinus disease or infertility. Therefore, α_1-antitrypsin deficiency testing would not be the most appropriate next diagnostic test in this patient with a clinical history suggestive of possible CF.

KEY POINT

- Negative sweat chloride testing does not exclude the diagnosis of cystic fibrosis in patients with high pretest probability of disease.

Bibliography

Farrell PM, White TB, Ren CL, Hempstead SE, Accurso F, Derichs N, et al. Diagnosis of cystic fibrosis: consensus guidelines from the Cystic Fibrosis Foundation. J Pediatr. 2017;181S:S4-S15.e1. [PMID: 28129811] doi:10.1016/j.jpeds.2016.09.064.

Item 62　　Answer:　C

Educational Objective: Screen for lung cancer in a patient at high risk.

The most appropriate test is a low-dose CT scan of the chest. Annual low-radiation-dose CT has been shown to reduce lung cancer mortality (20% relative decrease in lung cancer deaths) among high-risk individuals and is now recommended by the U.S. Preventive Services Task Force and other expert groups. Patients recommended for screening are those aged 55 to 74-80 years (range differs among expert groups) with a greater than 30-pack-year history of tobacco use within the prior 15 years, and without signs or symptoms suggestive of lung cancer. This patient fulfills these criteria and is, therefore, an appropriate candidate for a low-dose CT scan of the chest. Patients must also receive in-office counseling regarding the potential benefits and harms of screening, and documentation of shared decision making.

Monitoring respiratory parameters during exertion with the 6-minute walk test (6MWT) is helpful to assess disability and prognosis in chronic lung conditions. During a 6MWT, oxygen saturation, heart rate, dyspnea and fatigue level, and distance walked in 6 minutes are recorded. This relatively simple maneuver quantifies exercise tolerance, determines effective interventions, and helps predict morbidity and mortality. This patient has no indication for a 6MWT.

Chest radiography has been shown to be ineffective in screening for lung cancer and is not indicated in an asymptomatic patient such as this one.

Spirometry is warranted in any patient presenting with dyspnea, chronic cough, or sputum production. Screening for lung disease with spirometry should not be performed in asymptomatic patients, even those with a history of smoking.

Urinary cotinine is a metabolite of nicotine that is excreted in the urine and can be measured to assess if patients are using tobacco products. It is sometimes used while patients are actively attempting to quit smoking to assess adequacy of nicotine replacement therapy and monitor abstinence. This patient is high risk and a candidate for screening regardless of his current smoking status, and this test is not indicated.

KEY POINT

- Patients recommended for lung cancer screening are those aged 55 to 74-80 years with a greater than 30-pack-year history of tobacco use within the previous 15 years, and without signs or symptoms suggestive of lung cancer.

Bibliography

Mazzone PJ, Silvestri GA, Patel S, Kanne JP, Kinsinger LS, Wiener RS, et al. Screening for lung cancer: CHEST guideline and expert panel report. Chest. 2018;153:954-985. [PMID: 29374513] doi:10.1016/j.chest.2018.01.016

Item 63　　Answer:　D

Educational Objective: Manage oversedation in a patient in the ICU.

The most appropriate management is to stop sedation and analgesia. Clinicians at the bedside may resist stopping sedation and analgesia in a patient with a clear need for both, or because of concerns with ventilator synchrony or oxygenation. Protocolized care can help guide nursing and respiratory therapy if these problems arise. In addition, daily protocolized interruptions of sedation and analgesia have been shown to decrease the incidence of delirium, the need for diagnostic testing, and the amount of time spent on mechanical ventilation and in the ICU. Stopping sedation and analgesia, rather than gradually decreasing them, allows for a faster return to awareness and titration of infusions to achieve the sedation and analgesia goal. Analgesia and sedation can be restarted, at lower doses, if the patient requires them later.

Dexmedetomidine has pharmacological properties that may benefit this patient (analgesia, allows arousal). However, there is currently no evidence that it is superior to appropriately titrated propofol.

Ordering a CT scan is not the most appropriate first step in management of an unresponsive patient with nonfocal physical examination findings currently being treated with propofol and morphine. Moreover, a CT would expose the patient to the risks of being moved while critically ill and

CONT. unnecessary radiation. The rate of serious events during transport is important enough to warrant careful determination of need.

Ordering an electroencephalogram to assess his unresponsiveness would be part of the diagnostic evaluation if interruption of sedation did not lead to improved mental status. Nonconvulsive status epilepticus has been reported in up to 20% of patients with unexplained unresponsiveness. Current recommendations suggest continuous electroencephalogram as the diagnostic test of choice.

> **KEY POINT**
> - Daily protocolized interruptions of sedation and analgesia have been shown to decrease the incidence of delirium, the need for diagnostic testing, and the amount of time spent on mechanical ventilation and in the ICU.

Bibliography

Barr J, Fraser GL, Puntillo K, Ely EW, Gélinas C, Dasta JF, et al; American College of Critical Care Medicine. Clinical practice guidelines for the management of pain, agitation, and delirium in adult patients in the intensive care unit. Crit Care Med. 2013;41:263-306. [PMID: 23269131] doi:10.1097/CCM.0b013e3182783b72

Item 64   Answer: E

Educational Objective: Treat heat stroke with evaporative cooling techniques.

This patient should be sprayed with water, and fans should be used to lower his body temperature to a safe level (usually 38.5 °C (101 °F) through evaporative cooling. Heat stroke occurs with high ambient temperature and humidity and is defined by the presence of a temperature greater than 40.0 °C (104.0 °F) and encephalopathy. It is often associated with hypotension, gastrointestinal distress, and weakness. Patients with advanced heat stroke exhibit shock, multiorgan failure, rhabdomyolysis, and myocardial ischemia. Exertional heat stroke typically occurs in healthy individuals undergoing vigorous physical activity in warm conditions. In contrast, most patients with non-exertional heat stroke are older than 70 years of age or have chronic medical conditions that impair thermal regulation. Medications and recreational drugs with anticholinergic, sympathomimetic, and diuretic effects, including alcohol, pose added risk. The primary treatment of nonexertional heat stroke is evaporative, external cooling. This involves removing all clothing and spraying the patient with a mist of lukewarm water while continuously blowing fans on the patient. Evaporative and convective cooling techniques are generally the safest and most effective.

Acetaminophen and other centrally acting antipyretics are ineffective in the treatment of heat stroke. A cooling blanket could be used as an adjunct, but it is not as effective as evaporative cooling.

Alcohol would evaporate and provide cooling as effective as that from applying water, but it would also be absorbed through the vasodilated skin and could lead to

alcohol toxicity similar to that observed in patients who have ingested alcohol and is therefore contraindicated.

Although ice water immersion is sometimes used in younger patients with exertional heat stroke to lower the body temperature rapidly, there is evidence for increased mortality when this method is used in older patients. Also, this patient's core temperature of 40 °C (104 °F) is not so severe that more aggressive measures need to be considered.

The muscle relaxant dantrolene is ineffective in the treatment of heat stroke. It is used for malignant hyperthermia and sometimes for neuroleptic malignant syndrome, although this is an off-label application.

> **KEY POINT**
> - Patients with nonexertional heat stroke should be treated with evaporative cooling to lower their core temperature to a safe level.

Bibliography

O'Connor JP. Simple and effective method to lower body core temperatures of hyperthermic patients. Am J Emerg Med. 2017;35:881-884. [PMID: 28162872] doi:10.1016/j.ajem.2017.01.053

Item 65   Answer: A

Educational Objective: Treat septic shock with crystalloid infusion as the initial resuscitative therapy.

This patient should receive a 0.9% saline bolus. He has signs of septic shock from influenza (fever, tachycardia, hypotension, elevated leukocyte count, and exposure to influenza). In patients with septic or distributive shock, initial resuscitation efforts should be aimed at giving crystalloid fluids (0.9% saline, Ringer's lactate). The 2016 Surviving Sepsis guidelines recommend giving 30 mL/kg crystalloid solution within 3 hours of presentation in patients who demonstrate signs of tissue hypoperfusion. Judicious fluid administration is warranted thereafter, as intravascular volume overload can contribute to pulmonary edema and pleural effusions. This patient has several features of hypoperfusion, including hypotension, tachycardia, metabolic acidosis, and an elevated blood lactate.

Furosemide would be appropriate if the patient were in cardiogenic shock and presenting with signs of volume overload. The history, examination, and chest radiograph are not consistent with cardiogenic shock or volume overload. Therefore, furosemide is not recommended and would only promote further hypotension.

If hypotension does not rapidly correct with fluids, vasopressors should be titrated to maintain a mean arterial pressure of 65 mm Hg or greater. Norepinephrine is considered first-line therapy. This patient has not received crystalloid solution yet so initial therapy with norepinephrine is incorrect. However, in patients who are refractory to volume loading, vasopressor therapy is recommended to help improve hemodynamic stability.

In the absence of extenuating circumstances (myocardial ischemia, severe hypoxemia, or active hemorrhage), the

Surviving Sepsis guidelines recommend that red blood cell transfusion only be given if hemoglobin is less than 7 g/dL (70 g/L). Because this patient has a hemoglobin level above 7 g/dL, there is no direct role for packed red blood cell transfusion.

KEY POINT

- Initial treatment of septic or distributive shock should focus on aggressive fluid resuscitation with crystalloids within the first 3 hours of presentation.

Bibliography
Rochwerg B, Alhazzani W, Sindi A et al. Fluid resuscitation in sepsis: a systematic review and network meta-analysis. Ann Intern Med. 2014;161:347. [PMID 25047428]

Item 66   Answer: B

Educational Objective: Treat a patient in cardiac arrest due to accidental hypothermia with prolonged cardiopulmonary resuscitation and active internal rewarming.

Cardiopulmonary resuscitation (CPR) should be continued with active internal (core) rewarming. Conventional treatment of ventricular arrhythmias and asystole is often ineffective until the temperature is raised to greater than 30.0 °C (86.0 °F). Because severe hypothermia may appear clinically similar to death, aggressive rewarming is appropriate in all patients in the absence of obvious irreversible signs of death. A critical first step entails removing wet clothing and covering the patient with insulating material, especially the head and neck. For mildly hypothermic, healthy individuals capable of shivering, this strategy of passive external rewarming alone suffices. Active external rewarming using warm blankets or a forced heated air blanket is commonly used in hemodynamically stable patients with moderate hypothermia. Body cavity lavage with warm fluids is an option for patients with hypothermia that is severe or does not respond to external rewarming. The colon, bladder, and stomach are readily accessible for irrigation but have a small surface area for heat exchange. Rewarming by peritoneal or pleural space irrigation is supported by case reports. Extracorporeal support, including cardiopulmonary bypass, is recommended for patients in cardiac arrest because it maximizes the rewarming rate and can provide hemodynamic support.

Although this man has already received nearly an hour of CPR, there are reports of full recovery in patients with cardiac arrest in the setting of accidental hypothermia, sometimes even after CPR has been performed for many hours. Therefore, continued CPR is indicated until the patient can be rewarmed. Discontinuation of CPR is not appropriate because hypothermia prevents reaching a definite conclusion about the futility or possible effectiveness of continued resuscitation.

KEY POINT

- Cardiopulmonary resuscitation should be continued in patients with accidental hypothermia accompanied by cardiac arrest until the patient can be rewarmed.

Bibliography
Hilmo J, Naesheim T, Gilbert M. "Nobody is dead until warm and dead": prolonged resuscitation is warranted in arrested hypothermic victims also in remote areas—a retrospective study from northern Norway. Resuscitation. 2014;85:1204-11. [PMID: 24882104] doi:10.1016/j.resuscitation.2014.04.029

Item 67   Answer: B

Educational Objective: Treat high-altitude cerebral edema with dexamethasone.

The most appropriate treatment is dexamethasone. Hypoxia and hypocapnia associated with altitude alter cerebral blood flow and oxygen delivery to the brain. When autoregulatory mechanisms are overcome, symptoms may be mild, as with acute mountain sickness, or severe, as with life-threatening cerebral edema. Acute mountain sickness is characterized by nonspecific symptoms such as headache, fatigue, nausea, and vomiting, in addition to disturbed sleep. High-altitude cerebral edema is a more extreme manifestation of acute mountain sickness. Vascular leak leads to brain swelling, resulting in manifestations that range from confusion and irritability to ataxic gait to coma and death. Recognition of cerebral edema mandates immediate intervention. This patient is exhibiting signs and symptoms of encephalopathy indicative of high-altitude cerebral edema, the risk of which increases at more extreme elevations (higher than 3000 meters [9842 feet]). Although the most important intervention is descent to lower elevation, dexamethasone should be administered immediately upon recognition of high-altitude cerebral edema. Supplemental oxygen should also be administered.

High-altitude illness can be prevented by gradually ascending, which can generally be accomplished by spending one night at an intermediate altitude to allow acclimatization. Acetazolamide accelerates the acclimatization process to high altitude by inducing a slight metabolic acidosis to stimulate ventilation and enhance gas exchange; it can be used prophylactically in patients with a history of altitude illness. However, it isn't an effective treatment once symptoms develop; although it may be used as an adjunct to dexamethasone, it has no role in high-altitude cerebral edema as monotherapy.

Nifedipine is used as a preventive and therapeutic agent for high-altitude pulmonary edema.

Another vasodilator, sildenafil, may be used as an alternative to nifedipine in high-altitude pulmonary edema. However, neither is useful in the treatment of high-altitude cerebral edema.

KEY POINT

- Although the most important treatment of high-altitude cerebral edema is descent to lower elevation, dexamethasone should be administered immediately upon recognition of high-altitude cerebral edema.

Bibliography
Luks AM, Swenson ER, Bärtsch P. Acute high-altitude sickness. Eur Respir Rev. 2017;26. [PMID: 28143879] doi:10.1183/16000617.0096-2016

H **Item 68**   **Answer: C**

Educational Objective: **Treat a critically ill patient who has acute pain.**

This patient should receive an intravenous push of morphine. He has acute postoperative pain of the leg and is experiencing severe pain despite a morphine infusion. Analgesia should be titrated to a specific pain management goal while preventing and monitoring for side effects. A bolus dose of morphine will reach therapeutic levels faster than changing rates of infusion. The bolus dose should be repeated until the patient achieves the therapeutic goal, a protocol limit is reached, or side effects occur. He should be monitored closely while receiving acute pain treatment. Common side effects include somnolence, depression of respiratory drive, urinary retention, and nausea and vomiting.

Adding gabapentin is a good strategy for patients with neuropathic pain. Enteral gabapentin added to parenteral opioids can reduce the doses of opiates needed and improve pain control in mechanically ventilated patients. However, this patient is experiencing acute nonneuropathic pain and an intravenous opioid is the drug class of choice.

Epidural analgesia is an effective means to control pain in critically ill patients. This has been demonstrated in patients with cardiac or thoracic surgery or in the setting of rib fractures. It can lead to a reduction of opiate dosing and improved pain control during dressing changes in patients such as this one; however, it takes time to implement and the patient should receive acute pain control before consideration of alternatives to improve his baseline pain control.

Changing the medication to fentanyl is not appropriate as all intravenously administered opioids have equi-analgesic efficacy and are associated with similar clinical outcomes when titrated to similar pain intensity end points. The choice of opiate should be based on pharmacological properties. Fentanyl has a shorter half-life than morphine, and this patient was not having any adverse effect or contraindication to morphine.

KEY POINT

- Intravenous opioids are the first-line drug class of choice to treat nonneuropathic pain in critically ill patients; all intravenously administered opioids have equi-analgesic efficacy and are associated with similar clinical outcomes when titrated to similar pain intensity end points.

Bibliography

Barr J, Fraser GL, Puntillo K, Ely EW, Gélinas C, Dasta JF, et al; American College of Critical Care Medicine. Clinical practice guidelines for the management of pain, agitation, and delirium in adult patients in the intensive care unit. Crit Care Med. 2013;41:263-306. [PMID: 23269131] doi:10.1097/CCM.0b013e3182783b72

Item 69   **Answer: D**

Educational Objective: **Manage an asymptomatic patient with stage I pulmonary sarcoidosis.**

This patient should be managed with observation and clinical follow-up. She is incidentally discovered to have bilateral hilar lymphadenopathy likely representing pulmonary sarcoidosis.

Pulmonary sarcoidosis is classified based on the radiographic pattern: stage I, hilar lymphadenopathy with normal lung parenchyma; stage II, hilar lymphadenopathy with abnormal lung parenchyma; stage III, no lymphadenopathy with abnormal lung parenchyma; and, stage IV, parenchymal changes with fibrosis and architectural distortion. For patients such as this, a careful history and physical examination to rule out the possibility of lymphoma and infection are essential. In a series of 100 consecutive patients with bilateral hilar lymphadenopathy, none with either lymphoma or infection were asymptomatic. Furthermore, approximately 75% of patients with stage I pulmonary sarcoidosis, such as this patient, have spontaneous resolution of the hilar lymphadenopathy. Patients can, however, have extrapulmonary disease, and screening electrocardiography, assessment of serum calcium, and eye examination are appropriate initial tests in this population.

Endobronchial ultrasound is a bronchoscopic technique that involves the use of an ultrasound probe at the distal end of the bronchoscope. The ultrasound-tipped bronchoscope can identify mediastinal lymph nodes and increase the yield of a transbronchial needle aspiration by allowing direct visualization of the needle entering the lymph node. This can be used to visualize and biopsy structures adjacent to an airway. This patient has no need for endobronchial ultrasound and biopsy.

Obtaining a high-resolution CT of the chest in this patient may result in further findings of parenchymal lung disease; however, she is asymptomatic and the finding of parenchymal lung disease would not necessitate a change in management at this early stage.

Glucocorticoids are the mainstay of therapy for sarcoidosis. Treatment is usually limited to those with evidence of clinical symptoms from organ dysfunction. Because there is a high rate of spontaneous remission and stability, most treatment protocols favor a period of observation without therapy. The decision to initiate glucocorticoid therapy for sarcoidosis should be based on symptoms or physiologic impairment that is attributable to sarcoid disease. Therefore, treatment with prednisone is not indicated for this patient.

KEY POINT

- Treatment of pulmonary sarcoidosis should be based on symptoms rather than radiographic findings.

Bibliography

Baughman RP, Culver DA, Judson MA. A concise review of pulmonary sarcoidosis. Am J Respir Crit Care Med. 2011;183:573-81. [PMID: 21037016] doi:10.1164/rccm.201006-0865CI

Item 70   **Answer: D**   H

Educational Objective: **Prevent ventilator-associated lung injury.**

The most appropriate next step is to reduce the tidal volume. This patient fulfills the definition of acute respiratory distress syndrome (ARDS) with presentation within 1 week of known insult, arterial Po_2/Fio_2 ratio of 300 with positive end-expiratory pressure (PEEP) of 5 cm H_2O or greater, and bilateral otherwise unexplained opacities seen on frontal chest imaging. Common pulmonary causes of ARDS include pneumonia (most common), aspiration, inhalational injury, near drowning, and drugs. Although ARDS mortality remains high, significant reductions in mortality have been attributed to the use of lung protective ventilation strategies. These strategies generally include limiting the tidal volume given in mechanical ventilation to 6 mL/kg of ideal body weight, limiting the plateau pressure in the respiratory cycle to no more than 30 cm H_2O, and use of adequate PEEP to prevent the collapse of unstable alveolar units in the expiratory phase of the cycle. In the 2000 ARMA trial, low tidal volume ventilation (LTVV) was associated with a 9% absolute reduction in mortality when patients were ventilated at a goal of 6-8 mL/kg of ideal body weight compared with more liberal tidal volumes of 10-12 mL/kg. However, implementation of LTVV remains challenging for several reasons. Among them, patients who receive LTVV often demonstrate signs of air hunger. This can lead to ventilator dyssynchrony and increased sedation requirements.

Current recommendations are to use a PEEP level that achieves adequate oxygenation with an Fio_2 of less than 0.6 and does not cause hypotension. These parameters are being met with the current level of PEEP; therefore, adjustment of PEEP is not the most appropriate next step.

If the respiration rate remains constant, a lower tidal volume will reduce the total minute ventilation and thus reduce CO_2 removal. This results in higher arterial Pco_2 and lower arterial pH. In the ARMA trial, LTVV-related hypercapnea was permitted, provided the arterial pH did not go below 7.3. In cases where the pH did drop below 7.3, respiration rate was increased to improve minute ventilation and decrease the Pco_2. The patient's Pco_2 and pH are acceptable and adjustment of the respiration rate is not the most appropriate next step.

KEY POINT

- The use of low tidal volume ventilation and positive end-expiratory pressure is associated with prevention of ventilator-associated lung injury and a reduction in mortality related to acute respiratory distress syndrome.

Bibliography

Thompson BT, Chambers RC, Liu KD. Acute respiratory distress syndrome. N Engl J Med. 2017;377:562-572. [PMID: 28792873] doi:10.1056/NEJMra1608077

Item 71   Answer: D

Educational Objective: Recognize an emergently placed central venous catheter as a potential source of sepsis.

The most appropriate management for this patient is removal of the central venous catheter. Morbidity and mortality in patients with sepsis are heavily influenced by the care delivered during the first several hours after sepsis onset. Once sepsis is recognized, interventions focus on adequate fluid resuscitation. Crystalloid is recommended at a volume of 30 mL/kg of body weight. In septic shock, mortality increases with each hour that appropriate antibiotic therapy is delayed. Two sets of blood cultures should be obtained before antibiotic infusion in addition to cultures from the suspected infection site. Empiric antimicrobial treatment should cover all suspected pathogens, with special attention to risk factors for resistant or opportunistic organisms, including methicillin-resistant *Staphylococcus aureus* and *Pseudomonas* species. Identification and control of the source of infection are critical steps in managing sepsis. This patient may have sepsis due to a central line-associated bloodstream infection. Removal of the emergently placed central venous catheter is the next critical management step.

Glucocorticoid administration is not recommended for patients without shock or who have responded to fluids and vasopressors because it offers no benefit. Some studies suggest that glucocorticoid therapy might benefit patients who remain hypotensive following adequate fluid resuscitation and vasopressor therapy. It is premature to consider administering glucocorticoids to this patient without first assessing the response to the initial resuscitation attempts.

If hypotension does not rapidly correct with fluids, vasopressors should be titrated to maintain a mean arterial pressure of 65 mm Hg or greater. Norepinephrine is considered first-line therapy. Because fluid resuscitation has just been initiated, it is premature to consider vasopressor therapy. If vasopressor therapy is needed, a new intravenous catheter should be placed rather than using the existing catheter, which is suspected as the source of infection.

The biologic marker procalcitonin may help differentiate between bacterial and nonbacterial pneumonia and help exclude a bacterial community-acquired pneumonia diagnosis in outpatients where there is already low suspicion. Procalcitonin level has no evidence-based role in the management of sepsis in the hospital.

KEY POINT

- Fluid resuscitation, administration of antibiotics, and infection source control are essential in the early sepsis management.

Bibliography

Rhodes A, Evans LE, Alhazzani W, Levy MM, Antonelli M, Ferrer R, et al. Surviving Sepsis Campaign: international guidelines for management of sepsis and septic shock: 2016. Crit Care Med. 2017;45:486-552. [PMID: 28098591] doi:10.1097/CCM.0000000000002255

Item 72   Answer: A

Educational Objective: Evaluate a patient with excessive daytime sleepiness with actigraphy.

The most appropriate management is testing with actigraphy. The initial step in the evaluation of the patient with excessive daytime sleepiness is to ensure adequate quantities (7 to 8 hours) of sleep on a regular basis. This patient's self-report of a variable bedtime and restricted sleep schedule during the workweek raises the possibility of insufficient sleep syndrome. Wrist actigraphy measures movement and ambient light to estimate nightly sleep periods during a 1 to 2 week time frame. Actigraphy is more accurate than patient reports of sleep duration and is likely more accurate than sleep diaries. When actigraphy isn't available, a sleep diary can be a useful alternative. Insufficient sleep syndrome suggested by either actigraphy or sleep diary should prompt a trial of sleep extension.

Modafinil is a stimulant medication used in hypersomnia syndromes such as narcolepsy. It would not be appropriate therapy without first excluding insufficient sleep syndrome.

Multiple sleep latency testing can be useful in the evaluation of pathologic daytime sleepiness (for example, narcolepsy) and may help establish a diagnosis of narcolepsy, but it is resource intensive and expensive. It should be performed only after addressing insufficient sleep quantities and polysomnography has ruled out common sleep disorders such as sleep apnea.

Polysomnography or home sleep testing would be indicated if the clinical history strongly suggested a primary sleep disorder such as obstructive sleep apnea. However, obstructive sleep apnea is unlikely in a young woman who is not overweight and does not have obvious upper airway abnormalities. In addition, the patient is suspected of having a restricted sleep schedule that should be evaluated first with actigraphy.

> **KEY POINT**
>
> - The initial step in the evaluation of the patient with excessive daytime sleepiness is to ensure adequate quantities of sleep on a regular basis using either actigraphy or a sleep diary.

Bibliography

Watson NF, Badr MS, Belenky G, Bliwise DL, Buxton OM, Buysse D, et al; Consensus Conference Panel. Recommended amount of sleep for a healthy adult: a joint consensus statement of the American Academy of Sleep Medicine and Sleep Research Society. J Clin Sleep Med. 2015;11:591-2. [PMID: 25979105] doi:10.5664/jcsm.4758

Item 73   Answer: A

Educational Objective: Diagnose a complicated parapneumonic effusion.

This patient has community-acquired pneumonia and complicated parapneumonic effusion. A complicated parapneumonic effusion is defined as an effusion associated with a pneumonia that has a pH less than 7.2 and glucose less than 60 mg/dL (3.3 mmol/L). Complicated parapneumonic effusions occur when bacteria invade the pleural space. However, because bacteria may be cleared rapidly from the pleural space, the Gram stain is typically negative and cultures are usually sterile. Complicated parapneumonic effusions have a variable response to antibiotics alone. Pleural effusions greater than 10 mm in depth on

chest radiograph and associated with a pneumonic illness should be sampled. In general, these require thoracostomy tube drainage when the pH is less than 7.2 or the pleural fluid glucose level is less than 60 mg/dL (3.3 mmol/L). The American College of Chest Physicians consensus guidelines concur as thoracostomy drainage speeds clinical recovery and hospital discharge.

An empyema is defined as a bacterial infection of the pleural space that results in frank pus on visual inspection of the pleural fluid or a positive Gram stain. A positive pleural fluid culture is not required for diagnosis as cultures are less sensitive than Gram stain in the detection of bacteria. The management of empyema includes early thoracic surgical consultation because thoracoscopic or open debridement and drainage is often required to successfully manage this condition. However, this patient's pleural fluid was described as serous and the Gram stain was negative making empyema an unlikely diagnosis.

Pleural fluid acidosis (pH less than 7.3) is seen in complicated parapneumonic effusions, tuberculous pleuritis, rheumatoid and lupus pleuritis, esophageal rupture, and malignancy. A low pleural fluid glucose level results from either increased utilization within the pleural space (bacteria, malignant cells) or decreased transport into the pleural space (rheumatoid pleurisy), and a concentration less than 60 mg/dL (3.3 mmol/L) narrows the differential diagnosis significantly. Although a malignant effusion can have a low pH and glucose, this patient's presentation is more consistent with a parapneumonic effusion.

An uncomplicated parapneumonic effusion is characterized by a pH greater than 7.2 and glucose greater than 60 mg/dL (3.3 mmol/L). These effusions do not require drainage and typically resolve with antibiotic therapy alone.

> **KEY POINT**
>
> - In general, parapneumonic effusions associated with a pH less than 7.2 or pleural fluid glucose level less than 60 mg/dL (3.3 mmol/L) require thoracostomy drainage in addition to antibiotics.

Bibliography

Colice GL, Curtis A, Deslauriers J, Heffner J, Light R, Littenberg B, et al. Medical and surgical treatment of parapneumonic effusions: an evidence-based guideline. Chest. 2000;118:1158-71. [PMID: 11035692]

Item 74   Answer: B

Educational Objective: Provide recommended vaccinations for patients with COPD.

This patient should receive the pneumococcal polysaccharide vaccine and an annual influenza vaccine. Influenza vaccination has been shown to reduce serious illness (such as lower respiratory tract infections that require hospitalization) and death in patients with COPD. These vaccines should be administered annually in all patients with COPD. There are currently three different types of influenza vaccine available in the United States:

inactivated influenza vaccine, live attenuated influenza vaccine, and recombinant trivalent influenza vaccine. Inactivated influenza vaccine is approved for use in all adults, including immunosuppressed persons and pregnant women.

A high-dose inactivated influenza vaccine is approved for use in adults age 65 years and older; it has been shown to be modestly more effective than the standard-dose inactivated influenza vaccine in this patient population.

Pneumococcal vaccination is indicated for all adults aged 65 years and older and for high-risk persons younger than 65 years. Two vaccines are currently available: pneumococcal polysaccharide vaccine (PPSV23) is composed of polysaccharide capsular material from 23 pneumococcal subtypes, whereas pneumococcal conjugate vaccine (PCV13) contains capsular material from 13 subtypes conjugated to a nontoxic protein, which increases its immunogenicity. For pneumococcal vaccine–naïve adults between the ages of 19 and 65 years with certain immunocompromising conditions or who are otherwise at high risk, a single dose of PCV13 should be given. These conditions include functional or anatomic asplenia, cerebrospinal fluid leaks, cochlear implants, and conditions causing immunosuppression. All patients should also receive the 13-valent pneumococcal conjugate vaccine at age 65 years, although the polysaccharide and conjugate vaccines should be given sequentially at least a year apart for immunocompetent adults over age 65 rather than together for optimal effect. COPD alone is not an indication for PCV13 vaccination.

PPSV23 has the same indications as the PCV13 vaccine, plus it is indicated in immunocompetent people with certain chronic medical conditions such as heart, liver, and lung disease (COPD, emphysema, asthma) and diabetes, as well as in cigarette smokers. PPSV23 revaccination should be given at age 65 years if 5 years have elapsed since the previous pneumococcal immunization. When possible, the PCV13 vaccine should be administered first, followed by a dose of PPSV23 at least 1 year later for most immunocompetent patients. Some patients with immunocompromising conditions, cochlear implants, or cerebrospinal fluid leaks should receive the dose of PPSV23 at least 8 weeks after the first dose of PCV13. If a patient has already received the PPSV23 vaccine, a single dose of PCV13 should be given at least 1 year after the administration of PPSV23.

KEY POINT

- Annual influenza vaccination and the pneumococcal polysaccharide vaccine are recommended for all patients with chronic lung disease (COPD, emphysema, asthma).

Bibliography

Kim DK, Riley LE, Hunter P; Advisory Committee on Immunization Practices. Recommended immunization schedule for adults aged 19 years or older, United States, 2018. Ann Intern Med. 2018;168:210-220. [PMID: 29404596]

Item 75   Answer: D

Educational Objective: Treat a patient with chronic thromboembolic pulmonary hypertension.

This patient has chronic thromboembolic pulmonary hypertension (CTEPH) and the preferred treatment is pulmonary thromboendarterectomy. There are two diagnostic criteria for CTEPH: (1) mean pulmonary artery pressure of 25 mm Hg or higher by right heart catheterization in the absence of left heart pressure overload and (2) compatible imaging evidence of chronic thromboembolism. CT pulmonary angiography (CT-PA) may demonstrate proximally located abnormalities such as vascular webs, intimal irregularities, and luminal narrowing but has limited sensitivity in more distal lesions. Ventilation-perfusion scanning is a more sensitive indicator of CTEPH and is generally the preferred first imaging modality. Once CTEPH is suggested by noninvasive testing, conventional pulmonary angiography should be performed to characterize the extent and distribution of organized thrombus and to determine suitability for surgical intervention. Surgical intervention is the only definitive therapy for CTEPH and can prevent irreversible remodeling of the pulmonary arterial vasculature. Surgical evaluation at an experienced center is warranted in all patients with CTEPH; however, only about half of patients will be surgical candidates and fewer than that will opt for surgery.

Lifelong anticoagulant therapy, traditionally with warfarin, is indicated in all patients to help prevent further thromboembolism. Experience with direct oral anticoagulants such as apixaban is limited in this patient population. Because this patient's INR is in the therapeutic range, there's no proved advantage of switching from warfarin to apixaban.

Inferior vena cava interruption is typically indicated in patients with venous thrombus for whom anticoagulation is ineffective or not tolerated. In patients with CTEPH and coexisting clot in the lower extremities, inferior vena cava interruption can be considered to help prevent further thromboembolism; however, its role in long-term outcomes is not known and of unclear benefit.

Calcium channel blockers such as nifedipine are used in the setting of pulmonary arterial hypertension when right heart catheterization reveals acute vasoreactivity. Their role in the treatment of CTEPH is unproved.

KEY POINT

- Surgical intervention is the only definitive therapy for chronic thromboembolic pulmonary hypertension (CTEPH), and most patients with CTEPH should be referred for evaluation at a specialty surgical center.

Bibliography

Edward JA, Mandras S. An Update on the management of chronic thromboembolic pulmonary hypertension. Curr Probl Cardiol. 2017;42:7-38. [PMID: 27989311] doi:10.1016/j.cpcardiol.2016.11.001

Item 76　　　**Answer:　A**

Educational Objective: Evaluate readiness to liberate from mechanical ventilation in a patient with COPD.

A 30-minute spontaneous breathing trial (SBT) should be performed using low levels of pressure support (8 cm H_2O or less). Weaning from mechanical ventilation can start when the precipitating event or underlying condition that caused respiratory failure has resolved or is resolving. Patients should be assessed daily for their readiness to be removed from mechanical ventilation by performing an SBT. There are several methods used to assess if an SBT is successful. One criterion is the ability to tolerate a weaning trial for 30 minutes (in most patients, SBT failure will occur within approximately 20 minutes). 2-hour SBTs and 30-minute SBTs have a similar ability to recognize patients who are unable to breathe spontaneously. However a 30-minute trial has the benefits of less time on mechanical ventilation and less risk of respiratory muscle fatigue. If the patient successfully completes an SBT, the ability to follow commands, clear secretions, and a patent upper airway are other criteria that should be met to increase extubation success.

A "cuff leak" refers to measurable airflow around the endotracheal tube after the cuff of the endotracheal tube is deflated. Absent or minimal cuff leak following deflation of the cuff indicates reduced space between the endotracheal tube and the larynx. Minimal or absent cuff leak may be due to laryngeal edema, laryngeal stenosis, and thick secretions. The test is not standardized and not performed routinely and is not an initial routine test in the process of liberating a patient from mechanical ventilation. It might be considered in a patient who has a successful SBT but is at high risk for edema and stridor following extubation.

The Glasgow Coma Scale is pertinent to the actual extubation process, in which lack of awareness and ability to clear secretions and follow simple commands may increase the risk of aspiration and cooperation in the postextubation period. However, this patient should be placed on an SBT before being evaluated for extubation.

Negative inspiratory force has been used as a marker of inspiratory muscle strength to identify patients who will be able to be liberated from mechanical ventilation. However, there are technical issues that lead to variable predictive performance. A low negative inspiratory force by itself is not useful; however, serial measurements (for example, in patients with Guillain-Barré or myasthenia gravis) along with other measures (FVC, maximum tidal volume) may give a better picture of muscle strength recovery.

> **KEY POINT**
> - Patients should be assessed daily for their readiness to be removed from mechanical ventilation by performing a spontaneous breathing trial; one criterion for success is the ability to tolerate a spontaneous breathing trial for 30 minutes.

Bibliography

Schmidt GA, Girard TD, Kress JP, Morris PE, Ouellette DR, Alhazzani W, et al. Liberation from mechanical ventilation in critically ill adults: executive summary of an official American College of Chest Physicians/American Thoracic Society Clinical Practice Guideline. Chest. 2017;151:160-165. [PMID: 27818329] doi:10.1016/J.chest.2016.10.037

Item 77　　　**Answer:　C**

Educational Objective: Treat a patient with empyema.

Instillation of intrapleural tissue plasminogen activator-deoxyribonuclease (tPA-DNase) is the most appropriate treatment to promote drainage. This patient has a community-acquired pneumonia complicated by an empyema. The diagnostic criterion for empyema is either visualization of frankly purulent pleural fluid or a positive Gram stain. The Gram stain supports the diagnosis of *group A pneumoniae* pneumonia. An empyema requires drainage to resolve the infection. A small-bore (14-Fr) tube can be placed to facilitate drainage. An empyema can become loculated (divided into small cavities or compartments) and will not resolve with simple thoracostomy drainage; loculated empyemas often require thorascopic or open surgical debridement. This patient has an incompletely drained empyema due to loculation. When performed twice daily for 3 days, intrapleural administration of tPA-DNase has been shown to decrease the radiographic pleural opacity, lower the rate of surgical intervention, and decrease hospital stay of patients with empyema (MIST-2 trial). It should be noted that the tPA-DNase has not been shown to decrease mortality. In addition, video-assisted thorascopic surgery has also been shown to effectively manage empyema in greater than 90% of cases, and a delay in surgery increases the risk of open thoracotomy. Given the lack of prospective data, a multidisciplinary discussion should be undertaken for any patient presenting with an empyema who is a good surgical candidate.

Instillation of intrapleural antibiotic solution may be used for postsurgical empyema but has no demonstrated efficacy in the initial management of a loculated empyema.

The MIST-1 trial compared the use of intrapleural instillation of streptokinase compared to saline and found no difference in mortality, need for surgery, radiographic outcome, or length of hospitalization. Consequently, use of fibrinolytics alone in empyema is not recommended.

Continued systemic antibiotic therapy without adequate drainage of the pleural space is inadequate therapy. Failure to adequately drain the pleural space of a complicated pleural effusion or empyema will result in failure to resolve the infection, increased morbidity, and the possibility of death by overwhelming infection.

> **KEY POINT**
> - Instillation of intrapleural tissue plasminogen activator-deoxyribonuclease has been shown to decrease the radiographic pleural opacity, lower the rate of surgical referral, and decrease hospital stay of patients with empyema.

Bibliography

Rahman NM, Maskell NA, West A, Teoh R, Arnold A, Mackinlay C, et al. Intrapleural use of tissue plasminogen activator and DNase in pleural infection. N Engl J Med. 2011;365:518-26. [PMID: 21830966] doi:10.1056/NEJMoa1012740

Item 78   Answer: D

Educational Objective: Diagnose asthma in a symptomatic patient with normal spirometry.

Methacholine challenge testing is the most appropriate test to perform next for this patient with persistent cough and wheezing following a presumed viral upper respiratory tract infection. These symptoms can be the initial presentation of asthma, which is common in patients older than 65 years, with a prevalence of 8.1%; this age group also has the highest mortality rate, particularly in low-income Hispanic and black women. However, asthma is currently underdiagnosed and undertreated in patients older than 65 years in the United States. In patients with clinical symptoms suggestive of bronchospastic disease (such as cough or unexplained dyspnea) but with normal spirometry, bronchial challenge testing may be diagnostically helpful. Bronchial challenge testing uses a controlled inhaled stimulus to induce bronchospasm in association with spirometry; a positive test is indicated by a drop in the measured FEV_1. This symptomatic patient's spirometry is normal; therefore, methacholine challenge testing to evaluate for bronchial hyperresponsiveness is indicated.

Echocardiography could help evaluate cardiac function but the patient does not have findings of heart murmur or heart failure so this test would not be indicated.

Exhaled nitric oxide testing is a noninvasive breath test. Nitric oxide is normally present in airways but is increased in certain types of airway inflammation (asthma, eosinophilic airway inflammation). When elevated, it supports the diagnosis of asthma in the appropriate clinical context. Other factors may affect nitric oxide values such as age, sex, atopy, and cigarette smoking so a normal level in an older adult would not rule out asthma. The sensitivity and specificity of exhaled nitric oxide in the diagnosis of asthma are not well defined, particularly in patients with confounding variables, and it is not the preferred next test for this patient.

High-resolution CT (HRCT) is indicated if diffuse parenchymal lung disease is suspected. HRCT can help narrow the differential diagnosis based on the distribution of the lung parenchymal abnormalities and the presence or absence of associated findings. HRCT scan of the chest would not help confirm a diagnosis of asthma.

Nasal swab for influenza polymerase chain reaction would not be indicated because the patient's symptoms of a viral infection have resolved; furthermore, influenza testing in immunocompetent adults should be performed within 5 days of symptom onset.

- The diagnosis of asthma requires demonstrating reversible airflow obstruction; for a patient with symptoms of asthma and normal spirometry, methacholine challenge testing to evaluate for bronchial hyperresponsiveness is indicated.

Bibliography

Al-Alawi M, Hassan T, Chotirmall SH. Advances in the diagnosis and management of asthma in older adults. Am J Med. 2014;127:370-8. [PMID: 24380710] doi:10.1016/j.amjmed.2013.12.013

Item 79   Answer: B

Educational Objective: Treat a patient who has anaphylaxis with epinephrine.

This patient should be treated with epinephrine. Anaphylaxis is defined as a severe, potentially life-threatening allergic or hypersensitivity reaction that occurs within seconds to a few hours of allergen exposure, most commonly food, medication, or an insect sting. Classically, anaphylaxis occurs when allergen-specific IgE coating the surface of mast cells and basophils comes in contact with the triggering allergen, thereby precipitating cellular degranulation. The resulting abrupt systemic release of a host of mediators has various effects, including vasoconstriction, vasodilation, increased vascular permeability, and bronchoconstriction. The presentation is variable and findings may include flushing, urticaria, and angioedema (85%); wheeze, stridor, and respiratory distress (70%); and hypotension and tachycardia (less commonly bradycardia) (45%). Initial symptoms and findings may be mild but predicting the ultimate severity of the episode is difficult. The first step in treatment is immediate intramuscular or intravenous administration of epinephrine. There are studies showing increased mortality from anaphylaxis if epinephrine is delayed. The dose may be repeated after 5-15 minutes, or administered continuously as an intravenous solution (although at a lower concentration), until the effects are apparent. Patients can also be given supplemental oxygen and monitored for signs of airway compromise, which may require intubation to maintain airway patency. Following recovery, patients should maintain home access to an epinephrine auto-injector and may benefit from evaluation for anaphylactic triggers.

Diphenhydramine, a histamine$_1$-blocker, is often given because of its effect on itching and urticaria, but it has never been shown to effectively treat distributive shock, airway edema, or outcome in anaphylaxis. It is not a substitute for epinephrine.

Although intravenous fluids are often needed to manage anaphylaxis, they are reserved for use in cases where hypotension persists despite treatment with epinephrine.

Glucocorticoids are often given to reduce the risk of recurrent or persistent symptoms. However, there are no randomized controlled trials that confirm the effectiveness of glucocorticoids in preventing symptom recurrence.

H

Answers and Critiques

CONT.

More clinically relevant, a study of emergency department patients with anaphylaxis treated with glucocorticoids did not demonstrate a reduction in return visits to the emergency department for recurrent symptoms.

KEY POINT

- Epinephrine is the appropriate initial treatment of anaphylaxis.

Bibliography

Commins SP. Outpatient emergencies: anaphylaxis. Med Clin North Am. 2017;101:521-536. [PMID: 28372711] doi:10.1016/j.mcna.2016.12.003

Item 80   Answer: D

Educational Objective: Treat a patient with severe acute respiratory distress syndrome using early prone positioning.

This patient should be ventilated in the prone position. In patients with acute respiratory distress syndrome (ARDS) low tidal volume ventilation (6-8 mL/kg ideal body weight) is optimal and is associated with significantly better outcomes than conventional, higher tidal volume ventilation (10-12 mL/kg). In patients with severe ARDS, several adjunctive therapies have been studied, but few have demonstrated additional improved outcomes beyond low tidal volume ventilation. However, in 2013, the PROSEVA trial evaluated patients with ARDS who had an arterial P_{O_2}/F_{IO_2} ratio of less than 150 (defining severe ARDS) despite significant ventilator support. Patients were randomized to conventional therapy or low tidal volume ventilation plus prone positioning within 36 hours of developing ARDS and respiratory failure. The results suggested a 16.2% reduction in 28-day all-cause mortality in the prone-position group. The 2017 American Thoracic Society, European Society of Intensive Care Medicine, and Society of Critical Care Medicine (ATS/ESICM/SCCM) guideline makes a strong recommendation that all patients with ARDS receive ventilation with lower tidal volumes (4-8 mL/kg of predicted body weight). Patients with severe ARDS should be also ventilated in the prone position for at least 12 hours per day. Proning should be considered standard management for patients with severe ARDS, not a form of "rescue" or "salvage" therapy.

Recruitment is the application of a high level of continuous positive airway pressure to open up collapsed alveoli (for example, continuous pressure to 35 cm H_2O for 40 seconds). The ATS/ESICM/SCCM guideline provides a conditional recommendation for recruitment maneuvers based on low to moderate confidence in the small to moderate magnitude of its effect on mortality. The guideline cautions that recruitment should not be used in patients with preexisting hypovolemia or shock due to hemodynamic deterioration, which can occur during the maneuver. This patient is hypotensive and, therefore, not a candidate for recruitment maneuvers.

Nitric oxide (NO) selectively dilates the pulmonary vasculature when administered by inhalation. Its use in acute hypoxemic respiratory failure is based on the rationale that inhaled NO may improve ventilation-perfusion mismatch. Studies of inhaled NO in patients with severe ARDS have demonstrated temporary improvement in oxygenation but no improvement in survival.

In 2013 two large, prospective randomized trials demonstrated that compared to low tidal volume ventilation, high-frequency oscillator ventilation was either no different or harmful to patients with ARDS. In light of this, the ATS/ESICM/SCCM guideline strongly recommends against routine use of high-frequency oscillatory ventilation.

KEY POINT

- Patients with severe acute respiratory distress syndrome have a demonstrated mortality benefit from low tidal volume ventilation in the prone position.

Bibliography

Fan E, Del Sorbo L, Goligher EC, Hodgson CL, Munshi L, Walkey AJ, et al; American Thoracic Society, European Society of Intensive Care Medicine, and Society of Critical Care Medicine. An official American Thoracic Society/European Society of Intensive Care Medicine/Society of Critical Care Medicine clinical practice guideline: mechanical ventilation in adult patients with acute respiratory distress syndrome. Am J Respir Crit Care Med. 2017;195:1253-1263. [PMID: 28459336] doi:10.1164/rccm.201703-0548ST

Item 81   Answer: A

Educational Objective: Diagnose bronchiectasis using chest CT imaging.

The most likely diagnosis is bronchiectasis. Bronchiectasis is irreversible pathologic dilation of the bronchi or bronchioles resulting from an infectious process occurring in the context of airway obstruction, impaired drainage, or abnormality in antimicrobial defenses. The pattern of lung involvement varies greatly with the underlying cause and may be focal or diffuse. Bronchiectasis causes a chronic or recurrent cough typically characterized by voluminous sputum production with purulent exacerbations. The vast majority of chest radiographs are abnormal, typically showing linear atelectasis, dilated and thickened airways, and irregular peripheral opacities. High-resolution CT (HRCT) of the chest is the definitive diagnostic test for bronchiectasis.

Typical findings (airway dilatation with lack of tapering [green arrow], bronchial wall thickening [yellow arrow], and cysts [red arrow]) may be seen on HRCT.

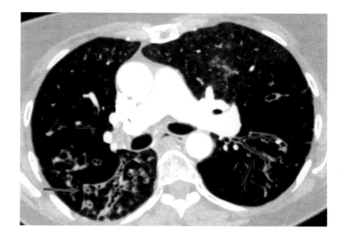

In addition to imaging, the cause of the bronchiectasis should be determined. This may involve testing for chronic bacterial or mycobacterial infections, assessing for the presence of connective tissue disease, and evaluating immune function. In selected patients, testing for cystic fibrosis or α_1-antitrypsin deficiency may be appropriate if suspected.

There is no evidence of emphysema on his chest CT imaging, which would typically appear as dilated airspaces, classified based on the distribution of abnormalities as centrilobular, panlobular, or paraseptal. Bullous or cystic changes may be seen.

Although the duration of his symptoms are consistent with chronic bronchitis, the chest CT scan shows evidence of bronchiectasis. In chronic bronchitis, the walls of the airways are thickened without dilation of the airways themselves.

Pulmonary Langerhans cell histiocytosis is a rare subacute interstitial lung disease of young, actively smoking adults. Patients may present with cough, fever, weight loss, and abnormal chest radiography. The chest CT findings include pulmonary nodules and cysts with midlung to upper-lung zone predominance and are not associated with bronchiectasis.

KEY POINT

- Chest CT is the definitive diagnostic study for bronchiectasis; typical findings are airway dilatation with lack of tapering, bronchial wall thickening, and cysts.

Bibliography

Milliron B, Henry TS, Veeraraghavan S, Little BP. Bronchiectasis: mechanisms and imaging clues of associated common and uncommon diseases. Radiographics. 2015;35:1011-30. [PMID: 26024063] doi:10.1148/rg.2015140214

Item 82   Answer: B

Educational Objective: Diagnose a patient with acute silicosis.

This patient most likely has acute silicosis, a fibrotic lung disease caused by the inhalation of silica dust. Silicosis is a spectrum of fibrotic lung diseases related to the inhalation of silica dust. Any occupation that disturbs the earth's crust involves potential risk. Workers in industries that process silica-containing rock or sand are also at risk. The typical disease course of simple silicosis can be accelerated (3 to 10 years after exposure) or latent (greater than 10 years after exposure). This patient has acute silicosis, a rare presentation characterized by onset of cough and dyspnea (but no fever) just a few weeks after intense exposure, patchy bilateral opacities on chest radiograph, and a milky effluent from bronchoalveolar lavage (BAL). Hydraulic fracturing, or fracking, is a process whereby large amounts of water and chemicals are injected into the ground; sand, which contains silica, is used to hold open the fissures created to enhance extraction of natural gas. Acute silicosis portends a

poor prognosis, as there is little evidence that any therapies can alter disease course. However, removal from the environment and smoking cessation will prevent further lung injury.

Acute interstitial pneumonia develops rapidly during days to weeks and results in progressive hypoxemic respiratory failure. Radiographic examination reveals bilateral alveolar opacities consistent with pulmonary edema. The findings on BAL are nonspecific. This patient's findings are not compatible with acute interstitial pneumonia.

Workers in the mining industry are at risk for asbestos exposure, but the typical latency period for asbestosis is decades rather than weeks, making this diagnosis unlikely. In addition, the most common radiographic finding of asbestosis is pleural plaques, which are not present on this patient's radiograph.

Patients with cryptogenic organizing pneumonia typically present with cough, dyspnea, fever, and malaise during 3 to 4 weeks that mimic community-acquired pneumonia. The chest radiograph reveals bilateral, patchy or diffuse, consolidative or ground-glass opacities and BAL effluent is not milky opaque.

KEY POINT

- Patients who work in industries that expose them to silica dust are at risk for silicosis.

Bibliography

Esswein EJ, Breitenstein M, Snawder J, Kiefer M, Sieber WK. Occupational exposures to respirable crystalline silica during hydraulic fracturing. J Occup Environ Hyg. 2013;10:347-56. [PMID: 23679563] doi:10.1080/15459624.2013.788352

Item 83   Answer: C

Educational Objective: Diagnose ICU-acquired weakness in a critically ill patient using the Medical Research Council muscle scale.

Although rarely used in practice, the most appropriate initial test to perform is the Medical Research Council (MRC) muscle scale. This patient has symmetrical quadriparesis and distal sensory neuropathy after sepsis and should be evaluated for ICU-acquired weakness. ICU-acquired weakness is the presence of profound muscles weakness in the setting of a current or recent critical illness. The MRC scale is most appropriately used in awake and cooperative patients. In such a patient, muscle strength of each extremity can be tested and graded from 0 (no movement) to 5 (normal). Summing the maximum score for 3 movements of each upper extremity (shoulder abduction, elbow flexion, wrist extension) and each lower extremity (hip flexion, knee extension, ankle dorsiflexion) can result in a maximum score of 60. In the absence of other known causes of muscular weakness, a score less than 48 is considered diagnostic of ICU-acquired weakness. The MRC muscle scale has several limitations; however, it is universally available, easy to perform, and can guide management decisions.

CONT.

Cervical spine MRI is an excellent imaging modality to detect a cervical epidural abscess in a patient with a history of bacteremia and supportive physical examination findings. However, the patient does not have numbness of the arms or increased tone and hyperreflexia of the lower extremities to support the diagnosis of a cervical myelopathy.

Electrodiagnostic testing can help establish the diagnosis of critical care polyneuropathy, critical care myopathy, or their combination, and provide clues to other causes of prolonged weakness (for example, acute inflammatory demyelinating polyneuropathy). However, the test is not universally available in all ICU centers, is invasive, may not affect management of patients with ICU-acquired weakness, and should not precede careful evaluation of the patient with the MRC scale.

Similarly, a muscle biopsy can also aid diagnosis of critical illness myopathy, especially in the setting of elevated serum creatine kinase levels, but it would not be an appropriate initial test.

KEY POINT

- Initial evaluation for ICU-acquired weakness can be done at the bedside using the Medical Research Council muscle scale.

Bibliography

Fan E, Cheek F, Chlan L, Gosselink R, Hart N, Herridge MS, et al; ATS Committee on ICU-Acquired Weakness in Adults. An official American Thoracic Society Clinical Practice guideline: the diagnosis of intensive care unit-acquired weakness in adults. Am J Respir Crit Care Med. 2014;190:1437-46. [PMID: 25496103] doi:10.1164/rccm.201411-2011ST

Item 84   Answer: C

Educational Objective: Diagnose cryptogenic organizing pneumonia.

The most likely diagnosis is cryptogenic organizing pneumonia. This patient has a subacute history of progressive dyspnea and persistent cough after an initial history consistent with community-acquired pneumonia. Despite treatment with appropriate antibiotic therapy, she now has clear evidence of new opacities that are located in different areas, are peripherally predominant, and coalesce along bronchovascular bundles. These findings are consistent with a diagnosis of organizing pneumonia, which involves proliferation of granulation tissue within alveolar ducts, alveolar spaces, and surrounding areas of chronic inflammation. There are many known causes of this pattern, including acute infections and autoimmune disorders like rheumatoid arthritis. The term *cryptogenic organizing pneumonia* is reserved for individuals who have this pattern but do not have a clear associated cause. Patients with cryptogenic organizing pneumonia will typically present with a 6-to-8-week history of symptoms that mimic community-acquired pneumonia. Typically, an initial empiric treatment of infection is given but fails; subsequently, noninfectious causes are considered. This patient has a subacute illness that began with viral symptoms, persistent and progressive cough and dyspnea that are not responsive to past

antibiotics, and radiographic findings typical of cryptogenic organizing pneumonia. Patients with cryptogenic organizing pneumonia respond well to glucocorticoids. Glucocorticoids are slowly tapered during the subsequent 6 months.

Acute HIV is unlikely in this patient who initially presented with symptoms of community-acquired pneumonia and whose fever has resolved. Although acute HIV symptoms are not specific, the most common presentation includes persistence of symptoms including fever.

Recurrent community-acquired pneumonia is also unlikely in this patient who was appropriately treated with azithromycin and whose symptoms have partially improved with resolution of the fever and sputum production.

Idiopathic pulmonary fibrosis (IPF) is a disease that affects older patients (the mean age of presentation is in the mid- to late 60s) and presents with chronic (longer than 6 months) symptoms of dry cough and shortness of breath. This patient's presentation is not consistent with these criteria, making a diagnosis of IPF unlikely.

KEY POINT

- A typical presentation of cryptogenic organizing pneumonia includes cough, fever, and malaise for 6 to 8 weeks that does not respond to antibiotics; patchy opacities on chest radiograph; and ground-glass opacities on CT scan that are peripherally distributed; glucocorticoids are first-line therapy.

Bibliography

Lazor R, Vandevenne A, Pelletier A, Leclerc P, Court-Fortune I, Cordier JF. Cryptogenic organizing pneumonia. Characteristics of relapses in a series of 48 patients. The Groupe d'Etudes et de Recherche sur les Maladies "Orphelines" Pulmonaires (GERM"O"P). Am J Respir Crit Care Med. 2000;162:571-7. [PMID: 10934089]

Item 85   Answer: A

Educational Objective: Treat a patient with a hemodynamically unstable pulmonary embolism using thrombolytic therapy.

The most appropriate treatment is thrombolytic therapy with a recombinant tissue plasminogen activator (rtPA). This patient has a large pulmonary embolism and is most likely becoming hypotensive from acute right ventricular (RV) failure. RV failure is the leading cause of death among patients with acute pulmonary embolism. In patients with hemodynamic collapse, treatment with thrombolytics is associated with decreased mortality and improvement in clinical and echocardiographic parameters. Although this patient has no contraindications to rtPA, thrombolytics carry a significant side effect profile, including an up to 2% risk of intracranial hemorrhage, but this should be considered relative in patients with life-threatening, high-risk pulmonary embolism. In patients with contraindications to thrombolysis, and in those in whom thrombolysis has failed to improve the hemodynamic status, surgical or catheter-based embolectomy should be considered if surgical expertise and resources are available.

According to the Apixaban for the Initial Management of Pulmonary Embolism and Deep-Vein Thrombosis as First-line Therapy (AMPLIFY) study, apixaban is an equivalent option to conventional heparin therapy for the initial treatment of pulmonary embolism. In this patient with hemodynamic collapse, it would not be more beneficial than low-molecular-weight heparin (LMWH) and is less beneficial than rtPA therapy.

In patients with acute pulmonary embolism, unfractionated heparin, LMWH, a new oral anticoagulant such as apixiban, or fondaparinux (a factor Xa inhibitor) should be started immediately unless otherwise contraindicated. Because this patient is experiencing hemodynamic collapse despite therapy with LMWH, continuing that treatment alone would not be appropriate.

Treatment of patients with acute pulmonary embolism with unfractionated heparin infusion appears to be associated with increased risk of adverse effect compared to LMWH administration. The 2014 European Society of Cardiology guidelines for diagnosis and management of pulmonary embolism recommends LMWH or fondaparinux rather than unfractionated heparin in hemodynamically stable patients because they are associated with a lower risk of heparin-induced thrombocytopenia and major bleeding events. However, the guidelines caution that LMWH and fondaparinux have not been tested in the setting of hypotension and shock and thus are not preferred modes of initial anticoagulation in that patient population.

> **KEY POINT**
>
> - In patients with pulmonary embolism and hemodynamic collapse, treatment with thrombolytics is associated with decreased mortality and improvement in clinical and echocardiographic parameters.

Bibliography

Konstantinides SV, Torbicki A, Agnelli G, Danchin N, Fitzmaurice D, Galiè N, et al; Task Force for the Diagnosis and Management of Acute Pulmonary Embolism of the European Society of Cardiology (ESC). 2014 ESC guidelines on the diagnosis and management of acute pulmonary embolism. Eur Heart J. 2014;35:3033-69, 3069a-3069k. [PMID: 25173341] doi:10.1093/eurheartj/ehu283

Item 86   Answer: D

Educational Objective: **Treat a malnourished, critically ill patient using parenteral nutrition.**

This patient should receive parenteral nutrition. Nutrition is an essential part of management for patients in the ICU and can be given enterally or parenterally, with the enteral route preferred. Initiation of enteral nutrition is recommended at 24 to 48 hours following admission if the patient is hemodynamically stable, with advancement to goal by 48 to 72 hours. Benefits include fewer infections and possibly reduced mortality. For patients with adequate nutritional status but who have contraindications to enteral nutrition or do not tolerate enteral nutrition, parenteral nutrition is delayed for 1 to 2 weeks based upon evidence that early parenteral nutrition may increase the risk of infection. For patients with inadequate nutrition (or who are at high risk for malnutrition) who have contraindications or intolerance of enteral nutrition, parenteral nutrition should be initiated as soon as possible. This practice is based on two meta-analyses showing early parenteral nutrition in poorly nourished patients is associated with fewer complications and decreased mortality. This patient has several features consistent with severe malnutrition (temporal wasting, edema, hypoglycemia, poorly healing wounds), as well as ileus and evidence of enteral nutrition intolerance (nausea, vomiting).

The patient is obviously not tolerating enteral nutrition, as evidenced by her clinical nutritional status, nausea, vomiting, and distended abdomen. Continuing enteral nutrition would not be appropriate.

Measurement of gastric residual volume is no longer recommended for routine monitoring of enteral nutrition because it does not affect outcomes. In this patient, it is clinically apparent that she is not tolerating enteral nutrition, and measurement of gastric residual volume will not add clinically useful information.

Metoclopramide improves enteral nutrition tolerance but does not affect patient outcomes and is associated with adverse events (diarrhea, QT prolongation, tardive dyskinesia, cardiac toxicity). Because of this patient's recent surgery, she should first be started on parenteral nutrition and evaluated for a mechanical cause of bowel obstruction. Metoclopramide and other prokinetic agents are contraindicated in the presence of mechanical small bowel obstruction.

> **KEY POINT**
>
> - Parenteral nutrition should be started as soon as possible for severely malnourished patients or those at high risk of malnutrition for whom enteral nutrition is not possible.

Bibliography

Taylor BE, McClave SA, Martindale RG, Warren MM, Johnson DR, Braunschweig C, et al; Society of Critical Care Medicine. Guidelines for the provision and assessment of nutrition support therapy in the adult critically ill patient: Society of Critical Care Medicine (SCCM) and American Society for Parenteral and Enteral Nutrition (A.S.P.E.N.). Crit Care Med. 2016;44:390-438. [PMID: 26771786] doi:10.1097/CCM.0000000000001525

Item 87   Answer: D

Educational Objective: **Diagnose respiratory bronchiolitis-associated interstitial lung disease.**

The most likely diagnosis is respiratory bronchiolitis-associated interstitial lung disease (RB-ILD). Evidence of RB-ILD is found on approximately 5% to 25% of cancer-screening CT scans. RB-ILD is used to describe disease in active smokers who have imaging findings of centrilobular micronodules with a pathologic finding of respiratory bronchiolitis and tan-pigmented macrophages (smokers' macrophages) on biopsy. Patients with RB-ILD are often asymptomatic. Symptomatic patients are typically smokers presenting in their fourth and fifth decades of smoking with cough and dyspnea and bibasilar inspiratory crackles. There are two other disorders that generally only develop in individuals who have an active smoking history. These are desquamative interstitial pneumonia and pulmonary Langerhans cell histiocytosis. Pulmonary function tests usually reveal an obstructive pattern with a decreased D$_{LCO}$ in individuals with more severe disease. For those with milder disease, pulmonary function tests can be normal, restrictive, or obstructive. Cessation of smoking is the primary management.

Desquamative interstitial pneumonia is due to extensive, diffuse macrophage filling of alveolar spaces with predominant cough and dyspnea symptoms and bilateral ground-glass opacities on chest imaging. This patient's symptoms and CT findings are not compatible with this disease.

CT scan findings of idiopathic pulmonary fibrosis include basal- and peripheral-predominant septal line thickening with traction bronchiectasis and honeycomb changes. This is the usual interstitial pneumonia pattern and can be seen in connective tissue disease, asbestosis, and chronic hypersensitivity pneumonitis; idiopathic pulmonary fibrosis is a diagnosis of exclusion. The CT scan findings are not consistent with this diagnosis.

Pulmonary Langerhans cell histiocytosis is characterized by middle and upper zone thin-walled cysts with accompanying nodules and is often associated with pulmonary hypertension. Patients tend to be young adults with cough and dyspnea. Thin-walled cysts are not present in this patient's CT scan, making this diagnosis unlikely.

KEY POINT

- Respiratory bronchiolitis–associated interstitial lung disease is found in active smokers who have chest CT scan findings of centrilobular micronodules.

Bibliography

Chung JH, Richards JC, Koelsch TL, MacMahon H, Lynch DA. Screening for lung cancer: incidental pulmonary parenchymal findings. AJR Am J Roentgenol. 2017:1-11. [PMID: 29231759] doi:10.2214/AJR.17.19003

Item 88   Answer: D

Educational Objective: Manage a patient with chronic silicosis and likely tuberculosis infection.

The most appropriate management is a sputum sample for acid-fast bacillus. This patient has constitutional symptoms that include night sweats, unintentional weight loss, hemoptysis, and upper-lobe cavitary disease on chest radiograph. Reactivation tuberculosis most commonly involves the apical-posterior segments of the upper lobe; cavitation is present in up to 40% of cases. Tuberculosis should be strongly considered when a patient with silicosis develops constitutional symptoms, worsening respiratory impairment, hemoptysis, or changes in the chest radiograph, particularly cavities. Chronic silicosis adversely affects macrophage function and is clearly associated with the development of infection with

tuberculosis. Concomitant silicosis and tuberculosis is associated with a substantially increased risk of mortality. Therefore, a high index of suspicion for this complication of chronic silicosis is essential to ensure early and appropriate medical therapy.

Aspergilloma is generally a consequence of colonization of a preexisting pulmonary cavity or cyst or in areas of devitalized lung. Symptoms include cough, hemoptysis, dyspnea, weight loss, fever, fatigue, and chest pain. Radiographic images show a round mass within a pulmonary cavity or cyst. Sputum cultures or IgG antibody are usually positive. This patient's chest radiograph is not consistent with an aspergilloma, and aspergillosis IgG antibody testing is not necessary.

Mine workers are often exposed to radon and several kinds of dust, and they have high rates of tobacco use; however, the development of silicosis is also an independent risk factor for the development of lung cancer. Nevertheless, bronchoscopy with transbronchial biopsy would not be appropriate for this patient. Although he has a substantially increased risk of lung cancer, the chest radiograph does not clearly demonstrate a target for biopsy. Furthermore, pursuing bronchoscopy without first ensuring there is not an active tuberculosis infection potentially places health care workers at risk for infection.

A high-resolution CT scan of the chest may identify additional findings not visible on the chest radiograph, but it will not change the need to rule out tuberculosis, which is a common comorbidity of chronic silicosis.

KEY POINT

- Tuberculosis should be strongly considered when a patient with silicosis develops constitutional symptoms, worsening respiratory impairment, hemoptysis, or changes in the chest radiograph, particularly cavities.

Bibliography

Nasrullah M, Mazurek JM, Wood JM, Bang KM, Kreiss K. Silicosis mortality with respiratory tuberculosis in the United States, 1968-2006. Am J Epidemiol. 2011;174:839-48. [PMID: 21828370] doi:10.1093/aje/kwr159

Item 89   Answer: C

Educational Objective: Diagnose upper airway obstruction using a flow-volume loop.

The most likely diagnosis is fixed upper airway obstruction. Flow-volume loops graphically plot pulmonary airflow during exhalation and inspiration, with characteristic patterns associated with specific clinical conditions. The normal expiratory portion of the flow-volume loop (above the x-axis) is characterized by a rapid rise to the peak flow rate, followed by a nearly linear fall in flow as the patient exhales. The inspiratory curve (below the x-axis) appears as a semicircle. Flattening of both the inspiratory and expiratory curve of the flow-volume loop suggests this patient has a fixed intrathoracic lesion, such as tracheal stenosis, which can be seen postintubation.

Spirometry is relatively insensitive to all but severe (greater than 71%) intrathoracic airway obstruction. Therefore, if intrathoracic airway obstruction is suspected, appearance of a normal flow-volume loop should not discourage further evaluation.

Patients with asthma would be expected to have this obstructive pattern, although patients without active symptoms can have a completely normal loop.

Patients with COPD demonstrate an obstructive pattern of the flow-volume loop. This is typically manifested by a fairly normal initial portion of the expiratory flow loop, with increased concavity of the terminal portion, indicating airway narrowing during exhalation.

The flow-volume loop demonstrates reduced inspiratory and expiratory volumes, and not the normal pattern described above.

KEY POINT

- Flattening of both the inspiratory and expiratory curve of the flow-volume loop suggests a fixed intrathoracic lesion; direct examination of the airways is indicated to confirm the finding and identify the cause.

Bibliography

Murgu SD, Egressy K, Laxmanan B, Doblare G, Ortiz-Comino R, Hogarth DK. Central airway obstruction: benign strictures, tracheobronchomalacia, and malignancy-related obstruction. Chest. 2016;150:426-41. [PMID: 26874192] doi:10.1016/j.chest.2016.02.001

Item 90   Answer: D

Educational Objective: Treat asthma during pregnancy.

This patient's previous medications of albuterol and budesonide should be restarted. Asthma management during pregnancy should consist of optimization of anti-inflammatory therapy, management of gastroesophageal reflux, and smoking cessation. Inhaled glucocorticoids are considered safe in pregnancy, and abundant long-term safety evidence exists for budesonide. With the exception of zileuton, most leukotriene receptor antagonists are also considered safe in pregnancy. The treatment of asthma in pregnancy is very similar to treatment in nonpregnant patients. This patient has mild persistent asthma, with symptoms more than twice weekly, and use of low-dose inhaled glucocorticoids plus a short-acting β_2-agonist is the recommended therapy. The risks to the fetus of untreated asthma are significantly greater than the risks of asthma medications. Maternal asthma increases the risk of perinatal mortality, preterm birth, low-birth-weight infants, and preeclampsia. Budesonide is the preferred inhaled glucocorticoid to use in pregnant asthma patients because there are more data available concerning budesonide use in pregnancy than the other inhaled glucocorticoid formulations. However, there are no studies indicating that other inhaled glucocorticoid formulations are unsafe in pregnancy, so if a patient's asthma is well controlled on another inhaled glucocorticoid, it is not necessary to change to budesonide during pregnancy.

Combination fluticasone/salmeterol is not the recommended treatment regimen for mild persistent asthma and would be inappropriate for this patient.

Prednisone is used to treat asthma exacerbations, and all patients with asthma should have a written asthma action plan to manage an exacerbation and begin self-treatment. Therefore, although prednisone may be part of this patient's asthma management plan, it is not indicated for treatment of her current symptoms of mild persistent asthma.

This patient is experiencing frequent symptoms of asthma and would benefit from treatment. Therefore, peak flow monitoring alone is not appropriate without initiation of pharmacotherapy.

KEY POINT

- Treatment of asthma during pregnancy is similar to treatment in nonpregnant patients.

Bibliography

Bonham CA, Patterson KC, Strek ME. Asthma outcomes and management during pregnancy. Chest. 2018;153:515-527. [PMID: 28867295] doi:10.1016/j.chest.2017.08.029

Item 91   Answer: B

Educational Objective: Evaluate a patient with diffuse parenchymal lung disease using high-resolution chest CT scan.

High-resolution CT (HRCT) scan of the chest is the most appropriate test. The choice of imaging modality in the evaluation of pulmonary disease is dependent on the information being sought based on the differential diagnosis. HRCT scan is indicated if diffuse parenchymal lung disease (DPLD) is suspected. The diagnostic approach to DPLD is grounded in the predominant pattern of abnormalities, distribution of disease, and associated findings (pleural plaques, calcifications, effusions, lymphadenopathy). HRCT scan provides more detail than either chest radiography or conventional CT scanning and can more accurately assess the pattern and distribution of DPLD. This patient's history, physical findings, pulmonary function tests, radiography results, and family history strongly suggest the diagnosis of idiopathic pulmonary fibrosis. An HRCT scan will allow for better characterization of pattern and distribution of the opacities on chest radiograph and will help diagnose the underlying disease.

Contrast-enhanced chest CT scan may be added to the study to better evaluate the mediastinal structures (for example, to assess for lymphadenopathy). However, there is no suggestion of mediastinal abnormality on the chest radiograph; rather, the patient's history, physical examination findings, and chest radiograph more strongly suggest DPLD, and HRCT is the preferred imaging modality in that situation.

Patients who meet criteria for lung-cancer screening should undergo imaging with low-dose chest CT scan to minimize radiation exposure. Low-dose chest CT images utilize a lower total radiation dose than standard CT chest protocols. The lower dose of radiation decreases the radiation to patients and is as effective as standard-dose CT in imaging lung nodules owing to the high inherent contrast between lung tissue and air. Low-dose CT scan is a good modality to screen for pulmonary nodules but not a good modality to assess DPLD.

Patients with a pulmonary nodule or other findings suggestive of malignancy may require PET/CT imaging. This test most commonly uses fluorodeoxyglucose (FDG) as a metabolic marker to identify rapidly dividing cells such as tumor cells. A nodule that demonstrates no FDG uptake is unlikely to be malignant. Any disease with metabolic activity, including infection, inflammation, and malignancy, can cause an FDG-avid nodule. PET/CT imaging would not be helpful in the evaluation of DPLD.

KEY POINT

- High-resolution chest CT scan is the preferred advanced imaging modality for suspected diffuse parenchymal lung disease; it can help narrow the differential diagnosis based on the character and distribution of the lung parenchymal abnormalities.

Bibliography
Walsh SL, Hansell DM. High-resolution CT of interstitial lung disease: a continuous evolution. Semin Respir Crit Care Med. 2014;35:129-44. [PMID: 24481766] doi:10.1055/s-0033-1363458

Item 92   Answer: D

Educational Objective: Evaluate recurrent unilateral exudative effusion for malignancy.

This patient should be referred for thoracoscopy and pleural biopsy. He has a recurrent exudative pleural effusion. The characterization of pleural fluid as a transudate or exudate helps narrow the differential diagnosis and direct subsequent investigations. An effusion is considered an exudate if any of the following criteria are met: pleural fluid total protein/serum total protein greater than 0.5; pleural fluid lactate dehydrogenase (LDH)/serum LDH greater than 0.6; pleural fluid LDH greater than 2/3 the upper limit of normal for serum LDH. This patient has an exudate. Despite the negative chest radiograph and CT scan, this exudate is concerning for malignancy considering his age, smoking history, and work in a shipyard with potential exposure to asbestos. The cytology of the pleural fluid was negative, but cytology is only 60% sensitive for malignancy.

Closed pleural biopsy is less sensitive than cytology and should not be performed.

A chylous effusion can be suspected by its milky appearance (seen in 50% of patients) and is associated with traumatic and nontraumatic etiologies. Nontraumatic chylous effusion is most commonly due to malignancy (lymphoma, chronic lymphocytic leukemia, metastatic cancer). Traumatic chylous effusions are most commonly associated with thoracic surgical procedures. A pleural fluid triglyceride level greater than 110 mg/dL (1.24 mmol/L) is characteristic of a

chylothorax. There is no reason to suspect a chylothorax at this point; thoracoscopic pleural biopsy will be of higher diagnostic yield.

The yield of sending more than two cytology specimens taken on different occasions is low. If cytology is negative and malignancy is still suspected, thoracoscopy with pleural biopsy allows for direct visualization of the pleural surface and has greater than 90% sensitivity for the diagnosis of malignancy.

KEY POINT

- For patients with negative cytology in whom malignancy is suspected, thoracoscopy with pleural biopsy allows for direct visualization of the pleural surface and has a diagnostic sensitivity for malignant disease of greater than 90%.

Bibliography
Hooper C, Lee YC, Maskell N; BTS Pleural Guideline Group. Investigation of a unilateral pleural effusion in adults: British Thoracic Society Pleural Disease Guideline 2010. Thorax. 2010;65 Suppl 2:ii4-17. [PMID: 20696692] doi:10.1136/thx.2010.136978

Item 93   Answer: C

Educational Objective: Diagnose interstitial lung disease with a high-resolution CT scan of the chest.

This patient should receive a high-resolution CT (HRCT) scan of the chest. He has symptoms of progressive dyspnea on exertion, inspiratory crackles, restrictive pulmonary function tests, and a chest radiograph demonstrating diffuse parenchymal lung disease. This constellation of findings suggests interstitial lung disease. Plain chest radiography findings may be highly variable in patients with diffuse parenchymal lung disease. Chest films may show increased interstitial reticular or nodular infiltrates in different patterns of distribution, but they may be normal in up to 10% of patients. Characteristics on HRCT of the chest have pulmonary pathology correlates that can help narrow the differential diagnosis. HRCT provides detailed resolution of the pulmonary parenchymal architecture. HRCT, clinical presentation (including time course of symptoms), physical findings, and, when necessary, lung biopsy and histopathology allow clinicians to reach selected diagnoses from an extensive list of diffuse parenchymal lung diseases.

In selected cases, bronchoscopic lung biopsy can provide enough tissue to demonstrate specific histopathologic features diagnostic of several specific disease processes, including carcinoma, sarcoidosis, and eosinophilic pneumonia. Bronchoalveolar lavage can provide additional diagnostic information, including culture, cytology, and cell differential. However, a lung biopsy and bronchoalveolar lavage would not be indicated until imaging studies confirmed the presence of diffuse parenchymal lung disease and have narrowed the differential diagnosis to entities that might be assessed with biopsy or bronchoalveolar lavage.

Cardiopulmonary exercise testing includes assessment of respiratory gas exchange during treadmill or bicycle exercise for a more detailed assessment of functional capacity and differentiation between potential causes of exercise limitation (cardiac, pulmonary, or deconditioning, versus volitional). It would not be the most appropriate next choice in a patient with increasing exercise limitation, pulmonary crackles, an abnormal chest radiograph, and restrictive findings on pulmonary function testing.

Methacholine challenge testing is used to evaluate bronchial hyperreactivity in patients with normal pulmonary function tests, and this patient's testing is abnormal, with a restrictive pattern, so such testing would not be indicated.

KEY POINT

- High-resolution CT scan of the chest is standard care for evaluating parenchymal opacities seen on a plain radiograph.

Bibliography

Meyer KC. Diagnosis and management of interstitial lung disease. Transl Respir Med. 2014;2:4. [PMID: 25505696] doi:10.1186/2213-0802-2-4

Item 94   Answer: D

Educational Objective: Treat disruptive snoring with weight loss.

The most appropriate next step in management is a trial of weight loss. In this obese but otherwise healthy patient without other sleep-related symptoms, weight loss is a reasonable first step that often relieves snoring. Obesity is the strongest risk factor for snoring and obstructive sleep apnea (OSA). Snoring occurs as the upper airway narrows during sleep, when inspired air collides with redundant soft tissue. Further airway collapse leads to OSA. Other treatments for snoring can include limiting time spent in the supine position (postural therapy) and curbing alcohol intake.

Home sleep testing should be reserved for patients with a high probability of moderate to severe apnea in whom positive airway pressure therapy is being considered. Although OSA hasn't been ruled out in this patient, his bed partner hasn't observed classic signs such as gasping or choking, nor does he exhibit strong indications for positive airway pressure therapy, such as excessive daytime sleepiness.

In-laboratory polysomnography allows more detailed analysis of the possible underlying sleep-related breathing disorder than out-of-center methods. Once the type of apnea is clarified during the diagnostic portion of the in-laboratory study, the technician may also then utilize the most appropriate mode of positive airway pressure therapy and assess the response to treatment. However, for this patient, testing of any kind should be preceded by a conservative approach that includes weight loss.

Upper airway surgical procedures, such as radiofrequency ablation of soft palate, are sometimes used to treat snoring and OSA but are variably effective and not considered first-line therapy.

KEY POINT

- Obesity is the strongest risk factor for snoring and obstructive sleep apnea, and in obese but otherwise healthy patients without other sleep-related symptoms, weight loss is a reasonable first step that often relieves snoring and improves mild obstructive sleep apnea.

Bibliography

Balachandran JS, Patel SR. In the clinic. Obstructive sleep apnea. Ann Intern Med. 2014;161:ITC1-15; quiz ITC16. [PMID: 25364899] doi:10.7326/0003-4819-161-9-201411040-01005

Item 95   Answer: A

Educational Objective: Manage a malignant pleural effusion.

This patient should be referred for an indwelling pleural catheter placement. Her diagnosis of a malignant pleural effusion signifies advanced disease and overall poor prognosis and the goal of management is the relief of symptoms. Several therapeutic options are available and should be made based on symptoms, prognosis, degree of lung reexpansion, and patient performance status. She has rapid reaccumulation of fluid and, therefore, should be offered more definitive management. Indwelling pleural catheters with intermittent drainage provide significant symptom relief, and 50% to 70% of patients achieve spontaneous pleurodesis after 2 to 6 weeks. In a recent randomized trial indwelling pleural catheters were found to be noninferior to talc pleurodesis, and patients who had an indwelling pleural catheter had a shorter hospital stay and less dyspnea at 6 months.

Pleurectomy is another management option but is rarely performed because it is invasive, associated with long recovery times, and appears to be no more effective than less invasive options.

Repeat therapeutic thoracentesis is appropriate for patients with poor prognosis (less than 3 months) and slow reaccumulation of fluid; given this patient's good performance status and rapid reaccumulation of pleural fluid, serial thoracentesis is not indicated.

Chemical pleurodesis refers to obliteration of the pleural space with a sclerosing agent (typically talc). Talc can be introduced through a thoracostomy tube (talc slurry) or during a thoracostomy or thoracotomy (talc poudrage). Talc pleurodesis is very effective, with a success rate of 60% to 90%, depending on the degree of lung reexpansion; however, it is associated with increased pain and longer initial hospital stay, so an indwelling pleural catheter would be preferable at this time.

KEY POINT

- For patients with a malignant pleural effusion and rapid reaccumulation of fluid, indwelling pleural catheters provide significant symptom relief, and 50% to 70% of patients achieve spontaneous pleurodesis after 2 to 6 weeks.

Bibliography

Feller-Kopman D, Light R. Pleural disease. N Engl J Med. 2018;378:740–751. doi: 10.1056/NEJMra1403503. [PMID: 29466146]

Item 96   Answer: D

Educational Objective: Diagnose serotonin syndrome.

The most likely diagnosis is serotonin syndrome. The features of hyperthermia, tremor, hyperreflexia, ocular clonus (slow, continuous, horizontal eye movements), other clonus (spontaneous or induced), and anxiety are classic features of this syndrome. Hyperreflexia and clonus help distinguish serotonin syndrome from other hyperthermic syndromes and toxic ingestions. This patient's history supports the diagnosis, which usually occurs after coingestion of several serotonergic medications—for example, fluoxetine and methylenedioxymethamphetamine ("ecstasy"). Treatment is mainly supportive, using benzodiazepines as needed to keep the patient calm and to control blood pressure and heart rate. Physical restraint can lead to agitated exertion and worsen hyperthermia. Autonomic instability is common, so close monitoring is recommended. Only in very severe cases of agitation or hyperthermia do patients need to be deeply sedated, intubated, paralyzed, and sometimes treated with cyproheptadine.

Anticholinergic toxicity is unlikely in this patient because he has no signs of mydriasis, dry mucus membranes, or urinary and bowel retention. He does exhibit hyperthermia and agitation, but has clonus and hyperreflexia, which are not associated with anticholinergic toxicity.

Malignant hyperthermia would be very unlikely without a history of inhaled anesthesia agents or neuromuscular blockade. Clinical features of malignant hyperthermia usually include higher fever, muscle rigidity, and, occasionally, hemorrhage but not hyperreflexia or clonus.

Neuroleptic malignant syndrome would be very unlikely without a history of neuroleptic medications, such as haloperidol. It usually develops subacutely during days or weeks, whereas serotonin syndrome typically develops within hours. Rigidity with hyporeflexia is more common, rather than hyperreflexia and myoclonus in serotonin syndrome. Hyperthermia, altered mental status, and rigidity are features of both syndromes. Neuroleptic malignant syndrome usually takes many days to resolve, whereas serotonin syndrome usually resolves within 24 hours.

> **KEY POINT**
>
> • Classic features of serotonin syndrome include hyperthermia, tremor, hyperreflexia and clonus; treatment is mainly supportive, using benzodiazepines as needed to keep the patient calm and to control blood pressure and heart rate.

Bibliography

Dobry Y, Rice T, Sher L. Ecstasy use and serotonin syndrome: a neglected danger to adolescents and young adults prescribed selective serotonin reuptake inhibitors. Int J Adolesc Med Health. 2013;25:193-9. [PMID: 24006318] doi:10.1515/ijamh-2013-0052

Item 97   Answer: A

Educational Objective: Treat a patient with acute hemorrhagic shock using volume resuscitation with blood products.

The most appropriate management for this patient is a transfusion of packed red blood cells. Clinicians should base decisions on blood transfusion on the full clinical picture, recognizing that overtransfusion may be as damaging as undertransfusion. A restrictive transfusion policy aiming for a hemoglobin level of 7 to 8 g/dL (70 to 80 g/L) is suggested in hemodynamically stable patients. More liberal blood transfusion thresholds lead to increased portal pressures and risk of further bleeding. This patient most likely is experiencing hemorrhagic shock from a recurrent variceal bleeding episode. Because the patient is hemodynamically unstable, initial guideline-based management includes volume resuscitation, and transfusion of blood products is the best method for achieving this. In patients who are bleeding and have a platelet count less than $50,000/\mu L$ $(50 \times 10^9/L)$ or who have an INR greater than 1.5, transfusion of platelets or fresh frozen plasma, respectively, is indicated.

Historically, uncontrolled variceal bleeding offered a compelling rationale for use of recombinant factor VII, but a 2014 meta-analysis of almost 500 patients from two randomized clinical trials evaluated the role of factor VII following variceal bleed. In both trials, there was no indication that factor VII improved outcomes. Therefore, it would not be appropriate for this patient.

Emergent upper endoscopy and consideration of placing a transjugular intrahepatic portosystemic shunt are indicated in this patient, but are pursued after initial resuscitation efforts are completed. Because this patient is hemodynamically unstable and these procedures take time to coordinate, they would not supersede initial resuscitative efforts with blood products.

> **KEY POINT**
>
> • In patients with hemorrhagic shock, initial management includes volume resuscitation with blood products to stabilize the patient.

Bibliography

Tripathi D, Stanley AJ, Hayes PC, Patch D, Millson C, Mehrzad H, et al; Clinical Services and Standards Committee of the British Society of Gastroenterology. U.K. guidelines on the management of variceal haemorrhage in cirrhotic patients. Gut. 2015;64:1680-704. [PMID: 25887380] doi:10.1136/gutjnl-2015-309262

Item 98   Answer: D

Educational Objective: Treat a patient intoxicated with isopropyl alcohol.

The most appropriate management is supportive care. Calculation of the plasma osmolal gap is helpful in assessing the presence of unmeasured solutes, such as ingestion of certain toxins (for example, methanol or ethylene glycol). The plasma osmolal gap is the difference between the measured and calculated plasma osmolality. Plasma osmolality can be calculated using the following formula:

$$\text{Plasma Osmolality (mOsm/kg } H_2O) = 2 \times \text{Serum Sodium} \\ \text{(mEq/L) + Plasma Glucose (mg/dL)} / \\ 18 + \text{Blood Urea Nitrogen (mg/dL)} / 2.8.$$

When the measured osmolality exceeds the calculated osmolality by greater than 10 mOsm/kg H_2O, the osmolal gap is considered elevated. This patient does not have an increased anion-gap metabolic acidosis, thus eliminating methanol and ethylene glycol poisoning. An elevated osmolal gap of 27 and absent blood ethanol support the diagnosis of isopropyl alcohol ingestion (rubbing alcohol), which does not cause a metabolic acidosis. It is metabolized by alcohol dehydrogenase (ADH) to acetone, which can cause a fruity odor on the patient's breath. There are no other toxic metabolites, and the main effect of isopropyl alcohol ingestion is central nervous system depression by both the isopropyl alcohol and the acetone.

There is no need to block the action of ADH with fomepizole. Administration of fomepizole would be advised for treatment of methanol or ethylene glycol ingestion, because these alcohols both have toxic metabolites that can lead to blindness, kidney failure, or death. Inhibiting ADH in patients who have ingested isopropyl alcohol only prolongs its elimination.

Hemodialysis is not normally needed to clear isopropyl alcohol from the blood, although it is a highly effective modality for eliminating all ingested alcohols. The risks of initiating hemodialysis in this patient who is inebriated but otherwise stable would not be justified.

Seizure prophylaxis with levetiracetam is not indicated for isopropyl alcohol ingestion, and this patient shows no clinical signs of withdrawal, a prelude to seizures. As long as he is closely monitored and treated appropriately with benzodiazepine medication for signs of withdrawal, antiepileptic medication should not be needed.

KEY POINT

- Patients with isopropyl alcohol poisoning can be treated effectively using supportive care.

Bibliography

Beauchamp GA, Valento M. Toxic alcohol ingestion: prompt recognition and management in the emergency department. Emerg Med Pract. 2016;18:1-20. [PMID: 27538060]

Item 99   Answer: B

Educational Objective: Evaluate potential lung cancer with the optimal diagnostic procedure.

The most appropriate diagnostic test for this patient with a lesion highly suspicious for lung cancer and PET-positive mediastinal lymphadenopathy is bronchoscopy with endobronchial ultrasound–guided transbronchial needle aspiration. The evaluation of a patient with suspected lung cancer aims to confirm whether the patient indeed has lung cancer, to determine the pathology (non-small cell lung cancer versus small cell lung cancer), and to assess the stage at presentation. Most patients undergo chest CT scan as the first imaging modality, either after an abnormal chest radiograph or in evaluation of a symptom. The findings on the chest CT scan determine whether a PET/CT scan is necessary. A PET/CT scan can help in staging and therefore also help guide where to biopsy. For example, if a patient has a solitary pulmonary nodule, a PET/CT scan may help determine if any lymph node involvement is present that was not visible on the chest CT scan.

The next step is to obtain tissue diagnosis. The choice of initial diagnostic testing should be aimed first at identifying potential lymph node involvement or metastatic disease. Tissue diagnosis should then be targeted at the lesion that would result in the highest potential staging. In this patient, sampling the mediastinal lymph nodes is critical to both diagnose and stage the patient and will affect the clinical decision making for this patient. Endobronchial ultrasound–guided transbronchial needle aspiration is a minimally invasive way and preferred to more invasive surgical techniques. Endobronchial ultrasound–guided transbronchial needle aspiration can sample most mediastinal and some hilar lymph node stations, although some of the more posterior lymph nodes are not accessible with this technique.

CT-guided needle biopsy has a high accuracy for diagnosis of lung cancers, but has higher risks of procedural complications than endobronchial ultrasound–guided transbronchial needle aspiration (mainly pneumothorax), and the patient would require a second procedure to sample the mediastinum if the lung lesion is a non-small cell lung cancer.

Sputum cytology has a lower sensitivity than endobronchial ultrasound–guided transbronchial needle aspiration for diagnosis of lung cancer, does not produce sufficient sample material for molecular studies, and will not provide needed staging information.

Thoracoscopic lung biopsy with lymph node dissection is less preferable than a minimally invasive approach, due to cost and risks of complications.

KEY POINT

- Endobronchial ultrasound–guided transbronchial needle aspiration is the procedure of choice for diagnosing and staging mediastinal and hilar lymphadenopathy in patients with suspected thoracic malignancy.

Bibliography

Silvestri GA, Gonzalez AV, Jantz MA, Margolis ML, Gould MK, Tanoue LT, et al. Methods for staging non-small cell lung cancer: diagnosis and management of lung cancer, 3rd ed: American College of Chest Physicians evidence-based clinical practice guidelines. Chest. 2013;143:e211S-e250S. [PMID: 23649440] doi:10.1378/chest.12-2355

Item 100   Answer: B

Educational Objective: Treat acute opioid overdose with naloxone.

The most appropriate management is continued observation for signs of recurrent respiratory failure. Patients with opioid overdose have findings that suggest the diagnosis including:

CONT. miosis, respiratory depression, lethargy, confusion, hypothermia, bradycardia, and hypotension. An early empiric trial of the opioid antagonist naloxone is warranted when opioid overdose is suspected. It is important to remember that naloxone has a very short half-life, and its antidote effects will usually wear off before the opioid effects are gone. Naloxone is given at higher doses to apneic patients, such as 2 mg intravenously (IV), which is larger than the typical starting dose of 0.4 mg IV usually given to overdose patients who are still breathing. The dose of naloxone is titrated to a respiration rate of at least 12/min, not to a normal mental status. Chronic opioid users require close monitoring for withdrawal.

Serial escalating doses of naloxone may be necessary in some patients, and patients who respond to serial dosing may require a continuous naloxone infusion. However, there is no immediate need for more naloxone because this patient has normal breathing and mentation. During the period of observation, more naloxone may be needed if her respiration rate slows or stops.

This patient cannot be discharged until it is known that her respiratory suppression will not return when the naloxone wears off. Patients should be observed for at least 60 minutes after the last dose of naloxone. Drug addiction resources should be accessed for this patient. It is also appropriate after overdose to rule out suicidal ideation or intent and refer the patient to a psychiatric clinician if needed.

Endotracheal intubation would not be appropriate because the patient is protecting her airway and is not in respiratory distress or failure. Intubation is required for patients whose respiratory suppression cannot be quickly reversed with naloxone.

KEY POINT

- In the treatment of opioid overdose the antidote effects of naloxone will usually wear off before the opioid effects are gone; observation and repeated dosing are often necessary.

Bibliography
Willman MW, Liss DB, Schwarz ES, Mullins ME. Do heroin overdose patients require observation after receiving naloxone? Clin Toxicol (Phila). 2017;55:81-87. [PMID: 27849133] doi:10.1080/15563650.2016.1253846

Item 101   Answer: C

Educational Objective: Diagnose pulmonary embolism as the cause of acute hypoxemic respiratory failure and shock.

This patient most likely has a pulmonary embolism. This patient has hypoxemic respiratory failure and shock. Severe hypoxemia is generally defined as an arterial P_{O_2} of 60 mm Hg (8.0 kPa) or less or an oxygen saturation of 89% or less while breathing ambient air. The most common causes of hypoxemic respiratory failure are conditions that lead to mismatch between the ventilation of inspired air in the alveoli and perfusion of adjacent alveolar capillaries by blood (called ventilation-perfusion [$\dot{V}/\dot{Q}$] mismatch). Conditions such as pulmonary embolism lead to $\dot{V}/\dot{Q}$ mismatch. Hypoxemia due to $\dot{V}/\dot{Q}$ mismatch should resolve with oxygen therapy. However, extremes of $\dot{V}/\dot{Q}$ mismatch (known as a shunt) do not fully resolve with supplemental oxygen because inspired gas does not interface with the shunted blood in the lungs. In addition, this patient has evidence of cardiogenic shock, including hypotension, elevated jugular venous pressure, fixed splitting of the second heart sound, and cool, mottled skin. Although cardiogenic shock can occur for many reasons, in this patient, it is the result of the pulmonary embolism causing a mechanical blockage in the pulmonary circulation, leading to impaired cardiac output from the right ventricle. Fat emboli following long-bone fractures can mimic pulmonary emboli.

Anaphylactic shock is a type of distributive shock, as might occur if a patient with an allergy to penicillin were given either penicillin or a related agent to which she reacted. Anaphylaxis is an IgE-mediated reaction and manifests within minutes to 1 hour after exposure to the implicated antigen. Anaphylactic shock would result in hypotension and warm extremities, typically with hives or rash. The patient is hypotensive, but does not have a rash. Respiratory failure could be present but would be associated with wheezing or stridor.

Opioid overdose can cause hypercapnic respiratory failure with hypoxemia occurring as the result of hypoventilation. Although the hypoxemia improves with oxygen, it does not improve the hypercapnea. Opioid overdose cannot account for the findings of obstructive shock.

Tension pneumothorax can cause respiratory failure and cardiogenic shock as a result of poor right ventricular filling. It should be suspected in patients with hypotension, diminished breath sounds on the affected side, distended neck veins, and tracheal deviation away from the affected side. Risk factors for tension pneumothorax include trauma, recent pulmonary procedure, mechanical ventilation, and underlying cystic lung disease. The patient has no risk factors for tension pneumothorax, and her lung findings do not support this diagnosis.

KEY POINT

- The most common causes of hypoxemic respiratory failure are conditions that lead to ventilation-perfusion mismatch or shunt; hypoxemia due to ventilation-perfusion mismatch with shunting does not improve with supplemental oxygen.

Bibliography
Wagner PD. The physiological basis of pulmonary gas exchange: implications for clinical interpretation of arterial blood gases. Eur Respir J. 2015;45:227-43. [PMID: 25323225] doi:10.1183/09031936.00039214

Item 102   Answer: C

Educational Objective: Diagnose obesity hypoventilation syndrome.

The most likely diagnosis is obesity hypoventilation syndrome. Obesity hypoventilation syndrome is characterized by daytime hypercapnia (arterial P_{CO_2} greater than 45 mm Hg [5.9 kPa]) that is thought to be a consequence of diminished ventilatory drive and capacity related to extreme obesity. Persons with a BMI of 35 or higher are considered at risk for obesity hypoventilation syndrome; it's estimated that more than half of patients with a BMI of 50 or higher have this condition. This patient's BMI of 44, compensated hypercapnic respiratory failure, hypoxemia during wakefulness but more pronounced during sleep, and polycythemia are all consistent with obesity hypoventilation syndrome. Positive airway pressure therapy (continuous positive airway pressure or bilevel positive airway pressure), sometimes with supplemental oxygen, is first-line therapy.

Neuromuscular diseases that can affect the respiratory system must be considered in the differential diagnosis of hypoventilation syndromes. Amyotrophic lateral sclerosis (ALS) often leads to hypercapnic respiratory failure. However, this patient has an unremarkable neurologic examination and none of the typical features of ALS, such as muscle weakness and fasciculations and hyperactive deep tendon reflexes.

Central sleep apnea (CSA) is defined by intermittent reduced central drive to breathe but is not a hypoventilation syndrome. In fact, the tendency to hyperventilate, as seen with the cyclic ventilatory pattern of Cheyne-Stokes breathing, is a key underlying mechanism of CSA. Patients with CSA are generally normocapnic or slightly hypocapnic on blood gas testing.

An apnea-hypopnea index (AHI) of 5 to 15 is indicative of mild obstructive sleep apnea (OSA). This patient has mild OSA based upon an AHI of 6. OSA is typically encountered on sleep testing in those with obesity hypoventilation syndrome, with upper airway collapse superimposed on obesity-related hypoventilation. Severe OSA is defined as an AHI of at least 30; OSA severity is not defined by degree or duration of hypoxemia.

KEY POINT

- Obesity hypoventilation syndrome is characterized by daytime hypercapnia, defined as an arterial P_{CO_2} greater than 45 mm Hg that is thought to be a consequence of diminished ventilatory drive and capacity related to extreme obesity.

Bibliography

Randerath W, Verbraecken J, Andreas S, Arzt M, Bloch KE, Brack T, et al. Definition, discrimination, diagnosis and treatment of central breathing disturbances during sleep. Eur Respir J. 2017;49. [PMID: 27920092] doi:10.1183/13993003.00959-2016

Item 103   Answer: E

Educational Objective: Treat an acute exacerbation of bronchiectasis with antibiotics.

The most appropriate treatment of this patient is levofloxacin. Oral antibiotic treatment is appropriate for clinically stable patients with an acute exacerbation of bronchiectasis. The choice of antibiotic therapy can be based on previous sputum culture results, if available. If not available, a reasonable empiric antibiotic choice is a respiratory fluoroquinolone such as levofloxacin or moxifloxacin. Although duration of therapy is not well defined, most experts treat for 10 to 14 days.

Amoxicillin or a macrolide such as azithromycin is a reasonable choice for patients in the absence of β-lactamase-positive *Haemophilus influenzae* or *Pseudomonas*. Initial empiric therapy can also be deescalated to amoxicillin based on the results of sputum culture and sensitivity. However, in the absence of bacteriologic data from sputum culture, amoxicillin is an inadequate choice for empiric therapy in patients with recurrent acute exacerbations previously treated with antibiotics due to the high risk of β-lactamase producing organisms and *Pseudomonas*.

For similar reasons, azithromycin is not an appropriate empiric antibiotic for this patient. There is likely a role for long-term azithromycin therapy to prevent recurrent exacerbations of bronchiectasis. The salutary effect on chronic macrolide therapy in these situations may not be entirely due to its antimicrobial properties but rather its well-known antiinflammatory properties. However, the development of antibiotic resistance is a potential risk.

Oral or inhaled glucocorticoids would seem to be reasonable adjunctive therapy for patients with acute exacerbation of bronchiectasis, but supporting evidence for their use is sparse. Some experts may employ glucocorticoids in patients with coexistent asthma and wheezing or allergic bronchopulmonary aspergillosis, but the risk of routine use is related to immunosuppression and promotion of bacterial and fungal colonization and is not recommended.

Inhaled aerosols of antibiotics, including inhaled tobramycin solution, are not recommended for an acute exacerbation of bronchiectasis. This recommendation is based on a multicenter randomized trial that demonstrated the addition of inhaled tobramycin to ciprofloxacin was not superior to ciprofloxacin alone but was associated with more wheezing. There may be a role of inhaled antibiotics in the prophylaxis of acute exacerbations of bronchiectasis.

KEY POINT

- If previous data on bronchiectasis exacerbations are not available, a fluoroquinolone should be started to ensure *Pseudomonas* coverage until the sputum culture is completed.

Bibliography

Smith MP. Diagnosis and management of bronchiectasis. CMAJ. 2017;189: E828-E835. [PMID: 28630359] doi:10.1503/cmaj.160830

Index